Desk Reference for
Neuroscience

Isabel Lockard

Desk Reference for Neuroscience

Second Edition

With 53 Illustrations

Springer-Verlag

New York Berlin Heidelberg London Paris
Tokyo Hong Kong Barcelona Budapest

Isabel Lockard, Ph.D.
Professor Emeritus
Department of Anatomy and Cell Biology
Medical University of South Carolina
Charleston, SC 29425-2204
USA

Library of Congress Cataloging-in-Publication Data
Lockard, Isabel, 1915–
    Desk reference for neuroscience / Isabel Lockard. – 2nd ed.
      p.   cm.
    Rev. ed. of: Desk reference for neuroanatomy. c1977.
    Includes bibliographical references (p.   ).
    ISBN 0-387-97629-9 (Springer-Verlag New York Berlin Heidelberg :
alk. paper). – ISBN 3-540-97629-9 (Springer-Verlag Berlin
Heidelberg New York : alk. paper)
      1. Neuroanatomy – Dictionaries.   2. Neurophysiology – Dictionaries.
    3. Neurology – Dictionaries.   I. Lockard, Isabel, 1915–   Desk
reference for neuroanatomy.   II. Title.
    QM451.L625   1991
    612.8′03 – dc20   91-28711

Printed on acid-free paper.

Camera-ready copy provided by the author.
Printed and bound by Braun-Brumfield, Ann Arbor, MI.
Printed in the United States of America.

9 8 7 6 5 4 3 2 1

ISBN 0-387-97629-9 Springer-Verlag New York Berlin Heidelberg (hardcover)
ISBN 3-540-97629-9 Springer-Verlag Berlin Heidelberg New York
ISBN 0-387-97715-5 Springer-Verlag New York Berlin Heidelberg (softcover)
ISBN 3-540-97715-5 Springer-Verlag Berlin Heidelberg New York

To my parents
Claude Wesley Lockard and Ethel Parker Lockard

Preface to the Second Edition

The DESK REFERENCE evolved from lists of terms and their definitions prepared for beginning students in neuroanatomy. So much of the nomenclature is new to beginners and so many common words have special meanings in a neurological context that to the neophyte it may seem almost like a new language. As the number of lists of terms increased and became cumbersome, they were assembled into a single glossary which also was gradually expanded. Eventually the glossary became the DESK REFERENCE FOR NEUROANATOMY.

In recent years the boundaries of the neurological fields have blurred, and students in all subdivisions of neuroscience require help not only with their own particular specialty but also with the related disciplines. In this edition of the DESK REFERENCE many terms from the first edition have been amplified and the text has been expanded to include many more terms from various NEUROSCIENCES-- neurophysiology, neuropathology, neuropharmacology, and the related clinical branches, in addition to neuroanatomy. As new discoveries in this as in other sciences are made, the researcher is confronted with the need to be familiar with the history and the development of the subject. Over the years terminology has changed. In this volume, as in the first edition, an attempt has been made to correlate older and newer neuroanatomical terminologies, to help those who wish to read the older literature. Most terms entered are those currently approved for the Nomina Anatomica (or the Nomina Histologica and Nomina Embryologica) and indicated by [NA], e.g., *ansa cervicalis* [NA], or the common English term with its Nomina Anatomica equivalent, if there is one, as *artery, common carotid [arteria carotis communis, NA]* and their synonyms are provided. Eponyms, so popular at one time, are falling into disuse. Most eponyms included here are given under the names of the individuals whom they commemorate, so that the *artery of Heubner* will be identified under *Heubner,* the name of the man for whom it was named and, where appropriate, described under its English equivalent, e.g., *artery, recurrent.* Even so, some still commonly used eponyms are cross referenced, e.g., *Sylvian fissure* for *lateral sulcus.*

Unless otherwise specified, all terms relate to the human nervous system. The references cited and provided in the bibliography do not cover any subject extensively. Some special references are included, but most, including reviews of many topics, are intended to provide a place to start if more information and references to the background literature are desired. Sources for most of the biographical and historical information are not included, but reference books containing historical accounts are added for the convenience of the reader.

Terms are entered in an order that, it is hoped, will make them most easily located by the reader. Compound terms, with two or more words, are usually entered according to the noun, as *body, cell*. Related terms, including subdivisions of a given topic, are grouped together, so that such compound terms as *aphasia, global; aphasia, jargon; aphasia, motor; aphasia, semantic; aphasia, sensory;* etc. are to be found in consecutive order after *aphasia*. For ease of access, singular and plural forms of the same terms are included together without regard to their number.

As a quick reference to the part of the central nervous system, eye, or ear, in which a structure is located, its location is usually given, e.g., CORD (for spinal cord), PONS, MEDULLA, HYPOTHALAMUS, FOREBRAIN, EYE, EAR.

The derivation of many terms is given: [Gr.] for Greek, [L.] for Latin, [Fr.] for French, and [Ger.] for German.

A simplified guide to the pronunciation of some words is given. Syllables having the major stress are followed by an accent (ʹ). Long vowels may be unmarked in a syllable without a final consonant or marked with a macron (ā). Short vowels may be unmarked when followed by a consonant or marked with a breve (ă)
a (long) for a as in *mate, aʹlar, ālar*
a (short) for a as in *mat, matʹter, mătter*
e (long) for e as in *meet, meʹter, mēter*
e (short) for e as in *met, metʹal, mĕtal*
i (long) for i as in *line, siʹnus, sīnus*
i (short) for i as in *lit, litʹter, lĭtter*
o (long) for o as in *go, oʹtic, ōtic*
o (short) for o as in *lot, otʹter, ŏtter*
ū (long) for u as in *cube, cuʹbic, cūbic*
ŭ (short) for u as in *cup, sulʹcus, sŭlcus*
oo (long) for oo as in *boot* or u in *ruin* (rooʹin)

Some consonants are pronounced as follows:
k (hard) for c as in *cat* (kat)
g (hard) for g as in *go*
j (soft) for g as in *germ* (jerm)
ch for ch as in *chin*
zh (voiced) for z as in *azure* (azhʹur)
sh (voiceless) for s as in *sure* or sh in *shine*

Isabel Lockard
Charleston, S.C.
1991

Preface to the First Edition

The main purpose of this book is to provide ready access to key information on parts of the nervous system. The student of neuroanatomy frequently encounters terms from such closely related anatomical fields as the gross anatomy of the peripheral nervous system, the histology and embryology of the nervous system and the anatomy of the eye and ear. Consequently many of the terms from these areas have been included. Although no complete listing of terms from cognate fields has been attempted, some of the more frequently encountered terms from neurophysiology, neuropathology and clinical neurology are also included.

References given for some entries are not intended to be exhaustive but to direct the reader's attention in some instances to places where the term has been introduced and in others to places where a more complete discussion of the subject is available.

Another purpose is to equate the terms that are synonyms and to differentiate between those that are not. In addition, an attempt has been made to include older terms and eponyms together with their newer counterparts.

Because not all authors agree on the precise meanings of many terms, some of the definitions given here may seem, and indeed often are, arbitrary. Although this author claims no special authority in the selection of preferred terms, some selection was necessary. If we are to use words that convey exactly the ideas that we intend, it is necessary to draw some semblance of order out of the overlapping and imprecise terminology of our field. When it comes to deciding on the meaning of a word, we are left with Humpty Dumpty's admonition to Alice—"The question is, which is to be master—that's all."

Isabel Lockard

"When *I* use a word," Humpty Dumpty said, in rather a scornful tone, "it means just what I choose it to mean—neither more nor less."

"The question is," said Alice, "whether you *can* make words mean so many different things."

"The question is," said Humpty Dumpty, "which is to be master—that's all."

—from "Through the Looking Glass"
by Lewis Carroll

Acknowledgments

I am deeply grateful for the suggestions and help I have received from my colleagues, particularly Drs. James A. Augustine, Hilda S. Debacker, Richard M. Dom, and Ludwig G. Kempe, to Dr. Robert M. Beckstead for allowing me access to the wordprocessing equipment I needed, and to Dr. Donald R. DiBona and for his support with time and place to continue this project. In addition I am indebted to Dr. Kempe for the illustrations which he kindly prepared especially for this volume. I also wish to thank Brooks Hart, who did the labeling on all the new illustrations, James Nicholson and Helen Braid for the photographs they prepared, including the illustrations borrowed from the literature and for the photomicrograph, Tina Moore for her endless patience and able help in controlling an obstreperous wordprocessing system, and, last but not least, the publishers, Springer-Verlag, for their patience and help.

Isabel Lockard

a

aba´sia [Gr. *a* not; *basis* step]   inability to walk.

aber´rant pyram´idal   *See* fibers, aberrant pyramidal.

acalcu´lia [Gr. *a* not; L. *calculare* to compute]   inability to complete simple arithmetical problems, associated with injuries in the region of the supramarginal gyrus of the dominant parietal lobe.

accommoda´tion   changes that occur in the adaptation of the eye for near vision: contraction of the ciliary muscle to increase convexity of the lens, of the circular muscle of the iris for constriction of the pupil, and of the medial rectus muscles for convergence of the eyes. *See also* reflex, accommodation.

acer´vulus cer´ebri [NA], EPITHALAMUS, [L. *acervulus* a little heap]   calcareous body in the pineal body. *Syn:* corpus arenaceum; brain sand.

acetylcho´line (ACh)   the primary neurotransmitter of the PNS, released at endings of preganglionic parasympathetic and sympathetic fibers, parasympathetic postganglionic fibers, postganglionic sympathetic fibers to sweat glands, and at motor end plates in skeletal muscle. It is also released in certain nuclei of the CNS, especially those in the basal region of the forebrain. *See also* neurotransmitters; muscarinic; nicotinic; plate, motor end.

acetylcholines´terase (AChE)   enzyme which inactivates (hydrolyzes) acetylcholine. *Syn:* cholinesterase.

ACh   acetylcholine.

AChE   acetylcholinesterase.

Achillini, Alessandro (1463-1512)   anatomist of Bologna who made original observations on the hippocampus. He also described the labyrinth of the internal ear, and the malleus and incus.

acou´stic [Gr. *akouein* to hear]   pertaining to the ear. *For* acoustic area, nerve, *and* tubercle, *see the nouns.*

ACTH   adrenocorticotropic hormone.

Adamkiewicz, Albert (1850-1921)   Polish pathologist of Krakow, noted for his description of the crescent-shaped cells under the neurolemma of medullated nerve fibers, and for his extensive study of the blood vessels of the spinal cord (1881, 1882). The *artery of Adamkiewicz* is the great anterior radicular (medullary) artery of the spinal cord, which he called the *great anterior spinal artery.*

adapta´tion   property of somatic receptors whereby the receptor potential decreases in amplitude in response to a constant stimulus.

adenohypoph´ysis   that part of the hypophysis derived from Rathke's pouch, an ectodermal evagination of the roof of the embryonic pharynx. It consists of three parts: pars distalis (anterior lobe), pars tuberalis (pars infundibularis) on the anterior surface of the infundibulum, and pars intermedia on the anterior surface of the pars nervosa. *See also* hypophysis cerebri; Rathke.

ADH   antidiuretic hormone, also called *vasopressin.*

adhe´sion, interthalam´ic [adhesio interthalamica, NA], DORSAL THALAMUS   median nuclear mass interconnecting the two dorsal thalami across the third ventricle. It is absent in about 30% of human brains. When present this mass contains the median nuclei of the dorsal thalamus (Figs. N-8, V-5). *Syn:* massa intermedia; interthalamic connexus; middle commissure; soft commissure.

adiadochokine´sia (adiadochokine´sis) [Gr. *a* not; *diadocho* succeeding; *kinesis* movement]   cerebellar disorder characterized by the inability to perform rapidly alternating contractions of antagonistic muscles, as in finger tapping or alternate pronation and supination of the hands. Although *dysdiadochokinesia* indicates a less severe disorder, the two terms are often used interchangeably.

Adie, William John (1886-1935)   British ophthalmologist, born in Australia, later a resident of England. *Adie's pupil* (1932) is one that reacts, unilaterally, slowly to accommodation and to light only after the patient has been in the dark a long time.

Adler, Alfred (1870-1937)   Viennese psychiatrist and psychologist, a follower of Freud's. He later disagreed with his mentor, for which Freud rejected him.

adrener´gic   releasing an epinephrine-like substance; pertaining to certain postganglionic sympathetic nerve endings.

adrenocorticotro´pic hor´mone (ACTH)   a polypeptide secreted by the anterior lobe of the hypophysis. It stimulates the adrenal cortex to release its hormones. *Syn:* adrenocorticotropin. *See also* neurotransmitters.

adrenocorticotro´pin   *See* adrenocorticotropic hormone (ACTH).

adren´aline   *See* epinephrine.

Adrian, Lord Edgar Douglas (1889-1977)   English neurophysiologist, noted for his studies of sensory phenomena. In 1932 he and Sir C.S. Sherrington were awarded the Nobel Prize for physiology and medicine for their discoveries regarding neuron function.

Af´fenspalte, CEREBRUM, [Ger. *Affe* ape; *Spalte* cleft, fissure]   *See* sulcus, lunate.

af´ferent   conducting toward.

af´terbrain   *See* hindbrain.

af´ter-nystag´mus   nystagmus in which the eye movements continue after the stimulus is removed.

agent, adrener´gic blocking   compound which selectively inhibits the responses of effector cells to adrenergic sympathetic nerve impulses and to epinephrine and related amines.

ageusia /ah-goo´zĭ-ah/ [Gr. *a* not; *geusis* taste]   neurologic disorder in which there is a loss of the sense of taste.

agnosia /ag-no´zĭ-ah/ [Gr. *a-*; *gnosis* knowledge]   loss of ability to recognize familiar sensory impressions or to interpret their significance. *For additional information on the agnosias and related disorders, see* Adams and Victor ('89, pp. 347-395).

agnosia, auditory   loss of the ability to recognize spoken words (auditory verbal agnosia or word deafness) or familiar sounds that can be recognized with another modality, e.g., the sound of water running which can be recognized when seen (auditory non-verbal agnosia) or music (amusia), without loss of hearing acuity. Auditory verbal agnosia and perhaps the non-verbal type of agnosia may be due to a lesion in the superior temporal gyrus bilaterally or in the dominant hemisphere. Amusia is said to occur with a lesion in the non-dominant hemisphere.

agnosia, tactile   inability to recognize an object by touch when it is placed in either or both hands, even though tactile sensibility is normal. The disorder occurs with a lesion of the parietal lobe posterior to the postcentral gyrus in the dominant hemisphere. *See also* astereognosis.

agnosia, visual   inability to recognize written words (alexia) or objects by sight, usually after a bilateral lesion in the inferior part of the occipitotemporal region. *See also* aphasia.

agraph´ia [Gr. *a-*; *graphein* to write]   loss of the ability to express language in written or printed form or to copy written words or pictures, caused by brain damage, sometimes in the region of the angular gyrus or in the middle frontal gyrus near the motor area for the control of hand movements. *See also* aphasia.

AICA   anterior inferior cerebellar artery.

akine´sia [Gr. *a-*; *kinesis* movement]   absence of the initiation, implementation, and facility of execution of movement. *See also* mutism, akinetic.

a´la al´ba lateral´is, PONS, MEDULLA, [L. *ala* wing; *alba* white]   *See* area, acoustic.

ala central´is [ala lobuli centralis, NA], CEREBELLUM   most rostral subdivision of the cerebellar hemisphere in the anterior lobe, between the precentral and postcentral fissures. It is continuous with the central lobule of the vermis (Fig. C-2).

ala ciner´ea, MEDULLA, [L. *cinereus* ashy]   *See* trigone, vagal.

ala lob´uli central´is [NA], CEREBELLUM   *See* ala centralis.

al´ba [L. white]   pertaining to the white matter of the brain.

alexia /ah-leks´ĭ-ah/ [Gr. *a* not; *lexis* word]   language disorder with loss of ability to interpret written or printed symbols, caused by damage usually in the occipital lobe cortex or its connections with the angular gyrus of the dominant hemisphere; word blindness, therefore inability to read. *Syn:* visual verbal agnosia. *See also* aphasia.

allocor´tex, CEREBRUM, [Gr. *allos* other; L. *cortex* bark]   nonlaminated or partly laminated cerebral cortex of the archipallium and paleopallium. *See also* cortex, heterogenetic.

all-or-none   principle according to which a nerve fiber always responds maximally to a threshold stimulus.

ALS   amyotrophic lateral sclerosis.

al´veus hippocam´pi [NA], CEREBRUM, [L. *alveus* trough or canal]   layer of myelinated fibers on the ventricular surface of the hippocampus. The fibers arise from nerve cells in the cornu ammonis and subiculum and, from the alveus, collect to form the fimbria (Fig. C-7).

Alzheimer, Alois (1864-1915)   German neuropathologist who first described the pathologic changes in the cerebral cortex characteristic of the dementia now known as *Alzheimer's disease* (1904). These changes consist of plaques containing high concentrations of aluminum, and neurofibrillary tangles, *Alzheimer's bodies*. Loss of nerve cells in the basal nucleus of Meynert is said to be a major feature of this disease. Certain abnormal proteins *(Alzheimer's Disease Associated Proteins,* ADAP), have been detected in brain regions related to cognitive function and memory in patients with this disease. If such changes can be detected elsewhere, as in cerebrospinal fluid, a diagnostic test for this condition may be possible (Ghanbari *et al.,* '90). The disease has been linked to a defective gene on chromosome 21 and possibly to a transmissible virus.

am´acrine, EYE, [Gr. *a* not; *makros* long; *is, inos* fiber]   *See* cell, amacrine.

amauro´sis [Gr. darkening]   blindness.

amic´ulum olivar´e [NA], MEDULLA, [L. *amiculum* little overcoat]   *See* capsule, olivary.

am´ine precur´sor uptake and decarboxyla´tion (APUD)   a class of nerve cells which belong to the diffuse neuroendocrine system. At least some of these cells are thought to be of neural crest origin. They produce certain peptides: neurotransmitters, hormones, and probably some endotoxins. Cells with these properties have been localized in the PNS, in the brain, and in many other areas, including the gastrointestinal and respiratory systems. *For a review of this subject, see* Pearse ('77).

aminobutyric acid /ah-me´no-bu-ter´ik/   *See* gamma-aminobutyric acid (GABA).

Ammon   Egyptian god whose symbol was the ram. He was represented with ram's horns, hence the term *Ammon's horn* or *cornu ammonis. For Ammon's formation, see* formation, hippocampal, *also* hippocampus. *Ammon's pyramids* are the pyramidal cells of the cornu ammonis.

amnesia   disturbance of memory.

am´phicyte [Gr. *amphi* two-sided, around; *kytos* cell]   satellite cell in the ectodermal capsule of ganglion cells.

ampul´la, mem´branous [ampulla membranacea, NA], EAR, [L. *ampulla* jug]   dilation at one end of each semicircular duct (anterior inferior end of the superior duct, posterior inferior end of the posterior duct, and anterior end of the horizontal duct) and containing the crista ampullaris, the sensory end organ of the duct.

ampulla, os´seous [ampulla ossea, NA], EAR   part of the bony labyrinth of the internal ear, which contains a membranous ampulla.

amu´sia [Gr. *amousia* lack of harmony]   inability to produce or to recognize music. *See also* agnosia, auditory.

amyelia /a-mi-e´ll-ah/ [Gr. *a* not; *myelon* spinal cord]   absence of the spinal cord, a condition which usually occurs in association with anencephaly and is not compatible for long with life.

amygdala /ah-mig´dă-lah/ [corpus amygdaloideum, NA], CEREBRUM, [Gr. *amygdale* almond]   subdivision of the basal ganglia located in the temporal lobe, anterior to the inferior horn of the lateral ventricle and partly beneath the uncus. Its two main parts are a corticomedial nuclear group (anterior amygdaloid area, nucleus of the lateral olfactory tract, and the medial cortical and central amygdaloid nuclei) with olfactory and subcortical connections, and a basolateral nuclear group (basal, lateral, and accessory basal amygdaloid nuclei) connected primarily with the overlying cortex. *For additional information, see* Crosby *et al.* ('62, pp. 388-393). *Syn:* archistriatum.

amygdala, extended cellular region consisting of the central and medial nuclei of the amygdala, cell columns traversing the sublenticular part of the substantia innominata, the bed nucleus of the stria terminalis, and part of the nucleus accumbens.

amyotro´phic lat´eral sclero´sis (ALS) *See* sclerosis, amyotrophic lateral.

analge´sia [Gr. *an* not; *algesis* sense of pain] insensitivity to pain without loss of consciousness.

Andersch, Carl Samuel (1732-1777) German anatomist of Göttingen, a pupil of Haller's. The *ganglion of Andersch* is the inferior (petrosal) ganglion of the glossopharyngeal nerve. *Andersch's nerve* is the tympanic branch of the glossopharyngeal nerve, which is also called *Jacobson's nerve.*

anenceph´aly [Gr. *an* not; *enkephalos* brain] a severe malformation of the brain in which the cerebral hemispheres and sometimes also the diencephalon fail to develop. It results from failure of the anterior neuropore to close. It is the most common serious malformation of the brain seen in stillbirths; it occurs in one of about 1000 live births but may occur even more frequently in some populations. It is always associated with rachischisis, an absence of the cranial vault, acrania, and often with a failure of the vertebral arches to fuse.

anesthe´sia [Gr. *an-; aisthesis* sensation] absence of sensation.

an´eurysm, berry [Gr. *aneurysma* an opening, from *ana* up, *eurys* wide] saccular dilation of a cerebral artery, usually located on or near the cerebral arterial circle.

angiog´raphy [Gr. *angeion* vessel; *graphein* to write] procedure in which a contrast medium is injected into a vessel, such as the common carotid artery, to render the vessel and its branches visible by radiography.

ang´le, cerebellopon´tine area on the ventrolateral surface of the brain stem where the cerebellum, pons, and medulla meet and where the facial and vestibulocochlear nerves attach to the brain. Early signs of a cerebellopontine angle tumor, all on the side of the lesion, consist of unilateral deafness (VIII nerve), corneal anesthesia (V nerve), and partial facial paralysis, with inability to close the eye completely (VII nerve). Additional signs may occur as the tumor enlarges.

angle, filtra´tion, EYE *See* angle, iridocorneal.

angle, iridocor´neal [angulus iridocornealis, NA], EYE area at the junction of the iris and the cornea where aqueous humor leaves the anterior chamber of the eye. *Syn:* filtration, iris, *or* iridial angle.

angle, ve´nous, FOREBRAIN point at the interventricular foramen where the superior thalamostriate (terminal) vein abruptly turns posteriorly to enter the internal cerebral vein (Fig. V-2).

anhidro´sis [Gr. *an* not; *hidros* sweat] absence of sweating.

animal, decerebrate /de-ser´ĕ-brāt/ one in which the brain has been severed at the level of the midbrain.

animal, spinal one in which the CNS has been severed at the junction of the brain and spinal cord.

animal, thalam´ic one in which the brain has been severed separating the cerebrum from the diencephalon.

anisocor´ia [Gr. *anisos* unequal; *kore* pupil] condition in which the pupils of the two eyes are unequal in size.

ankle jerk *See* reflex, Achilles tendon.

an´nulus *See* anulus.

ano´mia [Gr. *an* not; *onoma* name] word-finding difficulty usually associated with aphasia. There is an inability to recall or to recognize the names of people or objects, although the individual may recognize the people and may know how to use the object. It sometimes results from a lesion in the inferior temporal area in the dominant hemisphere, presumably area 37.

anosmia /an-oz´mĭ-ah/ [Gr. *an-* ; *osme* sense of smell] loss or lack of the sense of smell.

anosogno´sia [Gr. *a* not; *nosis* disease; *gnosis* knowledge] inability of a person to recognize a disease or bodily defect, such as paralysis, in himself.

an´sa cervical´is [NA] [L. *ansa* handle of a jug] loop of the cervical plexus, formed by the union of its radix superior (descendens hypoglossi) containing fibers from the C1 spinal nerve, and its radix inferior (descendens cervicalis), containing fibers from C2 and C3. Its branches supply the infrahyoid muscles. *Syn:* ansa hypoglossi.

ansa crural´is *See* ansa peduncularis.

ansa hypoglos´si *See* ansa cervicalis.

ansa lenticular´is [NA], MAINLY FOREBRAIN **1.** bundle of nerve fibers arising primarily from cells in the globus pallidus and putamen, emerging from the ventral surface of the lentiform nucleus, passing medially and dorsally into the diencephalon where some or most fibers synapse in the nucleus of the field of Forel. Some fibers end in the midbrain tegmental gray including the caudal red nucleus for relay to the spinal cord. Others continue into the thalamic fasciculus to end mainly in the ventral anterior nucleus of the dorsal thalamus.
2. several bundles of nerve fibers emerging from the lentiform nucleus and subdivided into three groups: a ventral division or ansa lenticularis proper (see *def.* 1. above), a dorsal division (the lenticular fasciculus), and an intermediate division (the subthalamic fasciculus). These three fiber bundles constitute the ventral peduncle of the lateral forebrain bundle of submammals.

ansa peduncular´is [NA], FOREBRAIN fiber bundle that bends medially around the posterior limb of the internal capsule. It includes the inferior thalamic peduncle, which interconnects the dorsomedial nucleus of the dorsal thalamus with the orbital cortex, amygdala, and temporal lobe cortex; and fibers of the ansa lenticularis and the lenticular fasciculus. *Syn:* ansa cruralis; Reil's ansa.

ansa sacral´is loop of nerve fibers interconnecting the caudal ends of the two sympathetic trunks.

ansa subcla´via [NA] bundle of nerve fibers that loops around the subclavian artery connecting the inferior and middle cervical sympathetic ganglia or sometimes the inferior ganglion and the recurrent nerve. It was first described by Raymond Vieussens in 1685. *Syn:* ansa or anulus of Vieussens.

an´siform describing an arc. *See* lobule, ansiform.

anticholines´terase (AChE) [Gr. *anti* against] substance which blocks the action of cholinesterase.

antidiuret´ic hormone (ADH) [Gr. *anti-*; *dia* throughout, completely; *ouresis* urination] neurohormone synthesized by the cells of the supraoptic (mainly) and paraventricular (to some extent) nuclei of the hypothalamus. Conjugated with a carrier protein, neurophysin, it is carried by axoplasmic flow in the fibers of the hypothalamohypophysial tract, and stored in terminal swellings (Herring bodies) in the neurohypophysis, from which it is released into the general circulation. Its main function is to conserve water and its lack results in diabetes insipidus, characterized by excessive thirst and drinking and the excretion of large volumes of urine. This hormone is also called *vasopressin* because administration, in amounts larger than necessary for antidiuretic action, will increase vasoconstriction and raise blood pressure.

antidro´mic [Gr. *anti-*; *dromos* running]   conducting impulses in the direction opposite the usual (dromic or orthodromic) direction of conduction.

an´trum, interventric´ular (of Wilder) [Gr. *antron* a cave]   anterior part of the third ventricle with which the two interventricular foramina communicate.

antrum, mas´toid [antrum mastoideum, NA], EAR   irregularly shaped space in the middle ear, located posterior to and somewhat superior and lateral to the tympanic cavity with which it communicates. The mastoid air cells, located within the mastoid process of the temporal bone, open into the antrum. *Syn:* tympanic antrum.

antrum, tympan´ic, EAR   *See* antrum, mastoid.

an´ulus of the aqueduct /ak´wĕ-dukt/, MIDBRAIN, [L. *anulus* ring]   *See* gray, periaqueductal.

ap´erture, lateral [apertura lateralis ventriculi quarti, NA]   opening between each lateral recess of the fourth ventricle and the subarachnoid space (Figs. V-3, V-4). *Syn:* foramen of Luschka; foramen of Key and Retzius.

aperture, median [apertura mediana ventriculi quarti, NA]   unpaired, median opening in the posterior medullary velum through which the caudal part of the fourth ventricle communicates with the subarachnoid space (Fig. V-3). *Syn:* foramen of Magendie.

apha´sia [Gr. *a* not; *phasis* speech]   language disorder involving a loss of ability to comprehend or express the signs and symbols by which man communicates with his peers. *For more information on this and related disorders, see* Benson ('79).

aphasia, auditory   *See* aphasia, sensory; agnosia, auditory.

aphasia, global   aphasia in which all aspects of speech and language are severely disturbed. It is usually due to a lesion in the dominant hemisphere caused by interruption of blood flow through the middle cerebral artery and its branches which supply the cortical *speech* areas. It can also occur with a relatively small lesion of the white matter in the posterior part of the cerebrum, between the lateral ventricle and the lateral sulcus. *Syn:* total aphasia.

aphasia, jargon   garbled speech with paraphasia, secondary to a sensory aphasia with lesions in the posterior part of the left superior temporal gyrus and adjoining middle temporal gyrus.

aphasia, motor   loss of the ability to express ideas by speech or writing. It is associated with a lesion, usually vascular, of the inferior frontal gyrus in the dominant hemisphere. *Syn:* Broca's aphasia.

aphasia, seman´tic   loss of the ability to understand the importance and relationship of things in the external environment.

aphasia, sensory   loss of the ability to understand spoken language (auditory aphasia, verbal auditory agnosia) or written language (visual aphasia) or both (Wernicke's aphasia). It is usually associated with a lesion in the temporal lobe in the dominant hemisphere in the region near the auditory area, or in the angular gyrus of the parietal lobe, or both. *See also* agnosia, auditory.

aphasia, total   *See* aphasia, global.

aphasia, visual   *See* aphasia, sensory.

aphe´mia [Gr. *a* not; *pheme* speech]   condition, not to be confused with motor aphasia, in which the patient is mute, although still able to write and to understand spoken and written words. There is no deterioration of intellectual function. The disorder is almost always transitory and language is restored within a few weeks. The anatomic basis for this syndrome has not been clearly established but it may result from a disconnection of the left inferior frontal gyrus (Broca's area) and subcortical motor centers.

apho´nia [Gr. *a-*; *phone* voice]   loss of voice; inability to phonate.

apparatus, retic´ular   organelle found in nerve cell cytoplasm, most highly developed in large nerve cell bodies, and frequently extending into the dendrites. It appears as a network of irregular, wavy strands when viewed by light microscopy. With electron microscopy it is seen as clusters of closely apposed, flattened cisternae arranged in stacks and surrounded by many small vesicles. *Syn:* Golgi apparatus or complex.

apparatus, subneu´ral   modified sarcolemma of a motor end plate.

aprax´ia [Gr. *a* not; *prassein* to do]   disturbance in the ability to carry out motor activities in their proper sequence on verbal command, although there may be no severe motor paralysis, sensory loss, or ataxia, and individual movements may be performed adequately. It is usually associated with a lesion in the dominant hemisphere involving the supramarginal gyrus or its connections.

APUD   amine precursor uptake and decarboxylation.

aqueduct, cer´ebral (mesencephalic) /ak´wĕ-dukt/ [aqueductus mesencephali (cerebri), NA], MIDBRAIN   narrow channel through the midbrain, connecting the third and fourth ventricles (Figs. P-1, V-3). *Syn:* iter; aqueduct of Sylvius.

aqueduct, coch´lear [aqueductus cochleae, NA], EAR   interconnected connective tissue spaces within the cochlear canaliculus of the temporal bone. Together they constitute a perilymphatic duct between the scala tympani of the cochlea and the subarachnoid space. *Syn:* perilymphatic duct; periotic duct.

aqueduct, mesencephal´ic [aqueductus mesencephali (cerebri), NA], MIDBRAIN   *See* aqueduct, cerebral.

aqueduct, vestib´ular [aqueductus vestibuli, NA], EAR   narrow channel in the petrous part of the temporal bone, containing the endolymphatic duct and sac.

arachnoid /ar-ak´noid/ [arachnoidea mater, NA] [Gr. *arachne* spider; resembling a spider's web]   outer layer of the leptomeninges, covering the brain and spinal cord smoothly without conforming to the irregularities of their surfaces.

arachnopia /ar-ak-nō´pī-ah/ [NA]   *See* leptomeninges.

Aranzio (Arantius), Giulio Cesare (1530-1589)   Italian physician and anatomist, a pupil of Vesalius at Padua. He wrote extensively in various anatomical fields, described the inferior horn of the lateral ventricle, and named the hippocampus. The *ventricle of Arantius* is the caudal, tapering part of the fourth ventricle.

arboriza´tion, terminal   *See* telodendron.

ar´bor vi´tae cerebel´li [NA], CEREBELLUM, [L. *arbor* tree; *vitae* of life]   vermis of the cerebellum, as viewed in a midsagittal section (Fig. V-6).

archaeo-, archeo-   *See* archi-.

Archambault, LaSalle (1879-1940)   American neurologist. *Archambault's loop* is the temporal loop of the optic radiation, more often called Meyer's loop.

archi- (archaeo-, archeo-) [Gr. *arche* beginning]   combining forms referring to the phylogenetically oldest part.

archicerebellum /ar-kī-sĕr-ĕ-bel´um/ [archeocerebellum, archaeocerebellum, NA], CEREBELLUM the oldest part of the cerebellum, that is, the flocculonodular lobe. Part of the lingula and the uvula of the vermis are sometimes also included (Figs. C-2, V-6). *Syn:* vestibulocerebellum.

archicor´tex [archeocortex (archaecortex), NA], CEREBRUM cortex of the hippocampal formation, comprising the dentate gyrus, cornu ammonis, and subiculum. It is the first part of the cerebral cortex to differentiate completely. *Syn:* archipallium.

archipal´lium, CEREBRUM *See* archicortex; formation, hippocampal.

archistria´tum, CEREBRUM *See* amygdala.

ar´cuate [L. *arcuatus* curved in the form of a bow] pertaining to any of several fiber bundles which follow a curved course, the nucleus of such fibers or a nucleus that is itself curved or C-shaped. *See also* fibers, nucleus, *and* fasciculus, arcuate.

area *See also* cortex.

area accli´nis, BRAIN STEM, [L. *acclinis* leaning against] area lateral to the medial longitudinal fasciculus in the dorsomedial region of the tegmentum throughout the brain stem. It contains large cells of the reticular formation and fibers which probably subserve a variety of functions.

area, acous´tic, PONS, MEDULLA area on the floor of the fourth ventricle, lateral to the sulcus limitans. It consists of the vestibular area overlying the vestibular nuclei and the acoustic tubercle containing the dorsal cochlear nucleus. *Syn:* ala alba lateralis.

area adolfac´tif, CEREBRUM *See* area, parolfactory.

area, agran´ular frontal, CEREBRUM cortical area of the frontal lobe in which the granular layers are reduced. *See* area, motor.

area, anterior hypothalamic, HYPOTHALAMUS *See* area, hypothalamic, anterior.

area, anterior perforated, CEREBRUM *See* substance, perforated, anterior.

area, apneustic /ap-noos´tik/, PONS, [Gr. *a* not; *pneusis* breathing] area in the pontine tegmentum concerned with the coordination of inspiration and expiration.

areas, Brodmann's, CEREBRUM *See* Brodmann; Fig. B-1.

area cingular´is anterior dorsalis, CEREBRUM *See* Brodmann, area 32.

area cingularis anterior ventralis, CEREBRUM *See* Brodmann, area 24.

area cingularis posterior dorsalis, CEREBRUM *See* Brodmann, area 31.

area cingularis posterior ventralis, CEREBRUM *See* Brodmann, area 23.

area cribro´sa [NA] [L. *cribrum* a sieve] *See* lamina cribrosa.

area, cuneiform /ku-ne´I-form/, CEREBRUM *See* area, parolfactory.

area, ectorhi´nal, CEREBRUM *See* Brodmann, area 36.

area, ectosple´nial, CEREBRUM *See* Brodmann, area 26.

area, entorhi´nal, CEREBRUM Brodmann's area 28, in the anterior part of the parahippocampal gyrus, comprising most of the gyrus (Fig. B-1). Although six-layered, it is not typical isocortex and is probably a transitional form of cortex. Brodmann included it as a part of his cortex striatus, a division of the heterogenetic cortex.

area entorhinal´is dorsal´is, CEREBRUM *See* Brodmann, area 34.

area fascic´ulata, CEREBELLUM *See* body, juxtarestiform.

area frontal´is agranular´is, CEREBRUM *See* Brodmann, area 6.

area frontalis granular´is, CEREBRUM *See* Brodmann, area 9.

area frontalis interme´dia, CEREBRUM *See* Brodmann, area 8.

area frontalis microcellular´is, CEREBRUM *See* Brodmann, area 12.

area frontopolar´is, CEREBRUM *See* Brodmann, area 10.

area gigan´topyramidal´is, CEREBRUM   Brodmann's area 4, part of the precentral and paracentral gyri containing giant pyramidal (Betz) cells (Fig. B-1).

area, hypothalam´ic, anterior [regio hypothalamica anterior, NA], HYPOTHALAMUS area immediately posterior to, but not sharply delimited from, the (medial) preoptic area. Its two most conspicuous nuclei are the supraoptic and paraventricular nuclei. Also in this area are the anterior hypothalamic and the suprachiasmatic nuclei. *Syn:* supraoptic region. *See also* hypothalamus.

area (nucleus), hypothalamic, dorsal [area (regio) hypothalamica dorsalis, NA], HYPOTHALAMUS   term often applied to the area dorsal to the dorsomedial hypothalamic nucleus, extending from a position lateral to the paraventricular nucleus caudally as far as the posterior hypothalamic area.

area, hypothalamic, intermediate [regio hypothalamica intermedia, NA], HYPOTHALAMUS **1.** zone between the anterior and posterior regions of the medial hypothalamic area. Its ventromedial, dorsomedial, and perifornical nuclei are concerned with parasympathetic control, eating, and emotional expression. Other nuclei in this region are the tuberal, posterior periventricular, and arcuate. *Syn:* tuberal region. **2.** Sometimes this term is used for the lateral part of the medial hypothalamic area, excluding the periventricular zone. *See also* hypothalamus.

area, hypothalamic, lateral [area hypothalamica lateralis, NA], HYPOTHALAMUS   area lateral to a sagittal plane through the column of the fornix. It is continuous anteriorly with the lateral preoptic nucleus and posteriorly with the ventral tegmental area of the midbrain. Its cells constitute the lateral tuberal nuclei and the tuberomamillary nucleus but the area consists largely of fine fibers, some of which are fibers of passage including some from the medial hypothalamic area. Lesions in the posterior part of this region usually disrupt the connections for temperature regulation so that body temperature varies with that of the environment, poikilothermism. *See also* hypothalamus.

area, hypothalamic, medial, HYPOTHALAMUS   that part of the hypothalamus medial to a sagittal plane through the column of the fornix. Most of the cell groups of the hypothalamus are in this region. This region is further subdivided, from anterior to posterior, into preoptic, anterior, intermediate, and posterior hypothalamic areas and sometimes a thin periventricular zone. *See also* hypothalamus.

area, hypothalamic, posterior [regio hypothalamica posterior, NA], HYPOTHALAMUS area in the posterior part of the hypothalamus including the posterior hypothalamic and the mamillary nuclei. This region is concerned with autonomic regulation, particularly sympathetic control, and with the regulation of body temperature against cold. Lesions result in the lowering of body temperature or, if extended laterally to include fibers from the anterior hypothalamic region, may result in poikilothermism. Bilateral lesions in the region lateral and dorsolateral to the mamillary bodies are said to result in pathological sleep or narcolepsy. *Syn:* mamillary region. *See also* hypothalamus.

area, motor, CEREBRUM   Brodmann's area 4 (Fig. B-1) in the precentral gyrus and anterior part of the paracentral lobule. It contains giant pyramidal (Betz) cells in layer V and is concerned with fine, skilled voluntary movements. *Syn:* motor strip; agranular frontal area; area gigantopyramidalis.

area occipital´is, CEREBRUM   Brodmann's area 18 (Fig. B-1), a visual association area, also concerned with optokinetic eye movements.

area occipitotemporal´is, CEREBRUM   *See* Brodmann, area 37.

area, olfac´tory, lateral, CEREBRUM   collective term used for the temporal lobe gray in which olfactory tract fibers end, and comprising the prepiriform area, the lateral part of the anterior perforated substance, and the corticomedial part of the amygdala.

area, olfactory, medial, CEREBRUM   collective term used for the septum pellucidum, subcallosal gyrus, parolfactory area, olfactory trigone, and the medial part of the anterior perforated substance.

area, oval (of Flechsig), CORD   lumbar part of the septomarginal fasciculus, along the dorsal median septum, between the two gracile fasciculi.

area, paracommis´sural, CEREBRUM, [Gr. *para* beside]   parolfactory area, near the anterior commissure.

area, parain´sular, CEREBRUM   *See* Brodmann, area 52.

area, parastri´ate, CEREBRUM   Brodmann's area 18 (Fig. B-1) in the occipital lobe cortex adjacent to the visual (striate) cortex. It is a visual association area and is also concerned with optokinetic eye movements.

area, parasubic´ular, CEREBRUM   *See* Brodmann, area 49.

area, parater´minal, CEREBRUM   *See* gyrus, paraterminal.

area parietal´is superior, CEREBRUM   *See* Brodmann, area 7.

area, parolfac´tory (of Broca), CEREBRUM   area on the medial surface of the frontal lobe anterior to the lamina terminalis. It consists of the anterior parolfactory gyrus between the anterior and posterior parolfactory sulci and the posterior parolfactory gyrus behind the posterior parolfactory sulcus and is the medial part of the septal area in the precommissural septum. *Syn:* carrefour olfactif; cuneiform area; area adolfactif; paracommissural area.

area, perirhi´nal, CEREBRUM, [Gr. *peri* around]   Brodmann's area 35 (Fig. B-1), along the rhinal fissure, a transitional zone between the entorhinal part of the parahippocampal gyrus and the adjoining neopallial cortex. Brodmann considered it a part of his cortex striatus, a subdivision of the heterogenetic cortex.

area, peristri´ate (preoccip´ital), CEREBRUM   Brodmann's area 19 (Fig. B-1), anterior and adjacent to the parastriate area, mostly in the parietal and temporal lobes. It is a visual association area, also concerned with optokinetic eye movements.

area, pir´iform (pyr´iform), CEREBRUM   *See* lobe, piriform.

area, pneumotaxic /nu-mo-tak´sik/, PONS   part of the pontine tegmentum concerned with the regulation of respiration.

area postcentral´is caudal´is, CEREBRUM   *See* Brodmann, area 2.

area postcentralis interme´dia, CEREBRUM   *See* Brodmann, area 1.

area postcentralis oral´is, CEREBRUM   *See* Brodmann, area 3.

area postre´ma [NA], MEDULLA   one of the ventricular organs, a highly vascular mound of tissue along the margin of the caudal part of the fourth ventricle (Fig. V-4). It consists of many large capillaries, many glial, and some small nerve cells. It receives fibers directly from the vagal and glossopharyngeal nerves. Its efferent fibers go directly to the nucleus solitarius and the parabrachial nuclei and indirectly to other areas. It appears to function as a chemoreceptor trigger zone for emesis. Unilateral or bilateral lesions in this region cause nausea and vomiting. *For additional information on this subject, see* Area postrema ('84).

area, postsubic´ular, CEREBRUM   *See* Brodmann, area 48.

area, precommiss´ural septal, CEREBRUM   *See* septum, precommissural.

area, prefron´tal, CEREBRUM   cortical area in the frontal lobe, anterior to the premotor area, including the frontal pole and presumably comprising all or parts of Brodmann's areas 9, 10, 11, and 12; the frontal association area.

area pregenual´is, te´nia tec´ti, CEREBRUM   *See* Brodmann, area 33.

area, premo´tor, CEREBRUM   Brodmann's area 6 (Fig. B-1), in the frontal lobe, anterior to the motor area. Stimulation produces gross movements.

area, preoccip´ital, CEREBRUM   *See* area, peristriate.

area, preop´tic [area preoptica, NA], HYPOTHALAMUS   area on each side of the third ventricle, anterior to a plane extending from the interventricular foramen to the anterior surface of the optic chiasm (Fig. N-4). This area has traditionally been regarded as a telencephalic derivative, but now is thought to develop from the diencephalon, as a part of the hypothalamus, to which it is functionally related (Kuhlenbeck, '69). The medial preoptic area, with the anterior hypothalamic nucleus, is concerned with temperature regulation, protecting the body against heat. A subdivision, designated the *sexually dimorphic nucleus,* is concerned with the regulation of gonadotropic hormones. A lesion in the medial preoptic area has been shown to cause hyperthermia. Lung edema (also called preoptic pulmonary edema) has also been reported. *See also* hypothalamus.

area preparietal´is, CEREBRUM   Brodmann's area 5 (Fig. B-1), sensory association cortex.

area, prepir´iform (prepyr´iform), CEREBRUM   the lateral olfactory gyrus, adjacent to the lateral olfactory tract (Fig. C-3C) on the ventral surface of the frontal lobe, and gyrus ambiens on the upper lateral surface of the uncus. Brodmann included it as a part of the cortex striatus, a subdivision of the heterogenetic cortex.

area, presubic´ular, CEREBRUM   Brodmann's area 27 (Fig. B-1), a cortical area on the ventromedial surface of the temporal lobe between the entorhinal area and the subiculum. Brodmann included it as a part of his cortex striatus, a subdivision of the heterogenetic cortex. *Syn:* presubiculum.

area, pretec´tal [area pretectalis, NA], DIENCEPHALON   In lower mammals, it is undifferentiated gray matter in the caudal part of the diencephalon, adjacent to the habenula, the pulvinar, and the pretectal nucleus of the midbrain. It receives some optic tract fibers. In primates, much of this area is contained in the pulvinar. *Syn:* pretectum.

area, pyr´iform (pir´iform), CEREBRUM   *See* lobe, piriform.

area retrolim´bica agranular´is, CEREBRUM   *See* Brodmann, area 30.

area retrolimbica granularis, CEREBRUM   *See* Brodmann, area 29.

area, retrosubic´ular, CEREBRUM   Brodmann's area 48 (Fig. B-1), cortical area (small in man) caudal to the perirhinal area on the medial surface of the temporal lobe. Brodmann included it as a part of his cortex striatus, a subdivision of heterogenetic cortex.

area, sen´sory association, CEREBRUM   usuallu the cortical area posterior to the postcentral gyrus and adjacent to the sensory projection cortex.

area, sep´tal, CEREBRUM   The major part of this area, the precommissural septum, is located anterior to the anterior commissure, between the medial surface of the frontal lobe and the anterior horn of the lateral ventricle, and consists of a number of nuclei. The posterior part, septum pellucidum or the postcommissural septum, is relatively thin with fewer cells. *See also* septum, precommissural.

area, silent, CEREBRUM   any cortical area which upon stimulation does not produce any detectable motor activity or sensory phenomenon, and in which a lesion may occur without producing detectable motor or sensory abnormalities, although such areas may serve cognitive or other important functions.

area, somesthet´ic, CEREBRUM   *See* cortex, somesthetic.

area, stri´ate (area striata), CEREBRUM   Brodmann's area 17 (Fig. B-1), visual projection cortex in the occipital lobe adjoining the calcarine sulcus, and containing 3 the macroscopic stripe of Gennari.

area, strip, CEREBRUM   area 4s, a narrow strip of cerebral cortex, lying between Brodmann's areas 4 and 6. It is a suppressor area which inhibits activity of area 4.

area, subcallo´sal [area subcallosa, NA], CEREBRUM   area ventral to the genu of the corpus callosum and anterior to the lamina terminalis. It consists primarily of the subcallosal gyrus and the parolfactory area (Fig. C-3B).

area, subcen´tral, CEREBRUM   *See* Brodmann, area 43.

area subgenual´is, CEREBRUM   *See* Brodmann, area 25.

area, supplemen´tary motor, CEREBRUM   any cortical area, other than the motor and premotor areas (Brodmann's areas 4 and 6), stimulation of which produces movements of the body, head, or limbs.

area, suppres´sor, CEREBRUM   any cortical area stimulation of which inhibits the motor activity elicited from another cortical area.

area temporal´is inferior, CEREBRUM   *See* Brodmann, area 20.

area temporalis media, CEREBRUM   *See* Brodmann, area 21.

area temporalis superior, CEREBRUM   *See* Brodmann, area 22.

area temporopolar´is, CEREBRUM   *See* Brodmann, area 38.

area triangular´is, CEREBRUM   area just lateral to the lateral geniculate nucleus and pulvinar and consisting of fibers mainly of the optic and auditory radiations, and pulvinar connections. *Syn:* field or zone of Wernicke.

area, ventral tegmen´tal (of Tsai), MIDBRAIN   part of the tegmental gray matter in the rostral part of the midbrain, ventral to the red nucleus. It is traversed by descending fibers from the hypothalamus and by fibers of the oculomotor nerve. Dopaminergic fibers from this region accompany those of the nigrostriate tract.

area, vestib´ular [area vestibularis, NA], PONS, MEDULLA   floor of the fourth ventricle lateral to the sulcus limitans, overlying the vestibular nuclei; part of the acoustic area (Fig. V-4).

area, vis´ual association, CEREBRUM   Brodmann's cortical areas 18 and 19 (Fig. B-1), adjacent to the visual projection cortex.

areflexia /a-re-flek´sĭ-ah/   absence of all reflexes.

Argyll Robertson, Douglas Moray Cooper Lamb (1837-1909)   Scottish ophthalmic surgeon. An *Argyll Robertson pupil* (1869) is a miotic pupil that does not react to light but constricts upon convergence-accommodation.

arhinenceph´aly   absence of the olfactory bulbs and tracts; originally this term was used to include other developmental defects of the face and head as well.

Ariëns Kappers, Cornelius Ubbo (1877-1946)   Dutch anatomist of Amsterdam, noted for his studies of comparative neuroanatomy. He introduced the tenet of neurobiotaxis in cell migration (1914) and published a comprehensive treatise on comparative neuroanatomy, later expanded and published in English (1936), with G.C. Huber and E.C. Crosby.

Arnold, Friedrich (1803-1890)   German anatomist who described many structures of the brain and ear. Named for him were: *Arnold's ganglion* (the otic ganglion) and *Arnold's nerve* (the auricular branch of the vagus nerve), both described in 1828; *Arnold's canal* (the channel in the petrous part of the temporal bone through which the nerve passes); *Arnold's recurrent nerve* (a branch connecting the ophthalmic and trochlear nerves); *Arnold's tracts* (both the frontal and the temporal corticopontine tracts); *Arnold's area* (the vagal trigone); Arnold's *ligament* (the suspensory ligament which connects the incus with the roof of the middle ear); and the *stratum zonale of Arnold* (the ventral external arcuate fibers on the surface of the medulla).

Arnold, Julius (1835-1916)   German pathologist, son of Friedrich Arnold. His description of the *Arnold-Chiari malformation,* was published in 1894, three years after that of H. Chiari.   In this developmental abnormality the cerebellum is elongated and extends through the foramen magnum into the spinal canal. The entire brain stem is stretched and displaced caudally and there is a hump on the posterior surface of the medulla. The upper cervical and lower cranial nerve roots slope upward to reach their foramina of exit.   The apertures of the fourth ventricle are closed and the subarachnoid space at the level of the foramen magnum is sealed off, resulting in an obstructive hydrocephalus. Various theories have been advanced for the etiology of this condition.   Most likely it does not result from caudal traction on the spinal cord secondary to a lumbosacral defect, as formerly supposed, but from overgrowth of the tissue in the region of the malformation or from an arrest in development of the hindbrain with failure of the pontine flexure to develop. *For a discussion of this syndrome and its possible causes, see* List and Schneider ('82, p. 894).

arteries   *For additional information on the arteries of the human brain and spinal cod, see* Stephens and Stillwell ('69), *and* Salamon and Huang ('76).

artery, angular [arteria gyri angularis, NA], CEREBRUM   branch of the middle cerebral artery which emerges from the posterior tip of the lateral sulcus. It overlies and supplies the angular gyrus and the area posterior to it (Fig. A-3). *Syn:* parieto-occipital branch of the middle cerebral artery.

arteries, anterolateral, CEREBRUM   *See* arteries, central, anterolateral.

arteries, anteromedial, CEREBRUM   *See* arteries, central, anteromedial.

artery, auditory, internal   *See* artery, labyrinthine.

artery, bas´ilar [arteria basilaris, NA], PONS   large single median artery on the ventral surface of the pons formed by the fusion of the two vertebral arteries, and supplying by way of its branches the pons and midbrain, and parts of the medulla, cerebellum, and forebrain.

artery, cal´carine [ramus calcarinus, NA], CEREBRUM   branch, which with the parieto-occipital artery arises from the medial occipital artery, a branch of the posterior cerebral artery (Fig. A-2).   It lies along the calcarine sulcus and supplies the adjoining (visual) cortex.

artery, callosomar´ginal [arteria callosomarginalis, NA], CEREBRUM   major branch of the anterior cerebral artery which usually arises anterior to the genu of the corpus callosum and follows the cingulate (callosomarginal]) sulcus (Fig. A-2).   Its branches supply much of the medial surface of the frontal and parietal lobes and their outer rim on the lateral surface.

artery, carot´id, common [arteria carotis communis, NA]   large paired vessel in the neck. The right common carotid artery arises from the bifurcation of the brachio-cephalic trunk; the left from the arch of the aorta.   At about the level of the upper border of the thyroid cartilage these vessels divide into the external carotid artery, which supplies extracranial structures, and the internal carotid artery, which supplies the brain.

artery, carotid, internal [arteria carotis interna, NA], CEREBRUM   branch of the common carotid artery which passes through the carotid canal and cavernous sinus (Figs. A-1, S-1) to enter the cranial cavity.   It and its counterpart of the other side form part of the cerebral arterial circle (of Willis) (Fig. C-5) on the ventral surface of the brain. Its main branches are the anterior and middle cerebral arteries, and the hypophysial, ophthalmic, posterior communicating, and anterior choroidal arteries. *See also* siphon, carotid; sinus, cavernous.

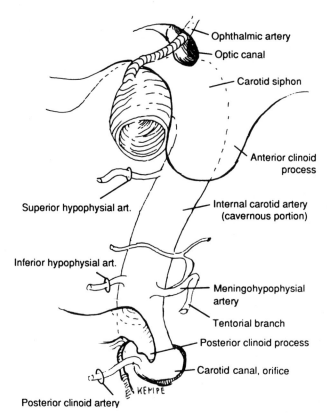

Fig. A-1.   Internal carotid artery in the cavernous sinus, as seen from above. Anteriorly the carotid siphon underlies the anterior clinoid process of the sphenoid bone. Drawing courtesy of Dr. L.G. Kempe.

arteries, central   1. MEDULLA, CORD   *See* arteries, sulcal.

2. FOREBRAIN   any of the small vessels which arise from the cerebral arterial circle (of Willis) or from the proximal parts of its major branches (Fig. C-5). They enter the brain near their origin and supply the deep structures within the forebrain. *Syn:* ganglionic arteries.

3. EYE   branch of the ophthalmic artery which runs through the center of the optic nerve into the eyeball and divides into the retinal arteries.

4. CEREBRUM   *See* artery (of the) central sulcus.

arteries, central, anterolateral [arteriae centrales anterolaterales, NA], FOREBRAIN   any of a series of 8 to 14 small arteries which arise from the proximal part of the middle cerebral artery and pass upward into the brain substance to supply the medial part of the head of the caudate nucleus, the globus pallidus and putamen, the anterior and medial parts of the dorsal thalamus, and most of the posterior limb of the internal capsule (Fig. C-5). *Syn:* lateral striate or lenticulostriate arteries.

arteries, central, anteromedial [arteriae centrales anteromediales, NA], FOREBRAIN any of a group of small vessels which arise from the anterior communicating artery and the proximal part of the anterior cerebral artery (Fig. C-5). They supply the anterior part of the hypothalamus, septum pellucidum, medial part of the anterior commissure, column of the fornix, and the anterior inferior part of the striatum. The recurrent artery, one of the larger of this group, supplies part of the caudate nucleus and putamen and part of the anterior limb of the internal capsule. *Syn:* medial striate or anteromedial arteries.

artery, central, long [arteria centralis longa, NA], CEREBRUM   *See* artery, recurrent.

arteries, central, posterolateral [arteriae centrales posterolaterales, NA], DIENCEPHALON any of several small branches which arise from the posterior cerebral artery lateral to its junction with the posterior communicating artery, as it passes around the cerebral peduncle, and which supply the pulvinar, the medial part of the lateral geniculate nucleus, and other posterior thalamic structures (Fig. C-5). *Syn:* thalamogeniculate arteries.

arteries, central, posteromedial [arteriae centrales posteromediales, NA], DIENCEPHALON, MIDBRAIN   any of the branches arising from the most proximal part of the posterior cerebral artery between the bifurcation of the basilar artery and the junction with the posterior communicating artery (Fig. C-5). They enter the brain through the rostral part of the posterior perforated substance and fan out to supply the medial parts of the diencephalon and upper midbrain. *Syn:* thalamo-perforating, posterior perforating, or retromamillary arteries.

artery (of the) central sulcus [arteria sulci centralis, NA], CEREBRUM   branch of the middle cerebral artery, which lies along the central sulcus on the lateral surface of the cerebral hemisphere and supplies the adjoining cortex (Fig. A-3). *Syn:* rolandic artery.

artery, cerebel´lar, anterior inferior (AICA) [arteria inferior anterior cerebelli, NA], PONS, MEDULLA, CEREBELLUM   branch arising from the basilar artery near its origin. It supplies some of the lateral part of the medulla and pons and the anterior and inferior surfaces of the cerebellum. *Syn:* middle cerebellar artery.

artery, cerebellar, middle, PONS, MEDULLA, CEREBELLUM   *See* artery, cerebellar, anterior inferior.

artery, cerebellar, posterior inferior (PICA) [arteria inferior posterior cerebelli, NA], MEDULLA, CEREBELLUM   branch of the vertebral artery which supplies the lateral part of the medulla, the inferior surface of the cerebellum, and the choroid plexus of the fourth ventricle. *Syn:* posterior cerebellar artery.

artery, cerebellar, superior [arteria superior cerebelli, NA], MIDBRAIN, PONS, CEREBELLUM branch which arises from the basilar artery just prior to the origin of the posterior cerebral arteries (Fig. C-5). It supplies the upper part of the pons, the middle and superior cerebellar peduncles, part of the tectum, and the superior surface of the cerebellum.

artery, cer´ebral, acces´sory middle, CEREBRUM   inconstant branch of the anterior cerebral artery which, when present, accompanies the main trunk of the middle cerebral artery and shares part of its territory of distribution.

artery, cerebral, anterior [arteria cerebri anterior, NA], CEREBRUM   one of the two main branches of the internal carotid artery. It gives off its ganglionic branches (the central anteromedial arteries) then passes dorsally onto the medial surface of the frontal lobe and curves up over the genu of the corpus callosum. Its cortical branches (the medial frontobasal, frontopolar, and callosomarginal arteries) supply the orbital surface of the frontal lobe and the medial aspect of the frontal and parietal lobes and their rim on the lateral surface (Figs. A-2, C-5). Some branches join the cortical branches of the middle cerebral artery laterally and the posterior cerebral artery posteriorly.

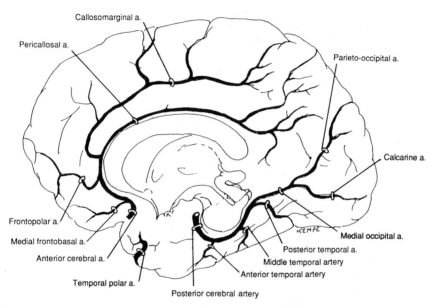

Fig. A-2.   The anterior and posterior cerebral arteries and their major cortical branches on the medial surface of the cerebral hemisphere. Drawing courtesy of Dr. L.G. Kempe.

artery, cerebral, middle [arteria cerebri media, NA], CEREBRUM   large terminal branch of the internal carotid artery. It gives off its ganglionic branches (the central anteromedial and anterolateral arteries and sometimes the anterior choroidal artery) (Fig. C-5) then enters the lateral sulcus of the cerebrum where its branches occupy the Sylvian triangle before they emerge onto the lateral surface of the cerebral hemisphere. These branches (the lateral frontobasal artery, the arteries of the precentral, central, and postcentral sulci, the supramarginal and angular arteries) distribute to almost the entire lateral surface of the cerebrum and the temporal pole (Fig. A-3). Some branches anastomose with those of the anterior and posterior cerebral arteries on the medial surface of the cerebrum. *Syn:* Sylvian artery. *See also* triangle, Sylvian.

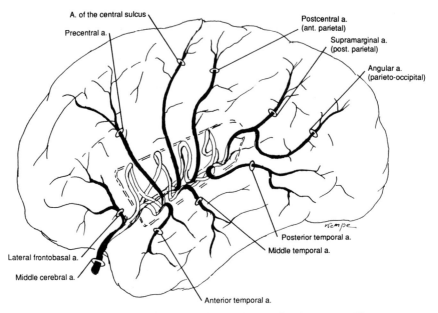

A. of the central sulcus

Precentral a.

Postcentral a.
(ant. parietal)

Supramarginal a.
(post. parietal)

Angular a.
(parieto-occipital)

Kempe

Posterior temporal a.

Middle temporal a.

Lateral frontobasal a.

Middle cerebral a.

Anterior temporal a.

Fig. A-3. The middle cerebral artery and its major cortical branches. The vessels on the lateral surface of the cerebral hemisphere are shown in black. Those shown in outline occupy the Sylvian triangle, the limits of which are outlined by the double line. Drawing courtesy of Dr. L.G. Kempe.

artery, cerebral, posterior [arteria cerebri posterior, NA], FOREBRAIN   large terminal branch of the basilar artery. After giving off its ganglionic branches (the postero-medial and posterolateral central and the posteromedial choroidal arteries) (Fig. C-5), it passes around the midbrain. Its cortical branches (the anterior, middle, and posterior temporal arteries and the medial occipital artery and its branches) supply the medial surface of the temporal and occipital lobes and their rim on the lateral surface (Fig. A-2). Some cortical branches anastomose with those of the anterior and middle cerebral arteries. Embryologically the posterior cerebral artery develops as a branch of the internal carotid artery by way of the posterior communicating artery, and occasionally this relationship is retained so that its main source of blood remains the internal carotid artery.

artery, choroiˊdal (chorioiˊdal), anterior [arteria choroidea anterior, NA], FOREBRAIN branch, usually of the internal carotid artery, sometimes of the middle cerebral artery (Fig. C-5). It passes posteriorly along the optic tract and enters the inferior horn of the lateral ventricle by way of the choroid fissure. In addition to the choroid plexus, it supplies the optic tract, amygdala, and much of the hippocampus, the genu of the internal capsule as well as the inferior and posterior parts of the posterior limb of the capsule, part of the globus pallidus, the posterior part of the putamen, the tail of the caudate nucleus, the lateral geniculate nucleus, and the optic radiation. A lesion involving this vessel may result in hemiplegia, hemianesthesia, and hemianopsia. *See also* artery, hippocampal; *and* artery, choroidal, posterolateral, *and* posteromedial.

arteries, choroidal posterolateral (posterior lateral) [rami choroidei posteriores laterales, NA], FOREBRAIN   two, sometimes three, branches which arise from the posterior cerebral artery after the origin of the posteromedial choroidal artery. They supply the choroid plexus of the lateral ventricle, the dorsal thalamus, and the fornix.

artery, choroidal posteromedial (posterior medial) [rami choroidei posteriores mediales, NA], FOREBRAIN   branch arising from the proximal part of the posterior cerebral artery (Fig. C-5). It passes around the midbrain then upward and forward in the roof of the third ventricle. It supplies the pineal body, the choroid plexus of the third ventricle, and to some extent the dorsal thalamus.

arteries, circumferen´tial   any of a class of arterial branches that arise from vessels on the ventral surface of the brain, pass laterally on the brain surface for a lesser (short circumferential arteries) or greater (long circumferential arteries) distance, and supply, directly or by their branches, much of the brain substance. *Syn:* lateral artery.

arteries, circumferential, long   any of the larger circumferential arteries of the brain. They arise from vessels on the ventral surface of the brain and pass laterally to supply parts of the brain at some distance from the ventral midline. The largest of these vessels are the anterior, middle, and posterior cerebral arteries and the superior, anterior inferior, and posterior inferior cerebellar arteries. *Syn:* long lateral arteries.

arteries, circumferential, short   any of the small arterial branches of the vertebral and basilar arteries, which pass laterally and supply an intermediate zone between the ventromedial and the dorsolateral portions of the brain stem. *Syn:* short lateral arteries.

artery, communicating, anterior [arteria communicans anterior, NA], CEREBRUM   short, usually single, median vessel connecting the two anterior cerebral arteries and completing the cerebral arterial circle anteriorly (Fig. C-5).

artery, communicating, posterior [arteria communicans posterior, NA], CEREBRUM   anastomotic vessel on the ventral surface of the brain connecting the internal carotid and posterior cerebral arteries and forming, on each side, a part of the cerebral arterial circle (Fig. C-5).

artery, frontal ascending, CEREBRUM   single trunk frequently arising from the middle cerebral artery at the base of the insula. It divides and gives rise to an anterior group of arteries: the lateral frontobasal, precentral, central, and postcentral arteries; and a posterior group: the anterior and posterior parietal, and angular arteries.

arteries, frontal, internal, CEREBRUM   branches of the callosomarginal artery which supply the posterior part of the superior frontal gyrus and much of the medial surface of the frontal lobe posterior to the territory supplied by the frontopolar artery.

artery, frontoba´sal, lateral [arteria frontobasalis lateralis, NA], CEREBRUM   branch of the middle cerebral artery which arises anterior to the insula and supplies the anterior inferior part of the lateral surface of the frontal lobe and anastomoses with the orbital vessels on the ventral surface (Fig. A-3). *Syn:* lateral orbitofrontal artery.

artery, frontobasal medial [arteria frontobasalis medialis, NA], CEREBRUM   branch of the anterior cerebral artery which arises ventral to the genu of the corpus callosum and supplies the anterior inferior part of the medial surface of the frontal lobe (Fig. A-2). It anastomoses with the orbital vessels on the ventral surface. *Syn:* medial orbitofrontal artery.

artery, frontopo´lar (frontal polar), CEREBRUM   artery which usually arises from the anterior cerebral artery near the genu of the corpus callosum but sometimes is a branch of the callosomarginal artery. It passes forward toward the frontal pole and supplies the anterior part of the superior frontal gyrus on the medial and lateral surfaces of the cerebrum and the anterior part of the middle frontal gyrus (Fig. A-2).

arteries, ganglion´ic (central), FOREBRAIN   *See* arteries, central, *def.* 2.

arteries, hippocam´pal, CEREBRUM   several branches (1 to 4) of the posterior cerebral artery which course along the hippocampal fissure into which they send branches in a rakelike pattern. These vessels contribute to the supply of all but the most anterior part of the hippocampal formation, which is supplied by branches of the anterior choroidal artery.

artery, hy´aloid [arteria hyaloidea, NA], EYE   terminal branch of the ophthalmic artery in the developing eye. It extends forward in the hyaloid canal of the vitreous body from the back of the eyeball to the lens and supplies the structures in the optic cup. Later the proximal part of the vessel becomes the central artery of the retina and the rest of the hyaloid artery degenerates.

artery, hypophysi´al, inferior   small branch of the internal carotid artery (Fig. A-1) which, with its counterpart of the other side, arborizes in the capsule of the hypophysis and sends branches mainly to the posterior lobe and partly to the anterior lobe of the hypophysis.

arteries, hypophysial, superior   several small branches arising from the internal carotid artery (Fig. A-1) which, with their counterparts of the opposite side, form a plexus around the base of the hypophysial stalk and supply the median eminence, the hypophysial stalk, and the anterior lobe of the hypophysis.

arteries, in´sular [arteriae insulares, NA], CEREBRUM   branches of the middle cerebral artery which overly the insula in the Sylvian triangle (Fig. A-3).

artery, internal auditory, EAR   *See* artery, labyrinthine.

artery (of) internal hemorrhage, CEREBRUM   one of the anterolateral central arteries (Fig. C-5), presumably the largest of the group which passes around the lateral border of the lentiform nucleus, so named by Charcot because he and others believed it to be frequently affected in cerebral hemorrhage. *Syn:* artery of Charcot.

artery, internal occipital, CEREBRUM   *See* artery, occipital, medial.

artery, labyrin´thine [arteria labyrinthi, NA], EAR   branch usually arising from the anterior inferior cerebellar artery, occasionally directly from the basilar artery, and passing through the internal auditory meatus with the facial and vestibulocochlear nerves to supply structures within the petrous part of the temporal bone. *Syn:* internal auditory artery; ramus meatus acustici interni.

arteries, lateral   *See* arteries, circumferential.

arteries, lenticulo-op´tic, FOREBRAIN   term sometimes applied to the most medial of the anterolateral central arteries (Fig. C-5).

arteries, lenticulostri´ate, FOREBRAIN   *See* arteries, central, anterolateral.

artery, medial occipital, CEREBRUM   *See* artery, occipital, medial.

arteries, median   any of the arterial branches which arise from vessels on the ventral surface of the brain and penetrate the surface near the median plane. Each vessel supplies a paramedian zone on one side only, not both. The sulcal arteries of the spinal cord correspond to the median arteries of the brain.

arteries, med´ullary, spinal, CORD *See* arteries, spinal medullary.

artery, menin´geal, acces´sory small branch of the internal maxillary artery which enters the cranial cavity through the foramen ovale and supplies the trigeminal ganglion and neighboring dura mater.

artery, meningeal, anterior [ramus meningeus anterior, NA] branch of the anterior ethmoidal artery which supplies the dura mater of the anterior cranial fossa.

artery, meningeal, middle [arteria meningea media, NA] branch of the internal maxillary artery which enters the cranial cavity through the foramen spinosum to supply much of the intracranial dura mater.

arteries, meningeal, posterior [arteria meningea posterior, NA] any of several small branches of the vertebral and occipital arteries and other small vessels which supply the dura mater of the posterior cranial fossa.

arteries, mesencephal´ic **1.** MIDBRAIN, [arteriae mesencephalicae, NA] any of the small posteromedial central branches of the posterior cerebral artery which supply the midbrain.
2. This term has also been applied to the proximal part of the posterior cerebral artery, from the bifurcation of the basilar artery to its junction with the posterior communicating artery.

artery, occipital, medial [arteria occipitalis medialis, NA], CEREBRUM branch of the posterior cerebral artery which gives rise to the parieto-occipital and calcarine arteries (Fig. A-2). *Syn:* internal occipital artery.

artery, occipitopari´etal, CEREBRUM *See* artery, parieto-occipital.

artery, ophthal´mic [arteria ophthalmica, NA], EYE branch arising from the internal carotid artery, usually just after it emerges from the cavernous sinus (Figs. A-1, C-5). It enters the orbit through the optic canal and supplies various orbital structures. Because of its connections with the external carotid system, it sometimes serves as a channel for collateral circulation for the anterior and middle cerebral arteries. Its main branches include: the central artery of the retina and the lacrimal, supraorbital, ethmoidal, and palpebral arteries.

artery, ophthalmic, acces´sory, EYE inconstant vessel arising from the anterior branch of the middle meningeal artery. It passes through the superior orbital fissure to supply structures in the orbit.

arteries, or´bital, CEREBRUM several branches which supply the orbital surface of the frontal lobe and the olfactory bulb and which anastomose with the medial and lateral frontobasal arteries, branches of the anterior and middle cerebral arteries.

artery, orbitofron´tal lateral [ramus orbitofrontalis lateralis, NA], CEREBRUM *See* artery, frontobasal, lateral.

artery, orbitofrontal medial [ramus orbitofrontalis medialis, NA], CEREBRUM *See* artery, frontobasal, medial.

artery, paracen´tral [arteria paracentralis, NA], CEREBRUM branch of the pericallosal or the callosomarginal artery which supplies the paracentral gyrus.

arteries, pari´etal, anterior and posterior [arteriae parietales anterior et posterior, NA], CEREBRUM branches of the middle cerebral artery which emerge from the lateral sulcus, separately or as a single vessel, then divide and supply the lateral surface of the parietal lobe (Fig. A-3). *Syn:* postcentral and supramarginal arteries, respectively.

artery, pari´eto-occip´ital, CEREBRUM **1.** the angular artery, a branch of the middle cerebral artery (Fig. A-3).

2. branch which arises with the calcarine artery from the medial occipital artery, a branch of the posterior cerebral artery, on the medial surface of the cerebral hemisphere. It supplies cortex adjacent to the parieto-occipital sulcus (Fig. A-2).

arteries, penetrating   any of the small vessels which arise from arteries on the surface of the brain and spinal cord, enter the substance of the CNS, and end there in capillary networks.

artery, pericallo´sal [arteria pericallosa, NA], CEREBRUM   terminal branch of the anterior cerebral artery which lies in the sulcus of the corpus callosum (Fig. A-2). It supplies the cingulate gyrus and the underlying corpus callosum and frequently gives rise to paracentral, precuneal, and posterior callosal branches.

arteries, pon´tine [arteriae pontis, NA], PONS   any of the small branches which arise from the basilar artery and supply the pons.

artery, postcentral [arteria sulci postcentralis NA], CEREBRUM   branch of the middle cerebral artery which lies along the postcentral sulcus on the lateral surface of the parietal lobe (Fig. A-3) and supplies the adjoining cortex. *Syn:* postrolandic artery; anterior parietal artery.

arteries, posterior perforating, DIENCEPHALON, MIDBRAIN   *See* arteries, central posteromedial.

arteries, posterolateral, DIENCEPHALON   *See* arteries, central posterolateral.

arteries, posteromedial, DIENCEPHALON, MIDBRAIN   *See* arteries, central posteromedial.

artery, postrolandic, CEREBRUM   *See* artery, postcentral.

artery, precentral [arteria sulci precentralis, NA], CEREBRUM   branch of the middle cerebral artery which lies along the precentral sulcus on the lateral surface of the frontal lobe (Fig. A-3) and supplies the adjoining cortex. *Syn:* prerolandic artery.

artery, precu´neal [arteria precunealis, NA], CEREBRUM   usually a branch of the pericallosal artery, sometimes a branch of the callosomarginal artery. It supplies the precuneus on the medial surface of the parietal lobe.

arteries, premam´illary, DIENCEPHALON   several arteries which arise from the posterior communicating arteries (rarely from the anterior choroidal artery), penetrate the hypothalamus anterior to the mamillary bodies, and supply the tuber cinereum and adjoining hypothalamus. *Syn:* thalamotuberal arteries.

artery, quadrigem´inal, MIDBRAIN   branch arising from the proximal part of the posterior cerebral artery. It passes around the brain stem to supply the posterior midbrain.

arteries, radic´ular, spinal, CORD   *See* arteries, spinal radicular.

artery, radicular (medullary), great anterior (ventral), CORD   unpaired large medullary artery which joins the anterior spinal artery, at a low thoracic or upper lumbar cord level (usually about L1 or L2), and supplies blood for the anterior two-thirds of the spinal cord below its level of entrance. *Syn:* artery of Adamkiewicz.

artery, radicular (medullary), great posterior, CORD   large radicular artery (not so large as its anterior counterpart) which joins the posterior arterial plexus at a low thoracic or upper lumbar level.

artery, recur´rent [arteria recurrens, NA], CEREBRUM   largest of the anteromedial central arteries, it arises from the anterior cerebral artery near its junction with the anterior communicating artery (Fig. C-5). Its branches penetrate the anterior perforated substance medial to the anterolateral central arteries and supply mainly the anterior, inferior part of the head of the caudate nucleus, putamen, and adjoining part of the anterior limb of the internal capsule. *Syn:* artery of Heubner; long central artery.

arteries, retromam´illary, DIENCEPHALON, MIDBRAIN *See* arteries, central, posteromedial.

artery, rolan´dic, CEREBRUM *See* artery (of the) central sulcus.

artery, spinal, anterior [arteria spinalis anterior, NA], MEDULLA, CORD unpaired median artery extending along the ventral surface of the medulla and the full length of the spinal cord. It receives tributaries at its cranial end from the vertebral arteries and at spinal cord levels from spinal medullary branches. It supplies by way of its sulcal (central) branches most of the ventral two-thirds of the spinal cord and the paramedian part of the medulla.

artery, spinal, anterior median, MEDULLA, CORD *See* artery, spinal, anterior.

arteries, spinal medullary, CORD any of the arterial branches that enter the intervertebral foramina, accompany the spinal nerve roots, and join the anterior spinal artery or the arterial plexus on the surface of the spinal cord. *See also* arteries, spinal radicular.

arteries, spinal, posterior [arteria spinalis posterior, NA], MEDULLA, CORD small branches of the vertebral arteries which descend, one on either side, along the dorsolateral surface of the medulla and upper spinal cord, then become continuous with a posterior arterial plexus.

arteries, spinal radic´ular, CORD any of the arterial branches that enter the intervertebral foramina, accompany and supply the spinal nerve roots, but do not reach the spinal cord. *See also* arteries, spinal medullary.

arteries, striate, lateral, FOREBRAIN *See* arteries, central, anterolateral.

arteries, striate, medial, FOREBRAIN *See* arteries, central, anteromedial.

arteries, sul´cal, MEDULLA, CORD any of the branches of the anterior spinal artery which enter the ventral median fissure on the ventral surface of the medulla and spinal cord and supply capillary beds on one side or the other. Only the most caudal of these vessels bifurcate to supply both sides. *Syn:* central arteries.

artery, supramar´ginal, CEREBRUM one of the parietal arteries arising from the middle cerebral artery and overlying the supramarginal gyrus (Fig. A-3). *Syn:* posterior parietal artery.

artery, Syl´vian, CEREBRUM middle cerebral artery, particularly the branches that make up the Sylvian triangle (Fig. A-3). *See also* triangle, Sylvian.

artery, temp´oral, anterior, CEREBRUM **1.** [arteria temporalis anterior, NA] branch of the middle cerebral artery on the lateral surface of the temporal lobe (Fig. A-3).
2. [rami temporales anteriores, NA] one or more branches of the posterior cerebral artery, on the medial, inferior surface of the temporal lobe, which frequently anastomose with corresponding branches from the middle cerebral artery (Fig. A-2).

artery, temporal, middle, CEREBRUM **1.** [arteria temporalis media, NA] branch of the middle cerebral artery on the lateral surface of the temporal lobe (Fig. A-3).
2. [rami temporales intermedii mediales, NA] one or more branches of the posterior cerebral artery, on the medial, inferior surface of the temporal lobe, which frequently anastomose with corresponding branches from the middle cerebral artery (Fig. A-2).

artery, temporal polar, CEREBRUM inconstant branch of the middle cerebral artery which supplies the temporal pole (Fig. A-2).

artery, temporal, posterior, CEREBRUM **1.** [arteria temporalis posterior, NA] branch of the middle cerebral artery on the lateral surface of the temporal lobe (Fig.

A-3).

2. [rami temporales posteriores, NA] one or more branches of the posterior cerebral artery, on the medial, inferior surface of the temporal lobe, which frequently anastomose with corresponding branches of the middle cerebral artery (Fig. A-2). *Syn:* temporo-occipital artery.

artery, temporo-occip´ital, CEREBRUM   *See* artery, temporal, posterior, *def.* 2.

artery, ter´minal   caudal continuation of the anterior spinal artery along the filum terminale.

arteries, thalamogenic´ulate, DIENCEPHALON   *See* arteries, central, posterolateral.

arteries, thalamoper´forating, DIENCEPHALON, MIDBRAIN   *See* arteries, central, posteromedial.

arteries, thalamostri´ate, anterolateral, FOREBRAIN   *See* arteries, central, anterolateral.

arteries, thalamostriate, anteromedial, FOREBRAIN   *See* arteries, central, anteromedial.

arteries, thalamotu´beral, DIENCEPHALON   *See* arteries, premamillary.

artery, trigem´inal   transitory branch of the internal carotid artery, which usually regresses as the posterior communicating artery develops but may persist as an anastomotic link between the cavernous portion of the internal carotid artery and the basilar artery.

artery, ver´tebral [arteria vertebralis, NA]   branch of the subclavian artery, which passes upward through the transverse foramina of the cervical vertebrae and enters the cranial cavity through the foramen magnum. It and its counterpart of the other side unite to form the basilar artery. Branches of the vertebrobasilar system supply the brain stem and cerebellum, the occipital and part of the temporal lobes, and certain basal forebrain structures.

Aschoff, Karl Albert Ludwig (1866-1942)   German pathologist. The *Aschoff-Tawara node* is the atrioventricular node.

aspar´tate (Asp)   an excitatory neurotransmitter found, along with glutamate, another excitatory transmitter, in high concentrations in the CNS, especially in corticostriate nerve fibers, parallel and climbing fibers of the cerebellum, and several of the hippocampal connections. *See also* neurotransmitters.

astasia /as-ta´zĭ-ah/ [Gr. *a* not; *stasis* standing]   inability to stand.

astereogno´sis [Gr. *a-*; *steros* solid; *gnosis* knowledge]   inability to identify objects by palpation, whether or not tactile sensation is impaired. *See also* agnosia, tactile.

aster´ion [NA] [Gr. *astron* star]   point at which the mastoid portion of the temporal bone meets the parietal and occipital bones. In the infant it is the site of the small posterolateral fontanelle. It is an important neurosurgical landmark, as it overlies the turn of the transverse into the sigmoid dural sinus.

asterixis /as-ter-ik´sis/ [Gr. *a* not; *sterixis* fixed position]   peculiar flapping, especially of the hands, with inability to maintain extension at the wrists and ankles. It is a feature of hepatic encephalopathy and impending hepatic coma but also occurs with other metabolic encephalopathies.

astrocyte /as´tro-sĭt/ [Gr. *astron* star; *kytos* cell]   neuroglial cell, of ectodermal origin, having a round nucleus, "star-shaped" body, and many long processes. Two types are distinguished by light microscopy: fibrous astrocytes (spider cells) and protoplasmic astrocytes (mossy cells). Processes from these cells end as vascular foot plates on the small blood vessels of the CNS and form the perivascular glial limiting membrane. Other processes, extending toward the external and ventricular surfaces of the CNS, fuse with the overlying pia mater or ependymal cell processes and form the superficial and periventricular limiting membranes. Under pathologic conditions these cells form scar tissue.

astrocyte, epen´dymal   *See* tanycyte.

astrocyte, fi´brous [astrocytus fibrosus, NA]   astrocyte with fine fibrils and scanty cytoplasm. These cells have straight and sparsely branched processes. They are located primarily in the white matter of the CNS. *Syn:* spider cell.

astrocyte, protoplas´mic [astrocytus protoplasmicus, NA]   astrocyte with few fibrils and numerous branched processes. These cells are located primarily in the gray matter of the CNS. *Syn:* mossy cell.

astrog´lia   astrocytes, collectively, as a tissue.

asyn´ergy [Gr. *a* not; *syn* with; *ergon* work]   motor disorder in which there is impairment of the sequence and degree of muscle contraction necessary for the execution of an act.

ataxia /ah-tak´sĭ-ah/ [Gr. *a-*; *taxis* order]   disorder of movement characterized by incoordination. *For additional information on the ataxias, see* Haymaker ('69, pp. 79-81, 286-291).

ataxia, fron´tal   incoordination of the extremities contralateral to a lesion of the frontal lobe cortex or of the anterior limb of the internal capsule, and resulting, presumably, from injury to the cells of origin or fibers of the frontal corticopontine tract.

ataxia, gait   disorder characterized by difficulty in walking. The individual staggers to either side, with a wide-based gait. Static equilibrium and coordination of voluntary movements of the extremities are normal. This type of ataxia is characteristic of a lesion of the vermis of the anterior lobe of the cerebellum, interrupting the connections from the spinal cord.

ataxia, pari´etal   incoordination of the extremities contralateral to a lesion of the parietal lobe. It is, perhaps, a form of apraxia.

ataxia, sen´sory   incoordination due to a deficit in position sensibility, as in lesions of the dorsal funiculi of the spinal cord or of the medial lemnisci.

ataxia, trun´cal   disorder characterized by impaired equilibrium. There is difficulty maintaining an upright position, either standing or sitting. The head wobbles on the body.   If fully supported, however, the patient can perform normally coordinated voluntary movements of the extremities. It is characteristic of a lesion of the flocculonodular lobe of the cerebellum (Brown, '67).

atheto´sis [Gr. *athetos* without position]   disorder in which there are slow, twisting or writhing, involuntary movements of the extremities, particularly of the fingers and hands. It is associated with lesions in the striatum, particularly the putamen.

a´trium (of the lateral ventricle)   *See* trigone, collateral.

at´rophy, progressive muscular   *See* sclerosis, amyotrophic lateral.

at´ropine   agent used to block parasympathetic discharge; an alkaloid drug capable, among other things, of blocking muscarinic cholinergic nerve endings.

auditory nerve   *See* nerve, vestibulocochlear.

Auerbach, Leopold (1828-1897)   German anatomist and neuropathologist of Breslau. *Auerbach's plexus* (1862) is the myenteric plexus. *Auerbach's ganglia* are the parasympathetic ganglia in the myenteric plexus.

aula /ow´lah/   median part of the prosencephalic ventricle, later the anterior part of the third ventricle.

aura /aw´rah/   some sensory phenomenon or involuntary movement that precedes the onset of an epileptic seizure, and which may indicate the trigger site from which the seizure arises.

auris /aw´ris/ [NA]   *See* ear.

autism, infantile /aw´tizm/   syndrome beginning in early childhood, characterized by severe emotional and behavioral disorders, impaired interpersonal relationships, inadequate language development, and resistance to change. Intelligence may or may not be affected. *Syn:* Kanner's syndrome. *For additional information, see* Infantile Autism ('87).

autonom´ic nervous system   *See* system, autonomic nervous.

av´alanche conduction   *See* conduction, avalanche.

Axelrod, Julius (b. 1912)   American neurophysiologist, noted for his work on catecholamines. He, U.S. von Euler, and B. Katz were awarded the Nobel Prize for physiology and medicine in 1970 for their work on humoral transmitters.

ax´ilemma   *See* axolemma.

ax´is, anatomical (of the eyeball) [axis bulbi externus, NA], EYE   line through the eyeball from the center of the convexity of the cornea (the anterior pole), through the pupil and the lens, to the center of the posterior convexity of the eyeball (the posterior pole). *Syn:* geometric axis; principal axis. *See also* axis, optic.

axis bulbi externus [NA], EYE   anatomical axis of the eyeball.

axis bulbi internus [NA], EYE   that part of the anatomical axis of the eye from the anterior pole to a point on the surface of the retina between the macula and the optic disk.

axis, cerebrospi´nal   *See* system, central nervous.

axis cylinder   long cytoplasmic extension of a nerve cell body; usually the axonal process of a neuron, but also the peripheral, dendritic process of a primary sensory neuron. *Syn:* neuraxon; neurite. *See also* axon.

axis, geometric, EYE   *See* axis, anatomical (of the eyeball).

axis, optic (optical) [axis opticus, NA], EYE   either the anatomical axis or the visual axis of the eye.

axis, orbital   longitudinal axis of the orbit that bisects the angle formed by its medial and lateral bony walls.

axis, principal, EYE   *See* axis, anatomical, of the eyeball.

axis, visual, EYE   line of vision from the focal point in the field of vision through the center of the pupil and of the lens to the center of the fovea centralis. *See also* axis, optic.

axolem´ma (axilemma) [Gr. *axon* axis; *lemma* husk]   **1.** cell membrane (plasmalemma) of an axis cylinder. *Syn:* Mauthner's sheath.
2. Originally this term was used to mean the inner membrane of the Schwann cell but this use is now obsolete.

ax´on   **1.** that process of a neuron which conducts impulses away from the cell body to other neurons, muscle fibers, or gland cells. *Syn:* obsolete terms: neuraxis, neuraxon, neurite.
2. The central and the peripheral processes of unipolar sensory neurons have the same histologic characteristics and some processes are indistinguishable from the motor fibers of peripheral nerves. Hence the term *axon* is sometimes used for the axis cylinder of any peripheral nerve fiber, regardless of the direction of conduction.

ax´oplasm   cytoplasm of the axis cylinder of a nerve cell.

Ayala, A.G. (1878-1943)   Italian neurologist. The *subputaminal nucleus of Ayala* is the lateral part of the substriatal gray. *See also* substantia innominata.

b

Babinski, Joseph François Félix (1857-1932)   French neurologist, born in Paris of Polish parents. He worked many years under Charcot at the Salpêtrière and was head of the neurological clinic at the Hôpital de la Pitié. The *Babinski reflex* or *sign* (1896) consists of extension of the great toe in response to stroking the sole of the foot, after injury to the corticospinal tract. The same response occurs normally in infants prior to medullation of the corticospinal fibers. *See also* Chaddock, Oppenheim, *and* Gordon for the same sign elicited in different ways.

bag, nuclear   mid-portion of one type of intrafusal muscle fiber in a muscle spindle, in which there is an aggregation of spherical, centrally placed nuclei (Fig. S-2).

Bailey, Percival (1892-1973)   eminent American neurologist, noted for his classification of brain tumors, for many other contributions in various related neurological fields, and as an outstanding teacher.

Baillarger, Jules Gabriel François (1809-1890)   French neurologist and psychiatrist of Paris, for many years at the Salpêtrière. He was the first to note that the cerebral cortex is made up of layers, and in 1840 described the two layers of fibers, the *external and internal striae of Baillarger,* in layers IV and V of the cerebral cortex.

Bainbridge, Francis Arthur (1874-1921)   British physiologist. A *Bainbridge reflex* is an increase in heart rate in response to an increase in blood pressure or to distention of the right atrium.

band, diagonal (of Broca) [stria diagonalis (Broca), NA], CEREBRUM   band of fibers that extends from the parolfactory area on the medial surface of the frontal lobe ventrally and along the lateral margin of the optic tract and marking the caudal boundary of the anterior perforated substance. *Syn:* olfactory radiation of Zuckerkandl; fasciculus hippocampi; diagonalis tenia.

Bandfasern   *See* fiber, band.

Bárány, Robert (1876-1936)   otologist of Hungarian origin who practiced in

Vienna and later at the University of Upsala. In 1914 he was awarded the Nobel Prize for medicine and physiology for his work on the physiology and pathology of the vestibular apparatus. He devised methods, widely used, for testing vestibular function. *Bárány's sign* consists of nystagmus following injection of warm or cold water into the external auditory meatus and varying with pathology of the internal ear.

Barnes, S.   *Barnes' tract* (1901), the anterolateral corticospinal tract, consists of fibers which do not decussate in the pyramidal decussation but descend directly in a superficial, ventrolateral position near the olivospinal tract fibers.

barorecep´tor   nerve ending in the wall of the carotid sinus and other parts of the vascular system which responds to changes in blood pressure.

Barr, Murray Llewellyn (b. 1908)   Canadian neuroanatomist. The *Barr body*, or nucleolar satellite, was first described in nerve cells of the cat (1949) and later in other cell types and species. It typifies females and contains a mass of sex chromatin, the second X-chromosome.

Barré, Jean Alexandre (1880-1967)   French neurologist. *For the Guillain-Barré syndrome, see* Guillain.

barrier, blood-brain   the barrier that prevents many substances, which pass easily through vessel walls in other parts of the body, from passing through blood vessel walls into CNS tissue. Blood is separated from brain tissue by the endothelium of its capillaries, an underlying basement membrane, and the footplates of astrocytes. Substances that do not penetrate the barrier do not pass through the endothelium in which contiguous cells, unlike those in other parts of the body, exhibit extensive tight junctions. There may also be a physiologic component. The exceptionally fast velocity of blood flow through brain blood vessels under normal conditions may reduce the pressure on capillary endothelium enough to render the barrier impermeable to many substances, and a reduction in the rate of flow under adverse conditions may permit their passage (Lockard, '82).

ba´sal   *For* basal ganglia, nucleus, *and* plate, *see the nouns.*

ba´sion [NA]   the center of the anterior margin of the foramen magnum.

ba´sis pedun´culi cer´ebri [NA], MIDBRAIN   ventral part of the cerebral peduncle of the midbrain, separated from its counterpart on the opposite site by the interpeduncular fossa (Fig. P-1). It is composed of a cellular portion (substantia nigra) and a fibrous portion (pes pedunculi) containing pyramidal and corticopontine tracts. Sometimes this term is used for just the fibrous part, the pes pedunculi. *Syn:* crus cerebri. *See also* peduncle, cerebral.

basis pon´tis, PONS   ventral part of the pons, composed of descending pyramidal and corticopontine tracts, transverse pontocerebellar fibers, and pontine gray.

Bauhin, Gaspar (Caspar) (1560-1624)   born in France, he later lived in Switzerland. He published extensively in the fields of anatomy and botany, revised much of their nomenclature, and named the phrenic nerve.

Beale, Lionel Smith (1828-1906)   English physician and microscopist. *Beale's cells* are nerve cells in the cardiac ganglia.

Beccari, Nello (1883-1957)   Italian comparative neuroanatomist, noted for his studies of the rhinencephalon and the rhombencephalon.

Bechterew   *See* Bekhterev.

Beevor, Charles Edward (1854-1907)   English neurologist and neurophysiologist, noted for his pioneer work on cortical localization.

Bekhterev (Bechterew), Vladimir Mikhailovich (1857-1927)   Russian neuropathologist, noted for his many contributions also in the fields of neuroanatomy, neurophysiology, and clinical neurology. Both the superior vestibular nucleus and the central superior nucleus of the raphe have been known as *Bechterew's nucleus.* *Bechterew's reticular nucleus* is the ventrolateral tegmental nucleus, and *Bechterew's bundle* is the spino-olivary tract.

Bell, Sir Charles (1774-1842)   Scottish neurologist and anatomist active in London. In 1811 he described experiments which demonstrated the motor function of the ventral roots. After Magendie's description of the sensory function of the dorsal roots, the *Bell-Magendie law* was formulated, according to which the ventral roots are motor in function and the dorsal roots are sensory, although there is now evidence that both dorsal and ventral roots probably carry antidromic fibers. In 1821 Bell described the motor branch of the facial nerve. *Bell's nerve* (1830) is the long thoracic nerve. *Bell's palsy,* idiopathic facial paralysis, results from an inflammatory reaction in or around the nerve near the stylomastoid foramen or in the facial canal. It sometimes occurs after exposure to cold, possibly with subsequent swelling and ischemia of the nerve within the bony facial canal. The onset tends to be sudden but frequently there is complete recovery. *Bell's phenomenon* (1823) is the palpebral-oculogyric reflex, in which the eyes invariably turn upward when the lids are closed.

Benedikt, Moritz (1835-1920)   Viennese physician, born in Hungary. *Benedikt's syndrome* occurs with a midbrain lesion of the oculomotor nerve and the red nucleus, causing an oculomotor paralysis and loss of the light and accommodation reflexes on the side of the lesion and an action tremor on the contralateral side. If the lesion is large enough to include the medial lemniscus, there is also a sensory deficit contralateral to the lesion.

Berengario da Carpi, Giacomo (ca. 1460-ca. 1530)   Italian surgeon and anatomist, noted for his great skill in both fields. He questioned, quite correctly, the presence of a *rete mirabile* in the human brain, although its presence was generally accepted from the writings of Galen. He described, among other things, the corpus striatum, pituitary gland, cerebrospinal fluid, and brain ventricles.

Berger, Johannes (Hans) (1873-1941)   German neurologist of Jena who was the first to record the electrical activity of the human brain, applying methods used in electrocardiography (1929) and, showed that electrical activity of the human brain could be recorded from the intact scalp. One of the basic electroencephalographic patterns bears his name.

Bergmann, Gottlieb Heinrich (1781-1861)   German physician. *Bergmann's cords* or *conductors* are the striae medullares of the fourth ventricle. *Bergmann's layer* is a layer of astrocytes, *Bergmann glial cells,* in the Purkinje cell layer of the cerebellar cortex, which hypertrophy with degeneration of the Purkinje cells and are thought to play a role in the development of the neurons.

Bernard, Claude (1813-1878)   French neurophysiologist, noted especially for his investigations of the ANS and the demonstration of vasomotor mechanisms.

Bernheimer, Stephan (1861-1918)   Austrian ophthalmologist. The *nucleus of Bernheimer* is the rostral part of the Edinger-Westphal (accessory oculomotor) nucleus and is concerned with pupillary constriction.

Betz, Vladimir Aleksandrovich (1834-1894)   Russian anatomist of Kiev. *Betz cells* (1874) are the giant pyramidal cells in layer V of the motor area (area 4) of the precentral gyrus.

Bezold, Albert von (1838-1868)   German physiologist. *Bezold's ganglion* is a cluster of nerve cells located in the interatrial septum of the heart.

Bichat, Marie François Xavier (1771-1802)   French anatomist and physician who described, among other things, the arachnoid membrane (1800). *Bichat's fissure* is the space below the splenium of the corpus callosum.

Bielschowsky, Max (1869-1940)   German neuropathologist. He developed a technique for staining nerve cells and fibers with silver, *Bielschowsky's method,* and investigated the pathology underlying many neurologic disorders.

bi´venter [lobulus biventer, NA], CEREBELLUM   two-part segment on the inferior surface of the cerebellar hemisphere, lateral to the tonsil and between the postpyramidal and prepyramidal fissures (Fig. C-2). It is continuous with the pyramis of the vermis. *Syn:* dorsal paraflocculus of comparative neuroanatomy.

bladder, atonic   bladder which lacks a sensory nerve supply, after degeneration of the sacral dorsal roots or dorsal root ganglia, as in tabes dorsalis. The bladder is greatly distended, and there is overflow incontinence.

bladder, automatic   *See* bladder, reflex.

bladder, autonomous   bladder which lacks any nervous control, after injury to the sacral spinal cord, cauda equina, or pelvic plexus or nerves. The bladder is distended, and empties irregularly and incompletely with much residual urine.

bladder, neurogenic   bladder characterized by some disordered function, resulting from injury to the nerves supplying the bladder or to related parts in the CNS.

bladder, reflex   bladder controlled by reflex function only, after injury to tracts between higher centers and the sacral spinal cord or to parts of the brain concerned with bladder function. Bladder capacity is reduced; micturition is sudden and uncontrolled. *Syn:* automatic bladder.

bladder, uninhibited   one which is controlled only by reflex action, as in normal infants or in adults with some brain damage or deficiency. Bladder capacity may be slightly decreased. Micturition occurs suddenly and without control.

blood-brain barrier   *See* barrier, blood-brain.

Blumenau, Leonid Wassiljewitsch (1862-1932)   Russian neurologist. *Blumenau's nucleus* is the accessory cuneate nucleus.

Bochdalek, Vincent Alexander (1801-1883)   Czech anatomist of Prague. *Bochdalek's ganglion* is a thickening in the superior dental plexus at the junction of the anterior and middle alveolar nerves. It is not a true ganglion but consists of interlacing bundles of nerve fibers and contains no nerve cells. The *flowerbasket* or *cornucopia of Bochdalek* (Bochdaleksches Blumenkörbchen) is a tuft of the choroid plexus which extends through the lateral aperture of the fourth ventricle into the subarachnoid space.

Bock, August Carl (1782-1833)   German anatomist and surgeon. *Bock's ganglion* is a ganglion on the carotid artery in the cavernous sinus.

body   *See also* corpus; gland; glomus; granule; nucleus; *and* paraganglion.

body, acces´sory (of Cajal)   small (about 1 μm in diameter), spherical, argyrophilic mass in the nucleus of many neurons. It is located between the nucleolus and the nuclear membrane and is distinct from the nucleolus and the nucleolar satellite.

body, amyg´daloid [corpus amygdaloideum, NA], CEREBRUM   *See* amygdala.

body, aor´tic [glomus aorticum, NA]   small cluster of cells on or near the arch of the aorta. It is a nonchromaffin paraganglion, similar in structure and function to the carotid body. Afferent fibers from the aortic body are carried by the vagus nerve. *Syn:* paraganglion aorticum. *See also* reflexes, respiratory.

body, carot´id [glomus caroticum, NA]   small collection of cells at the bifurcation of each common carotid artery. A nonchromaffin paraganglion, it serves as a chemoreceptor and functions in respiratory reflexes. Afferent fibers from this structure are carried by the glossopharyngeal nerve. *Syn:* ganglion intercaroticum.

body, cell [corpus neuroni, NA]   enlarged portion of the neuron, containing the nucleus of the cell and the surrounding cytoplasm, the perikaryon, with its chromophilic (Nissl) substance and other organelles, but excluding all the cell processes. *Syn:* nerve cell; cyton; soma. *See also* cell of origin.

bodies, chro´maffin   *See* paraganglia, chromaffin.

body, cil´iary [corpus ciliare, NA], EYE   structure which circles the iris, whose muscle contracts in accommodation and whose epithelium secretes aqueous humor. *See also* process, ciliary; crown, ciliary.

body, genic´ulate, external, DORSAL THALAMUS   *See* body, geniculate, lateral.

body, geniculate, internal, DORSAL THALAMUS   *See* body, geniculate, medial.

body, geniculate, lateral [corpus geniculatum laterale, NA], DORSAL THALAMUS   part of the metathalamus, it is a protuberance located lateral to the medial geniculate body, and contains the lateral geniculate nucleus. It serves as the thalamic center for the visual system. *Syn:* external geniculate body. *See also* nucleus, geniculate, lateral.

body, geniculate, medial [corpus geniculatum mediale, NA], DORSAL THALAMUS   part of the metathalamus, it is a protuberance on the posterior, inferior surface of the diencephalon, and the lateral surface of the rostral part of the midbrain. It contains the major part of the medial geniculate nucleus and serves as the thalamic center for the auditory system. *Syn:* internal geniculate body. *See also* nucleus, geniculate, medial.

body, juxtares´tiform, CEREBELLUM   inner part of the inferior cerebellar peduncle, composed primarily of uncrossed vestibulocerebellar and cerebellovestibular fibers. *Syn:* area fasciculata.

body, mam´illary [corpus mamillare, NA], HYPOTHALAMUS, [L. *mamilla* little breast] protuberance on the ventral surface of the hypothalamus containing the mamillary nuclei (Figs. C-3C, N-4, V-5).

body, parater´minal, CEREBRUM   *See* gyrus, paraterminal.

body (gland), pin´eal (pine´al) [corpus pineale (glandula pinealis), NA], EPITHALAMUS, [L. *pineus* relating to the pine, shaped like a pine cone]   an endocrine gland, located in the median plane, just posterior to the dorsal part of the dorsal thalamus and rostral to the superior colliculus (Fig. H-1). It is concerned with adjustment to circadian rhythms; light is thought to have an inhibitory effect on its secretory activity and darkness to be excitatory. Impulses are relayed from the retina to the suprachiasmatic nucleus, then to the pineal body by way of the thoracic spinal cord (Fig. N-7). *Syn:* conarium; epiphysis cerebri. *See also* nucleus, suprachiasmatic. *For a review of this subject, see* Erlich and Apuzzo ('85).

body (gland), pituitary   *See* hypophysis.

body, quadrigem´inal, inferior, MIDBRAIN   *See* colliculus, inferior.

body, quadrigeminal, superior, MIDBRAIN   *See* colliculus, superior.

body, res´tiform [corpus restiforme], PONS, MEDULLA, [L. *restis* rope; *forma* form] inferior cerebellar peduncle, but sometimes not including the vestibulocerebellar and cerebellovestibular fibers, which constitute the juxtarestiform body.

body, ti´groid   *See* substance, chromatophilic. *See also* tigroid.

body, trap´ezoid [corpus trapezoideum, NA], PONS   nerve fibers and cell bodies in the ventral and caudal part of the pontine tegmentum, a part of the auditory pathway between the cochlear nuclei and the medial geniculate and inferior collicular nuclei. It was so named because of its appearance in animals, such as the cat, in which it is located on the ventral surface of the brain stem, caudal to, and not covered by, the base of the pons.

body, vit´reous [corpus vitreum, NA], EYE, [L. *vitreum* glass]   transparent, semisolid gelatinous structure which fills the vitreous chamber of the eye behind the lens. It adheres to the inner surface of the retina, especially along the ora serrata.

Boettcher, Arthur (1831-1889)   German anatomist who described many anatomical features of the internal ear. *Boettcher's ganglion* is a small ganglion on the vestibular nerve. *Boettcher's cells* are small, polyhedral cells in the spiral organ, interposed between the basilar membrane and the cells of Claudius of the external spiral sulcus in parts of the basal coil of the cochlea. *Boettcher's canal* is the utriculosaccular duct.

bom´besin   a neuropeptide present in the CNS and in other body organs, a pressor substance which stimulates gastric secretion, pancreatic secretion, and gallbladder contraction. *See also* neurotransmitters.

Bourneville, Désiré Magloire (1840-1909)   French physician, in his time the leading continental authority on mentally abnormal children. *Bourneville's disease* (1880) is tuberous sclerosis.

bouton terminal /boo´to/ [*pl.* **boutons terminaux** /ter-min-o´/] [Fr. terminal button] *See* bulb, terminal.

Bowman, Sir William (1816-1892)   English ophthalmologist and anatomist of London, noted for his studies of the anatomy and physiology of the eye and of the kidney. *Bowman's membrane* is the anterior elastic membrane between the anterior epithelium and the substantia propria of the cornea. *Bowman's muscle* consists of the radial fibers of the ciliary muscle.

brachium /bra´kĭ-um/ [L. arm]   large bundle or trunk of nerve fibers in the CNS, consisting of one or more tracts. *See also* peduncle.

brachium (pe´duncle), collic´ulus, of the inferior [brachium colliculi inferioris (caudalis), NA]   fiber bundle on the lateral surface of the midbrain, consisting of fibers mainly from the inferior colliculus, and some from the lateral lemniscus, which end in the medial geniculate nucleus. *Syn:* brachium of the medial geniculate nucleus.

brachium, colliculus, of the superior [brachium colliculi superioris (rostralis), NA]   layer of fibers which passes over the surface of the medial geniculate body. It consists primarily of internal corticotectal fibers from the occipital and preoccipital cortices which end in the superior colliculus, for optokinetic eye movements in the vertical plane. Other fibers from the optic tract end in the pretectal nucleus for the light reflex.

brachium conjunctivum /kon-jung-ti´vum/ [L. *conjungere* to join together]   *See* peduncle, superior cerebellar.

brachium conjunctivum descendens   fibers of the superior cerebellar peduncle, probably arising from the dentate and emboliform nuclei, which, after crossing the median plane, leave the peduncle, descend with the central tegmental tract, and end primarily in the inferior olivary and accessory olivary nuclei (Fig. O-1).

brachium (peduncle) (of the) inferior colliculus   *See* brachium, colliculus, (of the) inferior.

brachium (of the) medial geniculate nucleus   *See* brachium, colliculus, (of the) inferior.

brachium pon´tis *See* peduncle, cerebellar, middle.

bradykinesia /bra-dĭ-ki-ne´zĭ-ah/ [Gr. *brady* slow; *kinesis* movement]   abnormal slowness of movements.

brain [encephalon, NA]   that part of the central nervous system contained within the cranium.

brain, end   *See* cerebrum; telencephalon.

Brain, Lord W. Russell (1895-1966)   distinguished British neurologist, author, through seven editions, of *Brain's Diseases of the Nervous System*, the last completed after his death by John N. Walton. *Brain's reflex* is a quadrupedal extensor reflex.

brain sand [acervulus cerebri, NA], DIENCEPHALON   calcareous bodies in the pineal body.

brain, split   one in which the corpus callosum, and sometimes other forebrain commissures, have been severed by an incision in the median plane.

brainstem   *See* stem, brain.

branchial ef´ferent /brang´ke-al/   pertaining to the special visceral efferent component of nerves conducting impulses from motor nuclei to striated muscle of branchiomeric (visceral arch) origin. *See* Tables C-1, C-2.

breg´ma [NA] [Gr. anterior part of the skull]   point on the skull where the coronal and sagittal sutures meet, at the juncture of the frontal bone with the two parietal bones. In infants it is the site of the anterior fontanel. It is used as a neuroradiological point of reference to determine the location of certain intracranial structures such as the middle cerebral artery and the venous angle.

Breschet, Gilbert (1784-1845)   anatomist in Paris. *Breschet's veins* or *spaces* are the diploic veins. *Breschet's hiatus* is the helicotrema of the cochlea and *Breschet's sinus* is the sphenoparietal sinus (1834).

Breuer, Josef (1842-1925)   Austrian physician and psychologist, noted for his studies of respiratory reflexes. *See also* Hering; reflexes, respiratory.

Broca, Pierre Paul (1824-1880)   French surgeon and anthropologist of Paris who described aphasia as a manifestation of injury to the left inferior frontal gyrus, and introduced the concept of cerebral localization (1861). *Broca's area* or *convolution* is the posterior part of the left inferior frontal gyrus (in the dominant cerebral hemisphere), Brodmann's area 44 and the adjoining part of area 45. *Broca's aphasia* is motor aphasia, in which spoken language is impaired, although speech comprehension may be relatively normal. It is attributed to injury in this general region. The *cap of Broca* is the triangular gyrus. The *parolfactory area (of Broca)*, on the medial surface of the frontal lobe, and the *diagonal band (of Broca)* were also named for him.

Brodmann, Korbinian (1868-1918)   German neurologist noted for his studies of the cytoarchitecture of the mammalian cerebral cortex, especially for his maps of the human cerebral cortex (´09). He divided the cortex, on the basis of its cytoarchitectural characteristics, into 11 principal regions and many smaller areas (Fig. B-1), numbered and named as follows:

1 (area postcentralis intermedia)   portion of the somesthetic cortex in the postcentral gyrus, a narrow strip along the border of the posterior lip of the central sulcus, between areas 3 and 2. It may be associated with fine tactile sensibility.

2 (area postcentralis caudalis)   portion of the somesthetic cortex in the postcentral gyrus, posterior to area l. It may be associated with joint or position sensibility.

3 (area postcentralis oralis)   portion of the somesthetic cortex in the postcentral gyrus, along the posterior wall of the central sulcus, deep to the surface. It is thought to be associated with the sense of pain.

4 (area gigantopyramidalis)   motor area in the precentral gyrus and paracentral lobule, containing giant pyramidal (Betz) cells.

5 (area preparietalis)   sensory association area in the superior parietal lobule, posterior to the postcentral gyrus.

6 (area frontalis agranularis)   premotor area in the frontal lobe, anterior to area 4.

7 (area parietalis superior)   sensory association area in the superior parietal lobule between areas 5 and 19.

8 (area frontalis intermedia)   frontal eye field in the frontal lobe anterior to area 6. Brodmann placed this area primarily in the superior frontal gyrus, but the frontal eye field, still called area 8, is now said to be mostly in the middle frontal gyrus and partly in the inferior frontal gyrus.

9 (area frontalis granularis)   area in the frontal lobe anterior to area 8.

10 (area frontopolaris)   area in the anterior part of the frontal lobe, including the frontal pole.

11 (area prefrontalis)   area in the frontal lobe, ventral to areas 10 and 47 laterally and to area 12 medially.

12 (area frontalis microcellularis)   area in the frontal lobe in the ventral part of the medial hemispheric wall.

13 (insula posterior)   area posterior to the central sulcus of the insula.

14 (insula anterior)   area anterior to the central sulcus of the insula.

15 (insula ventralis)   small area at the orbito-insular junction.

16 (insula olfactoria)   small area at the insulo-olfactory junction.

17 (area striata)   visual projection cortex adjoining the calcarine fissure in the occipital lobe, mostly on the medial surface of the cerebral hemisphere but including the occipital pole.

18 (area occipitalis)   parastriate area, adjacent to area 17 in the occipital lobe. It is a visual association area and also is concerned with optokinetic eye movements. *See also* cortex, visual association.

19 (area preoccipitalis)   peristriate area, adjacent to area 18 of the cerebral cortex. Brodmann put this area in the occipital lobe but it is now said to be in the most posterior parts of the parietal and temporal lobes. It is a visual association area and also concerned with optokinetic eye movements.

20 (area temporalis inferior)   area on the inferior surface of the temporal lobe, in the lateral occipitotemporal gyrus.

21 (area temporalis media)   area on the lateral surface of the temporal lobe, in the middle temporal gyrus, making up most of the gyrus.

22 (area temporalis superior)   auditory association cortex, mainly on the lateral surface of the superior temporal gyrus and adjoining areas 41 and 42.

23 (area cingularis posterior ventralis)   area in the posterior part of the cingulate gyrus, on the medial surface of the cerebral hemisphere.

24 (area cingularis anterior ventralis)   area in the anterior part of the cingulate gyrus.

25 (area subgenualis)   parolfactory area below the genu of the corpus callosum on the medial surface of the frontal lobe.

26 (area ectosplenialis)   small area in the isthmus of the fornicate gyrus adjoining the corpus callosum.

27 (area presubicularis)   area in the parahippocampal gyrus, adjacent to the hippocampal fissure, on the medial surface of the temporal lobe.

28 (area entorhinalis)   area which makes up most of the parahippocampal gyrus, in the temporal lobe.

29 (area retrolimbica granularis)   area behind the splenium of the corpus callosum, in the isthmus of the cingulate gyrus between areas 26 and 30.

30 (area retrolimbica agranularis)   area in the isthmus of the cingulate gyrus just posterior to area 29.

31 (area cingularis posterior dorsalis)   area in the cingulate gyrus just above area 23 and posterior to area 24.

32 (area cingularis anterior dorsalis)   area on the medial surface of the frontal lobe, above the cingulate sulcus, between area 33 posteriorly and areas 9 and 10 anteriorly.

33 (area pregenualis, tenia tecti)   area in the cingulate gyrus adjacent to the anterior part of the sulcus of the corpus callosum, a hippocampal rudiment.

34 (area entorhinalis dorsalis)   uncus of the temporal lobe.

35 (area perirhinalis)   area adjacent to the rhinal fissure in the temporal lobe.

36 (area ectorhinalis)   most of the medial occipitotemporal gyrus in the temporal lobe.

37 (area occipitotemporalis)   occipitotemporal transition area, on the medial and lateral cerebral surfaces.

38 (area temporopolaris)   temporal pole.

39 (area angularis)   angular gyrus.

40 (area supramarginalis)   supramarginal gyrus.

41 (area auditoria)   primary auditory area in the anterior transverse gyrus and part of the posterior transverse gyrus, on the opercular surface of the temporal lobe, within the lateral sulcus.

42 (area para-auditoria)   secondary auditory area in the posterior transverse temporal gyrus, posterior to area 41, mostly on the opercular surface of the temporal lobe within the lateral sulcus but extending slightly onto the exposed surface of the temporal lobe.

43 (area subcentralis)   small area at the base of the central sulcus.

44 (area opercularis)   opercular part of the inferior frontal gyrus.

45 (area triangularis)   triangular part of the inferior frontal gyrus.

46 (area frontalis media)   part of the frontal eye field, in the middle frontal gyrus.

47 (area orbitalis)   orbital part of the inferior frontal gyrus.

48 (area postsubicularis)   retrosubicular area posterior to area 35 on the medial aspect of the temporal lobe, presumably absent in man.

49 (area parasubicularis)   area in the parahippocampal gyrus next to and merged with areas 27 and 28.

50 (area gustatoria)   area on the upper wall of the lateral sulcus.

51 (area pyriformis)   small area at the base of the olfactory stalk.

52 (area parainsularis)   area on the opercular surface of the temporal lobe between area 41 and the insula, probably an association area for auditory and perhaps visceral functions.

Brown   the *vein of Brown* is the vein of the septum pellucidum.

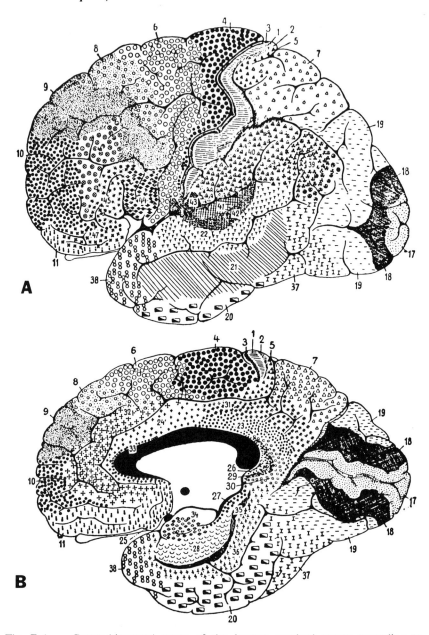

Fig. B-1.   Cytoarchitectural maps of the human cerebral cortex according to Brodmann (1909).   A. lateral surface.   B. medial surface.

Brown-Séquard, Charles Édouard (1817-1894)   British physiologist and neurologist. The *Brown-Séquard syndrome* (1850) results from a hemisection of the spinal cord and is characterized by a paralysis of the muscles supplied below the level of the lesion and a loss of position, vibration, and tactile discriminatory sensibilities, all on the side of the lesion. There is also a loss of pain and temperature sensibility on the contralateral side from about one segment below the level of the lesion down. These changes result from severing the fibers of the lateral corticospinal tract, the dorsal funiculus, and the lateral spinothalamic tract, respectively. If the injury occurs above the level of T1 there will also be a Horner's syndrome on the homolateral side, including a loss of sweating of the face, neck, and shoulder from section of the lateral reticulospinal tract, and miosis and ptosis from section of the lateral tectotegmentospinal tract (Fig. B-2).

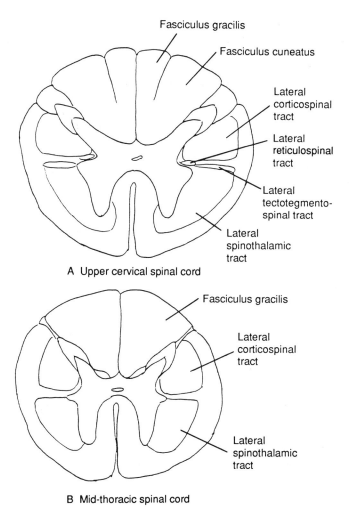

Fasciculus gracilis

Fasciculus cuneatus

Lateral corticospinal tract

Lateral reticulospinal tract

Lateral tectotegmento-spinal tract

Lateral spinothalamic tract

A Upper cervical spinal cord

Fasciculus gracilis

Lateral corticospinal tract

Lateral spinothalamic tract

B Mid-thoracic spinal cord

Fig. B-2. Diagram showing the position of the severed tracts underlying the signs and symptoms after a hemisection of the spinal cord at an upper cervical (A) or midthoracic (B) level. *See* Brown-Séquard.

Bruce, Alexander (1854-1911)   Scottish neurologist. *Bruce's tract* is the septomarginal fasciculus of the spinal cord.

Bruch, Karl Wilhelm Ludwig (1819-1884)   German anatomist of Basel and Giessen. *Bruch's membrane* (1844) is the basal layer of the choroid of the eye.

Brücke, Ernst Wilhelm Ritter von (1819-1892)   Viennese physiologist. *Brücke's muscle* consists of the meridional fibers of the ciliary muscle.

Brudzinski, Josef (1874-1917)   Polish pediatrician. *Brudzinski's sign* for meningitis (1909) consists of flexion at the knees and hips in response to passive flexion of the neck.

bulb [*adj.* **bulbar**]   the noun denotes the medulla oblongata but the adjective is used to denote any part of the brain stem, i.e., midbrain, pons, or medulla.

bulb, cer´ebral   *See* medulla oblongata.

bulb (si´nus), jug´ular   bulbous enlargement of the internal jugular vein just below the jugular foramen.

bulb, oc´ular [bulbus oculi, NA], EYE   eyeball.

bulb, olfac´tory [bulbus olfactorius, NA], CEREBRUM   enlargement on the orbital surface of the cerebrum in which olfactory nerve fibers terminate (Fig. C-3C).

bulb, ter´minal [bulbus terminalis, NA]   small, synaptic, bulblike nerve ending applied to the surface of the cell body and dendrites of many neurons. *Syn:* neuropodium; end foot; end bulb of Held; bouton terminal.

bul´bus   *See also* bulb.

bulbus cor´nus occipital´is (posterioris) [NA], CEREBRUM   ridge on the wall of the posterior horn of the lateral ventricle overlying the forceps major of the corpus callosum.

bundle   *See also* column, fasciculus, tract.

bundle, coch´lear, efferent, PONS   *See* bundle, olivocochlear.

bundle, comb, FOREBRAIN   fascicles of the nigrostriate tract which are separated into parallel strands and resemble the teeth of a comb as they pass through the internal capsule.

bundle, comma, CORD   *See* fasciculus interfascicularis.

bundle, forebrain, basal   combination of the medial and the lateral forebrain bundles.

bundle, forebrain, lateral   fiber bundle of lower vertebrates comprising a dorsal peduncle and a ventral peduncle. The dorsal peduncle consists of thalamostriate and striothalamic fibers. The ventral peduncle in submammals corresponds to the ansa lenticularis system of mammals and is not divided. *See also* ansa lenticularis, *def.* 2.

bundle, forebrain, medial [fasciculus prosencephalicus medialis, NA], FOREBRAIN   fiber bundle interconnecting the anterior perforated substance and septal area of the medial hemispheric wall with the preoptic and hypothalamic areas, especially the ventromedial hypothalamic nucleus. Other fibers, with brain stem connections, are considered by some to be a part of this bundle and by others to accompany it.

bundle, forebrain, medial [fasciculus prosencephalicus medialis, NA], FOREBRAIN   fiber bundle interconnecting the anterior perforated substance and septal area of the medial hemispheric wall with the preoptic and hypothalamic areas, especially the ventromedial hypothalamic nucleus. Other fibers, with brain stem connections, are considered by some to be a part of this bundle and by others to accompany it.

bundle, ground, CORD   *See* fasciculus proprius.

bundle, hook   *See* fasciculus, uncinate, *def.* 1.

bundle, longitudinal association, of the amygdala, FOREBRAIN   fibers which presumably arise from the central and perhaps other amygdaloid nuclei or the piriform cortex and which pass medially into the anterior hypothalamic area. *Syn:* ventral amygdalohypothalamic tract.

bundle, longitudinal, medial, BRAIN STEM   *See* fasciculus, longitudinal, medial.

bundle, longitudinal, posterior, BRAIN STEM   **1.** medial longitudinal fasciculus. **2.** Sometimes this term is used to mean the dorsal longitudinal fasciculus.

bundle, longitudinal, ventral   old term for the medial tectospinal tract.

bundle, olivococh´lear [tractus olivocochlearis, NA], PONS   bundle of nerve fibers which arise from cells in or adjoining the superior olive and pass dorsomedially as the peduncle of the superior olive. Most fibers cross the median plane and leave the brain stem with the vestibular nerve, then join the cochlear nerve and enter the cochlea. They cross the inner tunnel of the spiral organ as tunnel fibers and end primarily on the outer hair cells, presumably to modulate the function of the inner hair cells. These connections are thought to inhibit unwanted auditory impulses and sharpen frequency-resolving power.

bundle, oval, CORD   lumbar part of the septomarginal fasciculus. *Syn:* oval area of Flechsig.

bundle, pre´dor´sal (of Edinger)   medial tectospinal tract. This term is also used to include the tectobulbar fibers which end in the brain stem.

bundle, reflex, CORD   *See* fasciculus proprius.

bundle, respi´ratory (Gierke's), PONS, MEDULLA   *See* fasciculus solitarius.

bundle, tegmen´tal, central, MAINLY BRAIN STEM   *See* tract, tegmental, central.

Büngner, Otto von (1858-1905)   German neurologist. The *band of Büngner* is a multinuclear syncytial cord (band fiber) of regenerating peripheral nerve fibers.

Burdach, Karl Friedrich (1776-1847)   German anatomist and physiologist. The *nucleus* (1819) and *tract* (1826) *of Burdach* are the nucleus and fasciculus cuneatus.

C

C   cervical.

caecum   cecum.

Cajal, Santiago Ramón y (1852-1934)   great Spanish neurohistologist of Madrid, noted for innumerable contributions concerning the histology and pathology of the nervous system. He developed techniques using metallic stains to demonstrate neurons and in 1909/11 published a 2-volume text on the normal histology of the nervous system, illustrated profusely with his own drawings. Cajal was also the main protagonist in establishing the neuron doctrine. In 1906 he and C. Golgi were awarded jointly the Nobel Prize in medicine and physiology for their contributions. The *interstitial nucleus of Cajal* is the interstitial nucleus of the medial longitudinal fasciculus. *Cajal's basal nucleus* of th spinal cord occupies Rexed's lamina I.

cal´amus scriptor´ius, MEDULLA, [L. *calamus* reed, pen; pen point]   floor of the tapered caudal part of the fourth ventricle.

calcar a´vis [NA], CEREBRUM, [L. *calcar* spur; bird's claw]   eminence on the medial wall of the posterior horn of the lateral ventricle, overlying part of the calcarine fissure. *Syn:* hippocampus minor.

Calleja y Sanchez, Camilo (d. 1913)   Spanish anatomist of Madrid. The *islands of Calleja* are clusters of small nerve cells in the ventral striatum within the anterior perforated substance. They appear to be the site of receptors for estrogen and gonadotropic hormone-releasing hormone and perhaps serve as targets for hormones circulating in the vascular system (Alheid and Heimer, '90).

callo´sal   pertaining to the corpus callosum.

calva´ria [*pl.* **calvariae**]   upper part of the skull overlying the brain.

camera [NA]   *See* chamber.

Campbell, Alfred Walter (1868-1937)   Australian physician and anatomist, educated in Edinburgh, Vienna, and Prague. He was a pioneer, along with Brodmann and the Vogts, in the study of the cytoarchitecture of the cerebral cortex.

canal, carot´id [canalis caroticus, NA]   channel in the base of the skull through which the internal carotid artery and its accompanying carotid plexus pass to enter the cavernous sinus (Fig. A-1).

canal, central [canalis centralis, NA], MEDULLA, CORD   narrow channel extending the length of the spinal cord and the closed medulla and continuous with the caudal tip of the fourth ventricle (Fig. V-3). *Syn:* syringocele.

canal, coch´lear, EAR   *See* canal, spiral, of the cochlea.

canal, fa´cial [canalis facialis, NA]   channel in the petrous part of the temporal bone, from the internal auditory meatus to the stylomastoid foramen, through which the facial nerve passes. *Syn:* Fallopian canal or aqueduct.

canal, hy´aloid [canalis hyaloideus, NA], EYE   narrow channel through the vitreous body of the eye. It extends from the optic disk to the center of the posterior surface of the lens. The hyaloid artery, which passes through this canal in the fetus, normally disappears about six weeks before birth. *Syn:* Stilling's canal.

canal, hypoglos´sal [canalis hypoglossi, NA]   opening in the occipital bone just above each occipital condyle, through which the hypoglossal nerve passes.

canals, longitudinal, of the modi´olus [canales longitudinales modioli, NA], EAR   centrally placed channels that run lengthwise in the modiolus of the cochlea and contain its nerve fibers and blood vessels.

canal, neur´al [canalis neuralis, NA]   cavity extending through the neural tube of the developing CNS. *Syn:* neurocele.

canal, op´tic [canalis opticus, NA]   short channel in the sphenoid bone at the back of the orbit through which the optic nerve and the ophthalmic artery pass (Fig. A-1). *Syn:* optic foramen.

canal, sa´cral   caudal continuation of the vertebral canal into the sacrum.

canals, semicir´cular [canales semicirculares ossei, NA], EAR   three channels of the bony labyrinth, oriented at right angles to one another and containing the semicircular ducts of the membranous labyrinth.

canal, spinal   *See* canal, vertebral.

canal, spiral (of the cochlea) [canalis spiralis cochleae, NA], EAR   spiral tube of the bony labyrinth which winds around the modiolus. It is divided into the scala vestibuli and scala tympani and partially encloses the cochlear duct of the membranous labyrinth. *Syn:* cochlear canal.

canal, spiral (of the modiolus) [canalis spiralis modioli, NA], EAR   irregularly shaped cavity in the modiolus which contains the spiral ganglion.

canal, ver´tebral [canalis vertebralis, NA]   channel extending throughout the vertebral column and enclosing the spinal cord and its meninges. *Syn:* spinal canal.

canalic´uli, caroticotympan´ic [canaliculi caroticotympanici, NA]   one or two small openings in the carotid canal through which small fascicles of nerve fibers interconnect the internal carotid and tympanic plexuses.

canalic´ulus (of the) chorda tympani /kor´dah tim´pan-ĭ/ [canaliculus chordae tympani, NA]   narrow channel in the posterior wall of the tympanic cavity, for the chorda tympani, from the facial canal until it opens into the tympanic cavity.

canaliculus, coch´lear [canaliculus cochleae, NA], EAR   narrow channel within the temporal bone which contains the cochlear aqueduct.

canaliculus, mas´toid [canaliculus mastoideus, NA]   small opening in the temporal bone for the auricular branch of the vagus nerve.

Cannon, Walter Bradford (1871-1945)   American neurophysiologist, noted for his studies of the ANS and its chemical mediators, particularly in the control of the gastrointestinal tract and the responses of the body to stress.

cap´sule, external [capsula externa, NA], CEREBRUM   layer of nerve fibers between the putamen and the claustrum.

capsule, extreme [capsula extrema, NA], CEREBRUM   layer of nerve fibers between the claustrum and the insular cortex.

capsule (of the) inferior colliculus, MIDBRAIN   fibers from the lateral lemniscus which surround and end in the nucleus of the inferior colliculus.

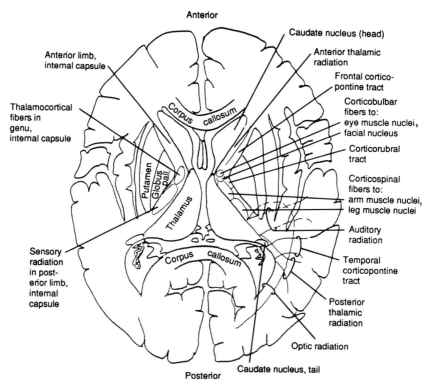

Fig. C-1.   Diagram of a horizontal section through the forebrain, to show the parts, relations, and tracts of the internal capsule. Overlapping tracts are shown separately on the two sides.

capsule, internal [capsula interna, NA], CEREBRUM   mass of nerve fibers between the caudate and thalamic nuclei medially and the lentiform nucleus laterally and connecting the cerebral cortex with various subcortical centers (Fig. C-1). Its major subdivisions are as follows:

  limb, anterior [crus anterior, NA]   that part of the internal capsule between the head of the caudate nucleus medially and the lentiform nucleus laterally. It comprises the frontal corticopontine tract and the anterior thalamic radiations.

genu [genu capsulae internae, NA]   the most medial part of the internal capsule between the anterior and posterior limbs. It is bounded anteromedially by the caudate nucleus, posteromedially by the dorsal thalamus, and laterally by the lentiform nucleus. It comprises the corticobulbar fibers of the pyramidal tract and the thalamocortical fibers which end in areas 4 and 6.

limb, posterior [crus posterior, NA]   those parts of the internal capsule between the dorsal thalamus and the body of the caudate nucleus medially and the lentiform nucleus laterally (thalamolenticular portion), posterior to the lentiform nucleus (postlenticular portion), and inferior to the lenticular nucleus (sublenticular portion). The thalamolenticular portion consists primarily of the corticospinal tract and the sensory radiations (including thalamocortical fibers to the parietal lobe); it also contains corticorubral and corticotegmental fibers. The postlenticular portion consists of visual and posterior thalamic radiations and the occipitotemporoparietal corticopontine tracts. The sublenticular portion contains auditory radiations and the temporal loop of the optic radiations.

capsule, lens [capsula lentis, NA], EYE   sheath which encloses the lens of the eye and into which the fibers of the suspensory ligament insert. Anteriorly the lens capsule overlies the lens epithelium, but posteriorly there is no intervening epithelial layer between the capsule and the body of the lens.

capsule, ol´ivary, MEDULLA   terminal portions of the fibers of the central tegmental tract as they enclose and enter the inferior olivary nucleus. *Syn:* amiculum olivae.

capsule, o´tic, EAR   layer of hard bone within the petrous part of the temporal bone which encloses the bony labyrinth.

carot´id [Gr. *karotides* from *karoun* to stupefy]   pertaining to the carotid arteries, their branches, or related structures, so named because pressure on the carotid arteries was known to cause an individual to fall into a stupor. *For the following:* common and internal carotid arteries; carotid body, canal, *and* siphon, *see the nouns.*

car´refour olfac´tif, CEREBRUM   *See* area, parolfactory.

CAT   computerized axial tomography, also called computed tomography (CT). *See also* tomography.

cat´aplexy   disorder characterized by the sudden relaxation of all muscles, particularly those of the lower limbs, in response to an emotional stimulus.

cat´aract   disorder characterized by loss of transparency of the lens of the eye or its capsule.

catecholamine /kat-ĕ-ko´lam-ĕn/   any of a class of monoaminergic neurotransmitters, comprising epinephrine, norepinephrine, and dopamine. *See also* neurotransmitters.

cauda cerebelli /kaw´dah ser-ĕ-bel´ī/, CEREBELLUM, [L. *cauda* tail]   old term for the cerebellar vermis.

cauda equi´na [NA] [L. *equus* horse]   lumbosacral nerve roots as they descend from the spinal cord through the subarachnoid space to emerge through their respective intervertebral or sacral foramina, so named for their resemblance to a horse's tail.

caudate /kaw´dāt/   *See* nucleus, caudate.

causalgia /koz-al´jī-ah/   severe, constant pain, often of a burning type, usually after injury to a major peripheral nerve. It was originally described in the last century by W. Mitchell and based on his observations during the American Civil War.

cavity   *See also* cavum.

cavity, cra´nial [cavitas cranii, NA]   large space in the skull which contains the brain, its meninges, and blood vessels.

cavity, epidu´ral [cavitas (cavum) epiduralis, NA]   *See* space, epidural.

cavity, lens [cavitas lentis, NA], EYE   space in the embryonic lens vesicle which later is obliterated as the lens completes its development.

cavity, neural   vertebral canal and cranial cavity.

cavity, optic [cavitas optica, NA], EYE   space partially enclosed by the optic cup of the developing eye, in which the vitreous body develops.

cavity, subarach´noid [cavitas (cavum) subarachnoidea, NA]   *See* space, subarachnoid.

cavity, tympan´ic [cavitas tympanica (cavum tympani), NA], EAR   largest space of the middle ear, not including the tympanic antrum and the auditory tube, and containing the ossicles and related structures.

ca´vum   *See also* cavity.

cavum sep´ti pellu´cidi [NA], CEREBRUM   median space between the two laminae of the septum pellucidum. It neither contains cerebrospinal fluid nor communicates with the ventricular system. The posterior part of this space is sometimes designated the sixth ventricle or ventricle of Vergae. *Syn:* fifth ventricle; Duncan's, Vieussens', or Wenzel's ventricle.

cavum trigeminal´e [NA]   invagination of the dura mater of the lateral wall of the cavernous sinus, containing the root, trigeminal ganglion, and proximal parts of the primary divisions of the trigeminal nerve. *Syn:* Meckel's cave, space, or cavity.

ce´cum [L. *caecus* blind]   any of several blind pouches.

cecum, cu´pular [cecum (caecum) cupulare, NA], EAR   blind pouch at the apical end of the cochlear duct. *Syn:* lagena.

cecum, vestib´ular [cecum (caecum) vestibulare, NA], EAR   blind pouch at the basal end of the cochlear duct, near the junction of the cochlear duct and ductus reuniens.

ce´liac [Gr. *koilia* belly]   *For* celiac ganglion *and* plexus, *see the nouns.*

cell, amacrine /am´ak-rin/ [neuronum amacrinum, NA], EYE, [Gr. *a* not; *makros* long; *is, inos* fiber]   retinal association neuron or interneuron with short branching processes and which appears not to have an axon. The cell bodies of these neurons are located in the inner part of the inner nuclear layer (layer 6), and the processes terminate in the inner plexiform layer (layer 7), synapsing with bipolar cells, other amacrine cells, interplexiform cells, and ganglion cells. These cells are thought to play a role both in the spatial aspects of vision and in color vision.

cell, basket [neuronum corbiferum, NA]   **1.** CEREBELLUM inhibitory cell located in the deep part of the molecular layer of the cerebellar cortex, with basketlike endings around the cell bodies of Purkinje cells (Fig. C-9). *Syn:* lower stellate cell.
2. CEREBRUM certain small, inhibitory cells in stratum oriens of the hippocampus.

cell, bipo´lar   *See* neuron, bipolar, *and* retina, layer 6.

cells, bor´der, EAR   cells which line the internal spiral sulcus of the cochlear duct.

cell, compound granular   round cell with granular cytoplasm and an eccentric nucleus found in areas of degeneration in the CNS, presumably a phagocytic cell derived from microglia. *Syn:* gitter cell.

cells, dorsal funic´ular, CORD   cells of nucleus proprius.

cell, effec´tor   muscle fiber or glandular cell on which a nerve fiber terminates.

cells, epen´dymal   ciliated, nonsecretory cells which line the ventricular spaces of the CNS.

cell, ependymo´glial   *See* tanycyte.

cell, feather, CEREBELLUM   elongated neuroglial cells in the molecular layer of the cerebellar cortex. They are characterized by numerous stubby processes which maintain close relations with the processes and body of Purkinje cells. *Syn:* Fañanás cells.

cell, ganglion   1. nerve cell body in a sensory or autonomic ganglion of the PNS.
2. EYE   one of the large cells of layer 8 of the retina, whose axons compose the optic nerve.
3. old term for any nerve cell body inside or outside the CNS.

cell, git´ter   *See* cell, compound granular.

cell, granule   1. [neuronum granuliforme, NA], CEREBELLUM   nerve cell having a diameter of 5 to 8 μm, in the granular layer of the cerebellar cortex. The dendrites of these cells synapse with mossy fibers. Their axons enter the molecular layer and branch as parallel fibers (Fig. C-9).
2. CEREBRUM   small nerve cell in the granular layers (layers II and IV) of the cerebral cortex. *See also* cell, compound granular.

cell group   *See* nucleus, *def.* 2.

cell, horizontal (of Cajal), CEREBRUM   neuron with a small, fusiform cell body and long processes within the molecular layer (layer 1) of the cerebral cortex.

cell, horizontal, EYE   retinal association neuron or interneuron. The cell bodies of these neurons are located in the outer part of the inner nuclear layer (layer 6) and their processes end in the adjoining part of the outer plexiform layer (layer 5). The dendrites of the horizontal cells are in contact only with cones, whereas their axons end on both rods and cones.

cell, interme´diate (of Lugaro), CEREBELLUM   fusiform, horizontal cell, present in the granular layer of the cerebellar cortex.

cell, interplex´iform, EYE   association neuron or interneuron having its cell body in the inner nuclear layer (layer 6) of the retina, among the bipolar cells. Presumably it constitutes a feedback mechanism between the inner and outer synaptic layers of the retina, conducting impulses from the amacrine cells to the horizontal and bipolar cells.

cell, lower stel´late, CEREBELLUM   *See* cell, basket, *def.* 1.

cells, mar´ginal, CORD   cells of the posteromarginal nucleus arranged tangentially on the apical surface of the dorsal horn of the spinal cord; Rexed's lamina I.

cells, midget, EYE   small, monosynaptic cells near the macula lutea of the retina. Each midget bipolar cell synapses with only one cone and one midget ganglion cell.

cells, mi´tral, CEREBRUM, [L. *mitra* turban]   large cells of the olfactory bulb, so named because of their resemblance to a bishop's miter. The olfactory nerve fibers synapse with these cells. Their axons enter the olfactory tract.

cell, mos´sy   *See* astrocyte, protoplasmic.

cell, multipo´lar   *See* neuron, multipolar.

cell, nerve   1. neuron.
2. *See* body, cell.

cell, neurog´lial   neuroglia.

cell, neurolem´ma sheath   part of the neurolemma sheath containing the nucleus and a small amount of cytoplasm. There is only one sheath cell per internodal segment. *Syn:* Schwann cell; lemmocyte.

cells, neurose´cretory, HYPOTHALAMUS   nerve cells of the supraoptic and paraventricular nuclei of the hypothalamus which produce either antidiuretic hormone or oxytocin and transport it to the neurohypophysis, where it is released.

cells, obscure   small, darkly staining, unipolar, sensory ganglion cells whose processes are nonmyelinated or thinly myelinated and which conduct impulses for pain from the periphery and impulses from the viscera.

cell, off-center, EYE   an inhibitory neuron in the ganglion cell layer (layer 8) of the retina. It is activated by stimulation of the central zone of its receptive field.

cell, on-center, EYE   an excitatory neuron in the ganglion cell layer (layer 8) of the retina. It is activated by stimulation of the central zone of its receptive field.

cell (of) origin   cell body of a neuron the axon of which contributes to some nerve fiber bundle or makes some neurological connection.

cells, parasol, EYE   neurons with a large cell body in the ganglion cell layer (layer 8) of the retina. These cells have large receptive fields and are most sensitive to the fine details needed for pattern vision.

cells, phalangeal /fah-lan´jī-al/, EAR   supporting cells for the hair cells of the spiral organ of the cochlea, their bases resting on the basilar membrane. The outer phalangeal cells are located between and adjacent to the outer hair cells. The inner phalangeal cells, next to the inner pillar cells, support the inner hair cells. *Syn:* cells of Deiters.

cells, pillar, EAR   supporting cells in the spiral organ of the cochlea. The bases of the inner and outer pillar cells rest on the basilar membrane and their tips are joined; they form the walls of the inner tunnel (of Corti). *Syn:* Corti's rods or pillars.

cell, pir´iform [neuronum piriforme, NA], CEREBELLUM   Purkinje cell of the cerebellar cortex. *See* Purkinje.

cell, pseudounipo´lar   *See* neuron, unipolar.

cell, pyram´idal, CEREBRUM   neurons of the cerebral cortex having a triangular shape, an apical dendrite extending toward the brain surface, basal dendrites extending laterally, and a long axon leading away from the cortex. Such cells are characteristic particularly of layers III and V of the neopallial cortex, and include the giant pyramidal (Betz) cells in layer V of the motor area.

cell, re´lay, EYE   bipolar cell of the retina.

cell, rod   1. EYE   rod (of the retina).
2. old term for microglia.

cell, sat´ellite   one of the cells which compose the ectodermal capsule of a ganglion cell and are continuous with the neurolemma.

cells, small intensely fluorescent (SIF)   small cells currently regarded as inter neurons. Many cells contain peptides which presumably act as modulators or transmitters at synapses.

cell, spider   *See* astrocyte, fibrous.

cell, stalked, CORD   neuron located at the border between the substantia gelatinosa (Rexed lamina II) and the overlying marginal cells (lamina I) of the spinal cord. Its dendrites extend ventrally; its axons enter lamina I. It may act as an excitatory interneuron for non-noxious impulses into lamina I.

cell(s), stel´late   1. any small neuron having a star-shaped cell body. Such cells serve as internuncial neurons in various parts of the CNS, including the cerebral cortex.
2. CEREBELLUM   various cells in the cerebellar cortex are called stellate cells

including: (1) [neuronum stellatum, NA] inhibitory cell in the outer part of the molecular layer of the cerebellar cortex; the axons of such cells synapse with and inhibit the dendrites of Purkinje cells. (2) [neuronum stellatum magnum, NA] large stellate cell in the granular layer of the cerebellar cortex; these cells synapse with and inhibit the dendrites of granule cells in the cerebellar islands in the granular layer. *Syn:* Golgi cell. (3) [neuronum corbiferum, NA] basket cell in the deep part of the molecular layer; they are sometimes called lower stellate cells (Fig. C-9). *See also* Golgi.

cell, T (T for transmission), CORD   cell in the dorsal horn of the spinal cord presumed, in the gate-control theory of pain, to provide a link for the transmission of pain to higher centers and also for local reflexes. *See* gate-control theory of pain.

cell, unipo´lar   *See* neuron, unipolar.

center   *See also* centrum.

center, storm, CEREBRUM   Steiner's Wetterwinkel. *See* Steiner.

central   *See* lobule, central *and* sulcus, central.

centrencephal´ic   pertaining to the central core of brain tissue extending through the brain stem to the diencephalon. *See* system, centrencephalic.

centrif´ugal   away from the central nervous system.

centrip´etal   toward the central nervous system.

cen´trum oval´e, CEREBRUM   *See* centrum semiovale.

centrum semioval´e, CEREBRUM   mass of white matter within the cerebrum, between the cerebral cortex and the basal ganglia, at the level of the body of the corpus callosum. It consists largely of fibers of the corona radiata and of the corpus callosum. *Syn:* centrum ovale.

ceph´alad   toward the head.

cephal´ic   pertaining to the head.

cephalocele /sef´ă-lo-sĕl/   hernia of the brain.

cerebel´lum [NA] [*adj.* **cerebellar**] [L. little brain, dim. of *cerebrum*]   part of the brain derived from the alar plates of the metencephalon. It is located in the posterior cranial fossa and consists of a median part, the vermis, and two laterally placed cerebellar hemispheres (Figs. C-2, V-6). It is concerned with equilibrium, coordination, and the regulation of muscle tone. Disorders resulting from cerebellar injury include: disorders of gait (vermis), of coordination, and a decrease in muscle tone (ipsilateral hemisphere), and impaired equilibrium (flocculonodular lobe). A cerebellar tremor is a coarse, ataxic tremor, also called an "action" or "intention" tremor, which occurs during voluntary movement, with lesions of the dentate nucleus or the fibers arising from it. *See also* tremor. Palatal myoclonus occurs with a lesion of the efferent fibers from the dentate nucleus to the inferior olivary nucleus (Figs. N-2, O-1). *For additional information on the cerebellum, see* Schneider and Crosby ('82, pp. 733-759). *See also* cortex cerebelli; vermis cerebelli. The lobes of the cerebellum, in rostral-to-caudal order, are as follows:

lobe, anterior [lobus anterior (rostralis), NA]   the paleocerebellum; the subdivision anterior to the primary fissure.

lobe, posterior [lobus posterior (caudalis), NA]   the neocerebellum; the subdivision between the primary fissure rostrally and the postnodular fissure of the vermis and the posterolateral fissure of the cerebellar hemispheres caudally. It is further subdivided into: lobulus simplex, superior and inferior semilunar lobules, gracile lobule, biventer, and tonsil. *See also* lobule, ansiform *and* paramedian; lobulus medianus *and* medius medianus.

lobe, flocculonodular [lobus flocculonodularis, NA]   the archicerebellum; the most caudal subdivision of the cerebellum, comprising the flocculus, nodule, and the peduncle of the flocculus connecting them.

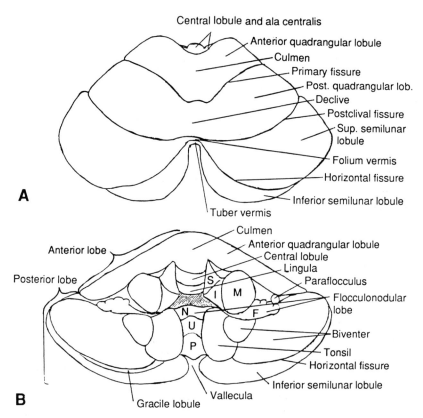

Fig. C-2.   Diagrams of the superior (A) and anterior (B) surfaces of the cerebellum, showing the divisions of the cerebellar vermis and hemispheres, and the superior (S), inferior (I), and middle (M) cerebellar peduncles. F-flocculus, N-nodule, U-uvula, P-pyramis.

cerebrum /ser ′ĕ-brum/ [NA] [*adj.* **cerebral** /ser ′ĕ-bral/] [L. brain]   part of the brain derived from the embryonic telencephalon and consisting of the cortex and white matter of the cerebral hemispheres (Fig. C-3), the basal ganglia, and certain other basal structures which are a part of the rhinencephalon. The term cerebrum has also been used loosely to mean the entire forebrain, i.e., the derivatives of both the telencephalon and the diencephalon. *Syn:* end brain. *See also* cortex, cerebral; lobe, fornicate, limbic, *and* piriform; *and* various cortical areas, including parolfactory and entorhinal. The cerebral hemispheres are subdivided as follows:

lobe, frontal [lobus frontalis, NA]   that part of the cerebral hemisphere anterior to the central sulcus.

lobe, parietal [lobus parietalis, NA]   that part of the cerebrum separated from the frontal lobe by the central sulcus, from the temporal lobe by the lateral sulcus on the lateral surface, and from the occipital lobe by the parieto-occipital sulcus on the medial surface of the hemisphere.

lobe, occipital [lobus occipitalis, NA]   posterior part of the cerebrum separated from the parietal lobe on the medial surface of the hemisphere by the parieto-occipital sulcus, and from the temporal lobe by a line from the parieto-occipital sulcus, to the preoccipital incisure.

lobe, temporal [lobus temporalis, NA]   that part of the cerebral hemisphere inferior to the lateral sulcus.

insula [lobus insularis (insula), NA]   that part of the cerebral cortex buried within and forming the floor of the lateral sulcus. *Syn:* island of Reil; central lobe.

cerebrum, lobules of the   *See* lobule, paracentral; lobule, parietal, inferior, *and* superior; cuneus; *and* precuneus.

cervical (C)   pertaining to one or more of the eight cervical spinal cord segments or nerves, or seven cervical vertebrae.

Chaddock, Charles Gilbert (1861-1935)   *Chaddock's sign* (1911) is dorsiflexion of the great toe in response to stroking the area of the lateral malleolus, after injury of the corticospinal tract, also called an external malleolar sign. *See also* Babinski.

chain, neuron   a series of two or more neurons, linked together consecutively so that an impulse may pass from one to the next throughout the series.

chamber, anterior [camera anterior bulbi, NA], EYE   space within the eyeball between the cornea and the iris.

chamber, posterior [camera posterior bulbi, NA], EYE   space within the eyeball posterior to the iris and in front of the lens and vitreous body. It communicates with the anterior chamber by way of the pupil.

chamber, vit´reous [camera vitrea bulbi, NA], EYE   space within the eyeball, behind the lens and containing the vitreous body.

Charcot, Jean Martin (1825-1893)   outstanding French neurologist. He established the famous Salpêtrière neurologic clinic in Paris. He is noted as the founder of clinical neurology and was a pioneer in neuropathology and psychotherapy as well. He founded the *Archives of Neurology* (1880) and published the first description of many neurologic disorders which subsequently were named for him. *Charcot's triad,* a common cerebellar manifestation in advanced cases of multiple sclerosis, consists of nystagmus, an intention tremor, and scanning speech. *Charcot-Marie-Tooth disease* is peroneal muscular atrophy, inherited as an autosomal dominant. It was so named following a description by Charcot and his pupil P. Marie in 1886, and by H.H. Tooth in a medical thesis the same year. The *artery of Charcot,* also known as the artery of internal hemorrhage, is the largest of the lateral striate arteries and passes around the lateral border of the lenticular nucleus. Among Charcot's outstanding pupils were Dejerine, Marie, Marinescu, and Babinski.

Charpy, Adrien (1848-1911)   French physician and anatomist. *Charpy's anastomotic vein* is the posterior communicating vein.

Chaussier, François (1746-1828)   French physician. *Chaussier's line* is the median raphe of the corpus callosum.

chemoreceptor /ke´mo-re-sep´tor/   nerve ending sensitive to chemical stimuli throughout the body. Included are the receptors for taste and smell, endings sensitive to special substances of the gastrointestinal tract, pH-sensitive receptors in the brain and blood vessels, and others.

Chiari, Hans (1851-1915)   German pathologist. His publication on the developmental defect now called the *Arnold-Chiari malformation* appeared in 1891, three years before that of Arnold. *See* Arnold, J.

chiasm (chiasma), optic /ki´azm, ki-az´mah/ [chiasma opticum, NA] [Gr. *chiasma* two crossing lines, from the Greek letter *chi* (χ)], DIENCEPHALON   structure on the ventral surface of the brain, first described and named by Rufus of Ephesus about 100 A.D. It is composed of crossing optic nerve fibers from the medial half of each retina. Fibers from the lateral half of each retina continue

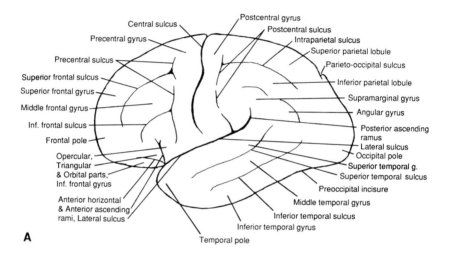

A

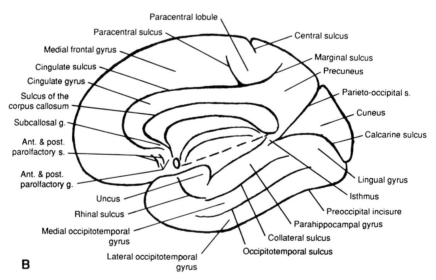

B

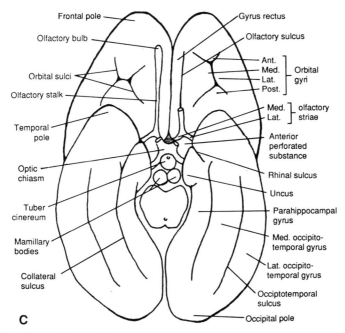

Fig. C-3. Illustrations to show the major named gyri and sulci on the lateral (A), medial (B), and inferior (C) surfaces of the cerebral hemispheres.

into the homolateral optic tract without crossing the median plane (Figs. C-3C, V-5). A lesion of the crossing fibers results in bitemporal hemianopsia.

cholinergic /ko-lin-er´jik/   pertaining to those nerve fibers which release acetylcholine at their axon terminals. Such fibers include many within the CNS, also autonomic preganglionic fibers, postganglionic parasympathetic fibers, those postganglionic sympathetic fibers that supply sweat glands, some sympathetic fibers for vasodilation and possibly some to uterine muscle. *See also* neurotransmitters; muscarinic; nicotinic.

cholinesterase /ko-lin-es´ter-ās/   enzyme which inactivates (hydrolyzes) acetylcholine. *Syn:* acetylcholinesterase (AChE).

chorda dorsalis /kor´dah dōr-sal´is/ [NA]   notochord.

chorda tym´pani [NA]   branch which leaves the facial (intermediate) nerve in the facial canal and enters the tympanic cavity through the tympanic aperture of the chorda tympanic canal. It passes between the short process of the incus and the neck of the malleus and leaves the tympanic cavity through the petrotympanic fissure to join the lingual nerve. It is composed of visceral sensory fibers for taste from the anterior two-thirds of the tongue and preganglionic parasympathetic fibers from the superior salivatory nucleus which, after synapse in the submandibular and Langley's ganglia, supply the sublingual and submandibular glands, respectively (Fig. C-4). *See also* nerve, facial.

chordo´ma   malignant growth derived from remnants of the notochord.

chore´a [Gr. *choros* a dance]   sudden, jerky, involuntary movements, together with

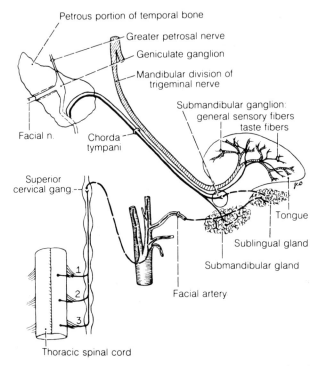

Fig. C-4. Diagram illustrating the distribution of the chorda tympani and the innervation of the submandibular and sublingual glands. Langley's ganglion, in the submandibular gland, is shown but not labeled. From R.T. Woodburne and W.E. Burkel, *Essentials of Human Anatomy,* 8th ed., 1988. Courtesy of the authors and Oxford University Press, Publisher, New York, Oxford.

      grimacing and faulty vocalization, resulting from a lesion of the caudate nucleus or its fibers. *See also* Huntington and Sydenham for the choreas named for them.

chore´iform   pertaining to chorea.

choriocapillaris /ko-rī-o-kap-il-lar´is/, EYE   *See* choroid, choriocapillary layer.

cho´roid (chorioid) [choroidea, NA], EYE, [Gr. *chorion* delicate membrane; *eidos* shape]   pigmented vascular tunic of the eye, interposed between the sclera and the retina. *See also* plexus *and* fissure, choroid. From the outside in, the layers of the choroid of the eye are as follows:

    suprachoroid layer [lamina suprachoroidea (fusca), NA] [L. *supra* above; *fuscus* dusky]   thin, outer, pigmented, nonvascular layer. This layer, structurally a part of the choroid, remains attached to the sclera when the sclera and choroid are torn apart, hence its name. *Syn:* epichoroid.

    vascular layer [lamina vasculosa, NA]   pigmented layer containing many small blood vessels and making up most of the thickness of the choroid. The outer part of this layer (Haller's layer) contains larger vessels (branches of the short posterior ciliary arteries and tributaries of the vorticose veins) and the inner part (Sattler's layer) contains somewhat smaller vessels.

choriocapillary layer [lamina choroidocapillaris, NA]   thin, nonpigmented layer
of closely packed, large capillaries in a single layer. From these vessels the
fovea and the outer layers of the retina receive their nourishment.   *Syn:*
membrane of Ruysch.

basal layer [lamina basalis (complexus basalis), NA]   thin, almost transparent,
refractile layer, formed from components of both the choroid and the retina.
It is semipermeable, permitting oxygen and nutrients to pass through it to reach
the rods and cones. *Syn:* Bruch's membrane; glassy membrane; lamina vitrea;
hyaline membrane.

chro´matin, sex   *See* satellite, nucleolar.

chromatol´ysis [Gr. *chroma* color; *lysis* loosening]   series of nuclear and cytoplasmic
changes which occur in the cell body of the neuron as a result of injury to one of
its processes or in response to other pathologic conditions.

chronaxie /kro-nak´sī/   minimum time during which a current twice the rheobasic
strength must flow in order to cause excitation.

ciliary /sil´ī-ar-ī/ [L. *cilium* eyelash]   pertaining to certain structures in or related
to the eyeball. *For* ciliary body, crown, epithelium, *and* ganglion, *see the nouns.*

cingulum /sing´gu-lum/ [NA], CEREBRUM, [L. girdle]   bundle of association fibers of
the cerebrum located mainly within the cingulate gyrus. It has connections all
along its course with adjacent frontal, parietal, and temporal lobe cortex. *Syn:*
fornix periphericus; longitudinal fasciculus of the fornicate gyrus.

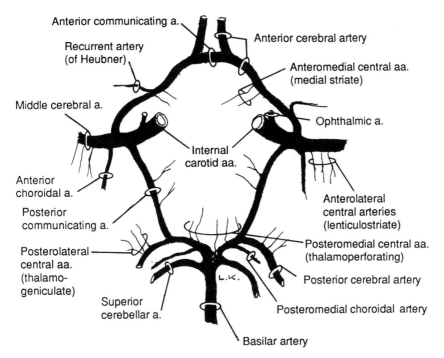

Fig. C-5. Cerebral arterial circle (of Willis) and its branches, on the base of the brain.
Drawing courtesy of Dr. L.G. Kempe.

cingulum ammonal´e, CEREBRUM   old term for the association fibers interconnecting
the hippocampus and parahippocampal gyrus.

cingulum lim´itans, CEREBRUM   old term for the cingulum.

circle, cerebral arterial [circulus arteriosus cerebri, NA], CEREBRUM   arterial circle on
the base of the brain formed by the internal carotid arteries, the anterior and
posterior cerebral arteries, and the anterior and posterior communicating arteries
(Fig. C-5). *Syn:* circle of Willis.

cis´tern [cisterna, NA]   widened part of the subarachnoid space, in the cranial
cavity in regions where the arachnoid spans irregularities on the surface of the
brain, and in the vertebral canal caudal to the spinal cord.

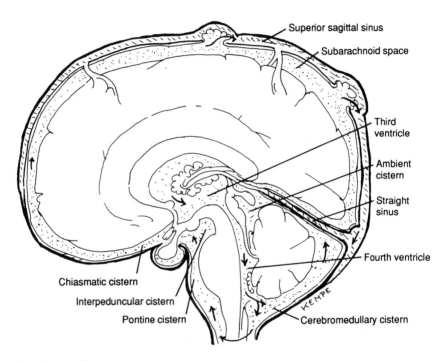

Fig. C-6.   Illustration to show the major subarachnoid cisterns and the flow of
cerebrospinal fluid. The chiasmatic and interpeduncular cisterns are subdivisions of the
basal cistern. Drawing courtesy of Dr. L.G. Kempe.

cistern, am´bient [cisterna ambiens, NA]   that part of the subarachnoid space that
surrounds the midbrain (Fig. C-6). The cistern of the great cerebral vein is
sometimes considered its dorsal part. *Syn:* circummesencephalic cistern.

cistern, ba´sal   that part of the subarachnoid space on the underside of the brain,
ventral to the hypothalamus and anterior to the midbrain. Sometimes the optic
chiasm is said to divide this cistern into an anterior part, the cistern of the optic
chiasm, and a posterior part, the interpeduncular cistern, which may or may not
include the interpeduncular fossa proper.

cistern, cerebellomed´ullary [cisterna cerebellomedullaris, NA]   that part of the subarachnoid space caudal to the cerebellum and posterior to the medulla, where the median aperture of the fourth ventricle communicates with the subarachnoid space (Fig. C-6). *Syn:* cisterna magna.

cistern (of the) cerebellopon´tine angle   that part of the subarachnoid space lateral to the brain stem in the region where the pons, medulla, and cerebellum meet and where the lateral aperture of the fourth ventricle communicates with the subarachnoid space.

cistern, chiasmat´ic [cisterna chiasmatis, NA]   that part of the subarachnoid space anterior to the optic chiasm, sometimes considered an anterior subdivision of the basal cistern (Fig. C-6).

cistern, circummesencephal´ic   *See* cistern, ambient.

cistern (of the) cor´pus callo´sum   that part of the subarachnoid space above the corpus callosum and between the two cerebral hemispheres.

cistern (of the) great cerebral vein   that part of the subarachnoid space dorsal to the superior colliculus and sometimes considered the dorsal part of the ambient cistern. It is located between the splenium of the corpus callosum above and the cerebellum below and contains the great cerebral vein and the pineal body. *Syn:* superior cistern; quadrigeminal cistern.

cistern, interpedun´cular [cisterna interpeduncularis, NA]   **1.** part of the subarachnoid space between the bases of the cerebral peduncles, i.e. the interpeduncular fossa, through which the oculomotor nerves pass (Fig. C-6). *Syn:* cisterna cruralis; Tarin's space or fossa.
2. This term is also sometimes used to include the space anterior to the midbrain between the temporal lobes, extending forward on the undersurface of the hypothalamus to the optic nerve and enclosing the cerebral arterial circle. *See also* cistern, basal.

cistern (of the) lam´ina terminal´is   that part of the subarachnoid space anterior to the lamina terminalis.

cistern (of the) lateral fos´sa [cisterna fossae lateralis cerebri, NA]   that part of the subarachnoid space anterior to the temporal lobe, at the entrance to the lateral sulcus and containing the proximal part of the middle cerebral artery.

cistern, lum´bar   that part of the subarachnoid space caudal to the conus medullaris of the spinal cord, from about the vertebral level of L1 to that of S2. It contains the lumbar and sacral nerve roots of the cauda equina and the filum terminale.

cistern, perimesencephal´ic   *See* cistern, ambient.

cistern, pontine   that part of the subarachnoid space anterior to the pons, and containing the basilar and pontine arteries (Fig. C-6).

cistern, quadrigem´inal   *See* cistern (of the) great cerebral vein.

cistern, superior   *See* cistern (of the) great cerebral vein.

cister´na crural´is   *See* cistern, interpeduncular.

cisterna mag´na   *See* cistern, cerebellomedullary.

Clark, Sir W.E. Le Gros (1895-1971)   *See* Le Gros Clark.

Clarke, Jacob Augustus Lockhart (1817-1880)   English physician and anatomist of London. The *dorsal nucleus of Clarke* or *Clarke's column* (1851) is the thoracic nucleus of the spinal cord.

Claudius, Friedrich Matthias (1822-1869)   Austrian anatomist of Marburg. The *cells of Claudius* compose a single layer of cuboidal cells lying in the base of the external spiral sulcus of the cochlear duct.

claustrum /klow´strum/ [NA], CEREBRUM, [L. an enclosed space or barrier]   thin sheet of gray matter interposed between the insula and extreme capsule laterally and the external capsule and putamen medially.

cla´va [L. club], MEDULLA   *See* tubercle, gracile.

cleft, synap´tic   narrow space (about 200 Å wide) between the pre- and the post-synaptic membranes of a synapse.

cli´vus [L. slope or hill]   **1.** CEREBELLUM   declive of the cerebellar vermis.

2. [NA] bony anterior wall of the posterior cranial fossa, part of the occipital bone.

3. EYE   slope of the fovea in the macula of the retina.

clo´nus [*adj.* **clonic**]   repetitive alternating contractions and relaxations of muscle.

Cloquet, Jules Germain (1790-1883)   French anatomist. The *canal of Cloquet* is the hyaloid canal of the developing eye.

coccygeal (Coc) /kok-sĭ-je´al/   pertaining to the coccyx, or to the most caudal segment of the spinal cord and its nerves.

cochlea /kok´le-ah/ [NA] [*pl.* **cochleae**], EAR, [L. snail shell]   that part of the internal ear concerned with hearing.

Coghill, George (1872-1941)   American anatomist and embryologist at the University of Kansas, later at the Wistar Institute of Anatomy. His experimental studies on salamanders established the relationship of the changing patterns of behavior to anatomical neuroembryology.

colliculus /kol-ik´u-lus/ [L. mound]   small protuberance.

colliculus, abdu´cent, PONS   *See* colliculus, facial.

colliculus, anterior, MIDBRAIN   *See* colliculus, superior.

colliculus axon´is [NA]   *See* hillock, axon.

colliculus, fa´cial [colliculus facialis, NA], PONS   elevation in the medial eminence, on the floor of the fourth ventricle, medial to the sulcus limitans and overlying the abducens nucleus and the genu of the facial nerve (Fig. V-4). *Syn:* abducent colliculus.

colliculus, inferior [colliculus inferior (caudalis), NA], MIDBRAIN   rounded elevation on the dorsal surface of the midbrain, on either side of the median plane in the caudal part of the tectum, and containing the nucleus of the inferior colliculus. It is a part of the auditory system. *Syn:* posterior colliculus.

colliculus, posterior, MIDBRAIN   *See* colliculus, inferior.

colliculus, superior [colliculus superior (rostralis), NA], MIDBRAIN   rounded elevation on the dorsal surface of the midbrain, on either side of the median plane in the rostral part of the tectum. *Syn:* anterior colliculus. It is composed of alternating layers of cells and fibers, which, from superficial to deep, are as follows:

strat´um zonal´e   most superficial layer of the superior colliculus, composed chiefly of fibers of the external corticotectal tract from auditory association cortex in the occipitotemporal region (Fig. R-3).

stratum gris´eum superficial´e   layer of small nerve cells just deep to the stratum zonale of the superior colliculus. It receives fibers from the adjoining fibrous layers and discharges to the deeper layers of the superior colliculus. *Syn:* stratum cinereum.

stratum op´ticum   layer of optic nerve fibers in the superior colliculus between the stratum griseum superficiale and stratum griseum intermediale. This layer is much reduced in primates, especially in man.

stratum lemnis´ci   the combined stratum griseum intermediale and stratum album intermediale of the superior colliculus.

stratum griseum intermedial´e layer of small nerve cells in the superior colliculus, just superficial to and associated with the stratum album intermediale, and part of the stratum lemnisci. *Syn:* stratum griseum medium.

stratum al´bum intermediale main receptive layer of the superior colliculus, composed mainly of nerve fibers of the internal corticotectal tract from the occipital (area 18) and preoccipital (area 19) cortex (Fig. R-2), supplemented by fibers of the spinotectal, nigrotectal, and thalamotectal tracts and collaterals of the ventral secondary ascending trigeminal tract. *Syn:* stratum album medium.

stratum griseum profun´dum layer of intermediate-sized and large nerve cells in the superior colliculus, just deep to the stratum album intermediale, and whose axons enter the underlying stratum album profundum.

stratum album profundum efferent layer of the superior colliculus at the edge of the periaqueductal gray, including fibers of the medial and lateral tectospinal, tectorubral, tecto-oculomotor, tectonigral, tectopontine, tecto-tegmental, and tectohabenular tracts.

stratum griseum et fibro´sum periventricular´e gray matter around the cerebral aqueduct of the midbrain, containing small to medium-sized neurons and thinly myelinated or nonmyelinated nerve fibers of the acoustico-optic tract and dorsal longitudinal fasciculus.

colobo´ma [Gr. *kolobos* mutilated, stunted, or imperfect] defect resulting from incomplete closure of the choroid fissure of the optic cup and consisting of a gap in the inferior part of the iris, ciliary body, retina, or choroid coat of the eye.

col´umn [columna, NA] *See also* horn; tract; bundle; fasciculus; nucleus.

column, anterior [columna ventralis (anterior), NA], CORD *See* column, ventral.

column, central magnocel´lular cell, CORD cells of nucleus proprius, in the dorsal horn of the spinal cord.

columns, cortical, CEREBRUM columnar organization of cells in the cerebral cortex, first noted in the somatosensory system by Mountcastle, and in the visual cortex by Hubel and Wiesel. *See also* columns, ocular dominance.

column, dorsal (posterior), CORD **1.** [columna dorsalis (posterior), NA] column of gray matter in the dorsal part of the spinal cord containing the cell bodies of secondary sensory and other neurons. In cross sections of the spinal cord, this area constitutes the dorsal horn. *See also* horn, dorsal.
2. *See* funiculus, dorsal.

column (of the) for´nix [columna fornicis, NA], FOREBRAIN *See* fornix, column.

column, intermediolat´eral [columna intermediolateralis, NA], CORD *See* nucleus, intermediolateral.

column, lateral, CORD **1.** [columna lateralis, NA] column of gray matter between the dorsal and ventral columns (horns) of some spinal cord segments (T1- about L3, S2-S4), and containing the cell bodies of preganglionic autonomic fibers. In the thoracolumbar region it includes the cells in the lateral horn. *See also* horn, lateral.
2. *See* funiculus, lateral.

columns, ocular dominance, CEREBRUM cortical columns that extend vertically from the surface of the visual cortex to the white matter, studied extensively by Hubel and Wiesel. Each column receives impulses from the retina of only one eye and adjoining columns relate to the opposite eye in a mosaic pattern. No such columns occur in the parts corresponding to the monocular retinal fields, nor is there any representation of the optic disk, the blind spot of the retina.

column, pericor´nual magnocellular, CORD   *See* nucleus, posterior marginal.

column, posterior [columna posterior, NA], CORD   *See* column, dorsal.

column, spinal   *See* column, vertebral.

column, ventral (anterior), CORD   1. [columna ventralis (anterius), NA]   column of gray matter in the anterior part of the spinal cord, containing the cell bodies of spinal cord motor neurons.   In cross sections of the spinal cord, this area constitutes the ventral horn.
2. *See* funiculus, ventral.

column, ver´tebral [columna vertebralis, NA]   series of vertebrae and intervertebral disks, forming the support of the neck and trunk and enclosing the spinal cord. *Syn:* spinal column; spine; backbone.

co´ma   unconsciousness from which a patient cannot be roused.

coma vigil /vī´jil/   *See* mutism, akinetic.

comb bundle, FOREBRAIN   *See* bundle, comb. *See also* tract, nigrostriate.

commissu´ra al´ba [NA] [L. *commissura*, from *con* or *com* together and *mittere* to put], CORD   *See* commissure, ventral white.

commissura ansulat´a, MIDBRAIN   *See* decussation, tegmental, ventral.

commissura in´fima [NA], CORD   fibers from fasciculus solitarius which cross the median plane dorsal to the dorsal gray commissure and central canal, in the rostral part of the spinal cord, mainly C1. *Syn:* dorsal white commissure; commissure of Haller.

commissura rostral´is [NA], CEREBRUM   *See* commissure, anterior.

commis´sural (commissu´ral)   pertaining to a commissure, particularly the anterior commissure.

com´missure [commissura, NA] [*adj.* **commissural**]   bundle of nerve fibers which crosses the median plane, sometimes but not always connecting similar structures on the two sides. *See also* decussation.

commissure, anterior [commissura anterior (rostralis), NA], CEREBRUM   bundle of nerve fibers which crosses the median plane in the upper part of the lamina terminalis (Fig. V-5) and which consists primarily of interconnections between the olfactory bulbs, amygdaloid nuclei, anterior perforated substances, parahippocampal gyri, and parts of the neopallial cortex of the temporal lobe.

commissure, anterior white, CORD   *See* commissure, ventral white.

commissure, cerebel´lar, anterior, CEREBELLUM   *See* commissure, cerebellar, superior.

commissure, cerebellar, inferior, CEREBELLUM   fibers which cross the median plane in the cerebellum in the region of the fastigial nucleus, and including (among others) cerebellovestibular and ventral spinocerebellar fibers. *Syn:* posterior cerebellar commissure.

commissure, cerebellar, posterior, CEREBELLUM   *See* commissure, cerebellar, inferior.

commissure, cerebellar, superior, CEREBELLUM   fibers which cross the median plane in the rostral part of the cerebellum and containing, at least in part, association fibers which interconnect the cerebellar hemispheres. *See also* decussation (of the) peduncles, cerebellar, superior.

commissure, dorsal gray, CORD   dorsal part of substantia intermedia centralis, dorsal to the central canal of the spinal cord, a part of Rexed's lamina X.   It includes, in its most rostral portion, the commissural nucleus.

commissure, dorsal white, CORD   *See* commissura infima.

commissure (of the) fibrae ansulatae, HYPOTHALAMUS   old term for the dorsal supraoptic decussation.

commissure (of the) fornix [commissura fornicis, NA], CEREBRUM   *See* commissure, hippocampal.

commissure, gray, DORSAL THALAMUS   *See* adhesion, interthalamic. *See also* commissure, dorsal *and* ventral gray.

commissure, haben´ular [commissura habenularum (habenularis), NA], EPITHALAMUS   bundle of nerve fibers which crosses the median plane through the upper attachment of the pineal body between the two habenulae, and through which the habenulae are connected mainly with subcortical centers of the opposite side (Figs. H-1, V-5).

commissure, hippocam´pal [commissura fornicis, NA], CEREBRUM   commissure between the crura of the fornix, just beneath the splenium of the corpus callosum. It consists mostly of fornix fibers from the hippocampus of one side which cross the median plane and enter the contralateral fornix for distribution with the fibers of the opposite side (Fig. P-2). *Syn:* fornix transversus.

commissure, hypothalam´ic, anterior, HYPOTHALAMUS   old term for the dorsal supraoptic decussation.

commissure, hypothalamic, superior, HYPOTHALAMUS   old term for the dorsal supraoptic decussation.

commissure (of the) inferior collic´ulus [commissura colliculorum inferiorum (caudalium), NA], MIDBRAIN   fibers which cross the median plane in the caudal part of the tectum, between the two inferior colliculi.

commissure (of the) lateral lemniscus, PONS   nerve fibers which arise from cells in the dorsal nucleus of the lateral lemniscus, cross the median plane in the rostral pons and end in the contralateral nucleus of the lateral lemniscus, or ascend as part of the lateral lemniscus of that side. *Syn:* commissure of Probst.

commissure, middle, DORSAL THALAMUS   *See* adhesion, interthalamic.

commissure, posterior [commissura posterior, NA], EPITHALAMUS, MIDBRAIN   bundle of nerve fibers which crosses the median plane at the junction of the midbrain and diencephalon (Fig. V-5). It is composed in part of fibers interconnecting the two pretectal nuclei (Fig. R-7) and fibers from certain midbrain nuclei into the contralateral medial longitudinal fasciculus (Fig. F-2). *See also* fasciculus, longitudinal, medial.

commissure (of the) superior colliculus [commissura colliculorum superioris (rostralis), NA], MIDBRAIN   fibers which cross the median plane in the rostral part of the tectum, between the two superior colliculi (Figs. R-2, R-3).

commissure, soft, DORSAL THALAMUS   *See* adhesion, interthalamic.

commissure, supramam´illary, HYPOTHALAMUS   *See* decussation, supramamillary.

commissure, supraop´tic, dorsal [commissura supraoptica dorsalis, NA], HYPOTHALAMUS   old term for the supraoptic decussations; a dorsal part corresponds to the dorsal supraoptic decussation and a ventral part to the ventral supraoptic decussation. *See also* commissure, supraoptic, ventral.

commissure, supraoptic, ventral [commissura supraoptica ventralis, NA], HYPOTHALAMUS   old term for the intrachiasmatic decussation when both the dorsal and ventral supraoptic decussations are considered subdivisions of the dorsal supraoptic commissure. *Syn:* commissure of Gudden.

commissure, ventral (anterior) gray, CORD   ventral part of substantia intermedia centralis, a thin layer of gray matter ventral to the central canal of the spinal cord, a part of Rexed's lamina X.

commissure, ventral (anterior) white [commissura alba, NA], CORD   fiber bundles which cross the median plane in the spinal cord, in the space between the central canal and the ventral median fissure.

complexus basalis /kom-plek´sus ba-sal´is/ [NA], EYE   *See* choroid, basal layer.

compo´nent, nerve   the sum of all neurons having like anatomical and physiological characters so that they could act in a common mode (Herrick, '15). Such neurons may be afferent (sensory) or efferent (motor) in type and innervate structures of visceral or of somite origin. *For the components of the brain stem nerves, see* Tables C-1, C-2, C-3. The nerve components are as follows:

> **general somat´ic af´ferent (sensory) (GSA, GSS)**   pertaining to those nerve fibers which conduct impulses to the CNS from cutaneous endings for pain, temperature, and touch (exteroceptive) and from muscles, tendons, and joints (proprioceptive).

> **somatic ef´ferent (motor) (SE, SM)**   pertaining to those nerve fibers which conduct impulses from motor nuclei of the spinal cord to striated muscle derived from somites and somatic mesoderm, and those from motor nuclei of the brain stem that supply the extraocular and the tongue muscles. Sometimes those fibers arising from the spinal cord are designated *general* somatic efferent, and those from the brain as *special* somatic efferent.

> **general vis´ceral afferent (sensory) (GVA, GVS)**   pertaining to those nerve fibers which conduct impulses to the CNS from structures derived from entoderm and splanchnic mesoderm, including thoracic, abdominal, and pelvic viscera, and certain viscera of the head, but excluding the fibers carrying olfactory and gustatory impulses.

> **general visceral efferent (motor) (GVE, GVM)**   pertaining to those nerve fibers which supply motor innervation of smooth muscle, cardiac muscle, and glands, and comprising the pre- and postganglionic fibers of the ANS.

> **special somatic afferent (sensory) (SSA, SSS)**   pertaining to those cranial nerve fibers which conduct visual and auditory impulses from the retina and the cochlea, respectively (exteroceptive), and from the vestibular apparatus (proprioceptive) to the brain.

> **special visceral afferent (sensory) (SVA, SVS)**   pertaining to those cranial nerve fibers which conduct olfactory and gustatory impulses from their sensory epithelium to the brain.

> **special visceral efferent (motor) (SVE, SVM)**   pertaining to those nerve fibers which conduct impulses from motor nuclei of the brain stem, and the accessory nucleus of the spinal cord, to striated muscle of branchiomeric (visceral arch) origin.

compu´terized (computed) tomog´raphy (CT) (computerized axial tomography, CAT)   *See* tomography.

cona´rium, EPITHALAMUS, [Gr. *konarion* small cone]   *See* body, pineal.

concus´sion   traumatic injury of the brain without demonstrable pathologic changes in the tissue, but sometimes with loss of consciousness for a short time or for hours.

conduc´tion, av´alanche   term introduced by Cajal ('11), describing a type of conduction in the cerebellar cortex in which stimulation of a single neuron was presumed to fire many secondary neurons, each of which, in turn, would fire many tertiary neurons.

conduction, sal´tatory [L. *saltatio* from *saltare* to jump]   conduction in which a

Table C-1
Nerve Components of the Medulla

Nerve	Component	Origin	Termination	Function
Glosso-pharyngeal (IX)	General visceral efferent	Inferior salivatory nucleus	Otic ganglion	Preganglionic parasympathetic for parotid gland
	Special visc. efferent	Nucleus ambiguus	Stylopharyngeus muscle	Motor
	General somatic afferent	Superior ganglion of IX	Spinal nucleus of V	Cutaneous sensibility from palate, post. ⅓ tongue, tonsils, ext. ear, pharynx
	General visc. afferent	Inferior ganglion of IX	Nucleus parasolitarius	Impulses from carotid body and carotid sinus
	Special visc. afferent		Dorsal visceral gray	Taste from the posterior ⅓ of the tongue
Vagus (X)	General visceral efferent	Dorsal efferent nucleus	Terminal ganglia in or near organs innervated	Pregang. parasympathetic for thoracic & most abdominal viscera
	Special visceral efferent	Nucleus ambiguus	Muscles of palate, larynx, pharynx, upper esophagus	Motor: swallowing, phonation, closure of nasal orifice
	General somatic afferent	Superior ganglion of X	Spinal ganglion of V	Cutaneous sensibility from part of external ear
	General visceral afferent	Inferior ganglion of X	Nucleus parasolitarius	Impulses from thoracic & abdominal viscera, aortic sinus & body
	Special visc. afferent		Dorsal visceral gray	Taste from epiglottis
Bulbar acc. (XI)	Visceral efferent	Supplements vagus nerve		
Spinal accessory (XI)	Special visceral efferent	Accessory nucleus (sp. cord)	Trapezius & sternocleidomastoid muscles	Motor
Hypoglossal (XII)	Somatic efferent	Hypo-glossal nucleus	Muscles of tongue, (all but palatoglossus)	Motor

Table C-2
Nerve Components of the Pons

Nerve	Component	Origin	Termination	Function
Trigeminal nerve (V)	Special visc. efferent	Motor nucleus of V	Chewing muscles	Motor
	General somatic afferent	Trigeminal ganglion	Spinal and pontine nuclei of V	Pain, touch & temperature from face & oral cavity
		Mesencephalic nucleus of V	Motor nucleus of V	Propriocep. from chewing musc. & temporomand. joint
Abducens nerve (VI)	Somatic efferent	Abducens nucleus	Lateral rectus muscle	Abducts the eye
Facial nerve (VII)	General visceral efferent	Lacrimal nucleus	Pterygopalatine ganglion	Parasymp. for lacrimal gland
		Superior salivatory nucleus		Parasymp. for nasal & palatine glands
			Submandibular ganglion	Parasymp. for sublingual gland
			Langley's ganglion	Parasymp. for submand. gland
			Ganglia near glands supplied	Parasymp. for glands ant. ⅔ tongue
	Special visc. efferent	Facial nucleus	Facial muscles	Motor
	General somatic afferent	Geniculate ganglion	Spinal nucleus of V	Pain, touch, temp. part of external ear
			Facial nucleus	Proprioception from facial muscles
	General visceral afferent		Nucleus parasolitarius	Impulses from mastoid air cells and middle ear
	Special visc. afferent		Dorsal visceral gray	Taste from anterior ⅔ tongue
Vestibulo-cochlear (VIII)	Special somatic afferent	Spiral ganglion	Dors/vent. coch. nuc.	Hearing
		Vestibular ganglion	Vestibular nuclei, cerebellum	Equilibrium

Table C-3
Nerve Components of the Midbrain

Nerve	Component	Origin	Termination	Function
Oculomotor (III)	Somatic efferent	Oculomotor nucleus	All extraocular muscles except lateral rectus & superior oblique	Motor
	General visceral efferent	Edinger-Westphal (accessory oculomotor) nucleus	Ciliary and/or episcleral ganglia	Preganglionic parasympathetic neurons for ciliary muscle and constrictor muscle of iris
Trochlear (IV)	Somatic efferent	Trochlear nucleus	Superior oblique muscle	Motor

nerve impulse jumps from one node of Ranvier to the next along a nerve fiber.

cone, EYE   photoreceptor of the retina, for color. *See also* rod.

con´fluence (of the) sinuses [confluens sinuum, NA]   place in the region of the internal occipital protuberance of the skull where the superior sagittal, straight, occipital, and transverse sinuses communicate. Usually the superior sagittal sinus continues into the right transverse sinus and the straight sinus continues into the left transverse sinus, with or without communication between the two systems. *Syn:* torcular Herophili.

connexus, interthalam´ic, DORSAL THALAMUS   *See* adhesion, interthalamic.

continuation, anterior, of the hippocampus, CEREBRUM   a hippocampal rudiment, consisting of a poorly developed strand of cells anterior to the lamina terminalis. Posteriorly it is continuous with the indusium griseum above and the septohippo-campal nucleus below the corpus callosum. Anteriorly it is sometimes continuous with cells of the anterior olfactory nucleus at the base of the olfactory stalk.

co´nus medullar´is [NA], CORD   caudal, tapering part of the spinal cord, comprising the lower sacral and coccygeal cord segments (S3-Coc1). Lesions of this region are characterized by impairment of bladder and bowel control, weakness or paralysis of the lower limb muscles, and sensory abnormalities. *Syn:* conus terminalis.

conus termina´lis, CORD   *See* conus medullaris.

convolu´tion, CEREBRUM, [L. *con* together; *volere* to roll]   elevation or ridge on the surface of the cerebral hemisphere, separated from other such elevations by a cerebral sulcus. *Syn:* gyrus.

convolution, abrupt, CEREBRUM   *See* cuneus.

convolution, anterior ascending, CEREBRUM   old term for the precentral gyrus.

convolution, callo´sal, CEREBRUM   *See* gyrus, cingulate.

convolution, fron´tal, ascending, CEREBRUM   old term for the precentral gyrus.

convolution, frontal, first, CEREBRUM   old term for the superior frontal gyrus.

convolution, frontal, second, CEREBRUM   old term for the middle frontal gyrus.

convolution, frontal, third, CEREBRUM   old term for the inferior frontal gyrus.

convolution, pari´etal, ascending, CEREBRUM   old term for the postcentral gyrus.

convolution, posterior ascending, CEREBRUM   old term for the postcentral gyrus.

convolution, subtem´poral, CEREBRUM   old term for the inferior temporal gyrus.

convolution, superfron´tal, CEREBRUM   old term for the superior frontal gyrus.

convolution, transisthmian /tranz-is´mĭ-an/, CEREBRUM   *See* isthmus (of the) gyrus, cingulate.

cop´ula, CEREBRUM, [L. a bond, tie]   *See* lamina rostralis.

cord, spinal [medulla spinalis, NA]   elongated, thick-walled, tubular subdivision of the CNS contained within the vertebral canal. *Syn:* myelon.

cordot´omy   surgical procedure in which a tract of the spinal cord is severed, usually the lateral spinothalamic tract in the anterior part of the lateral funiculus, for the relief of intractable pain.

Cormack, Allan MacLeod (b. 1924)   physicist, born in South Africa, later active in the United States. His studies were the basis for the imaging technique now used in computerized axial tomography (CAT). In 1979 he and G.N. Hounsfield were awarded the Nobel Prize for their contribution of this non-invasive technique for the study of the brain.

cor´nea [NA], EYE   transparent, avascular, anterior segment of the eyeball, about 0.5 mm in thickness. Its five layers, from anterior to posterior are:

anterior epithelium   layer of stratified squamous epithelium that rests on a smooth base without papillae.

anterior limiting membrane [lamina limitans anterior, NA]   thin layer, about 30 μm thick, essentially an outer part of the substantia propria but lacking cells. If destroyed it will not regenerate. *Syn:* Bowman's membrane; anterior elastic lamina.

substan´tia pro´pria [NA]   layer forming 90% of the cornea, the stroma, consisting mostly of collagenous fibers interspersed with flattened, modified fibroblasts.

posterior limiting membrane [lamina limitans posterior, NA]   thin layer, about 10 μm thick, a homogeneous membrane easily separated from both the substantia propria and the endothelium. After injury it can regenerate. *Syn:* posterior elastic membrane; Descemet's membrane; formerly also called Duddell's membrane or membrane of Demours.

endothelium   single layer of large squamous cells, a thinner layer than the adjacent posterior limiting membrane.

cor´nu [L. horn]   *See also* horn.

cornu ammo´nis, CEREBRUM, [L. horn of Ammon]   subdivision of the hippocampal formation usually regarded as a folded 3-layered cortex: a polymorphic layer next to the alveus on the ventricular surface, a layer of pyramidal cells, and a superficial, molecular layer apposed to the surface of the dentate gyrus in the depths of the hippocampal sulcus. Cajal ('11) subdivided this region into seven layers, from the ventricular surface to what was originally the external surface (Fig. C-7), as follows:

epen´dyma   ventricular layer.

al´veus   layer of myelinated fibers which continue into the fimbria.

strat´um or´iens   corresponds to the polymorph layer of the 3-layered subdivision. It includes cells of various shapes which distribute to other layers of the cornu ammonis. Some inhibitory basket cells of this layer have processes which end in the molecular layer.

stratum pyramidal´e   most conspicuous layer of the cornu ammonis, consisting of Ammon's pyramids or double pyramids. Axons of these cells enter the alveus. Their basal dendrites spread out in the same layer or in the stratum oriens and the alveus and their apical dendrites enter the more superficial layers, especially the stratum moleculare.

stratum radia´tum   often included as a part of the stratum pyramidale, it consists largely of the apical dendrites of the double pyramids interlacing in the radiating patterns for which the layer is named. Among the fibers are some association neurons and a few pyramidal cells.

stratum lacuno´sum   rich plexus of fibers, from the alveus and various cornu ammonis layers. Among the fibers are scattered cells, thought to be associative neurons.

stratum molecula´re   layer containing mainly dendrites of the double pyramids but also processes from cells in other layers of the cornu ammonis, including Schaffer collaterals, and axons from the alveus. The strata lacunosum and medullare correspond to the molecular layer of the 3-layered subdivision.

The cross-sectional area of the cornu ammonis was also secondarily subdivided into special fields CA1-CA4 by Lorente de Nó ('34), and H1-H5 by Rose ('27). *Syn:* hippocampus major; limbus corticalis. *See also* hippocampus.

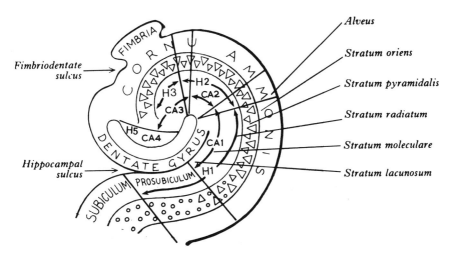

Fig C-7. Diagram to show the subdivisions of the hippocampus, the layers (strata) of the cornu ammonis, and its subdivisions into the C1-C4 fields of Lorente de Nó and the H1-H5 fields of Rose. From P.L. Williams and R. Warwick, *Functional Neuroanatomy of Man,* 1975. Courtesy of Churchill Livingstone, Publishers, Edinburgh.

cornuco´pia   tuft of choroid plexus that extends through the lateral aperture on each side of the fourth ventricle into the subarachnoid space. *Syn:* flower basket of Bochdalek.

coro´na [Gr. *korone* crown]   *See also* crown.

corona radia´ta [NA], CEREBRUM   fibers of the cerebral white matter which emerge from the internal capsule and fan out as they approach the cerebral cortex.

cor´pora   plural of *corpus*.

corpora albican´tia, HYPOTHALAMUS   old term for the mamillary bodies.

corpora quadrigem´ina, MIDBRAIN   the four protuberances on the dorsal surface of the midbrain; the superior and inferior colliculi. *See also* tectum.

cor´pus [*pl.* corpora] [L. body]   *See also* body; corpora.

corpus amygdaloi´deum [NA], CEREBRUM   *See* amygdala.

corpus arena´ceum [NA], EPITHALAMUS   *See* acervulus cerebri; brain sand.

corpus callo´sum [NA], CEREBRUM, [L. *callosus* hard]   thick band of commissural fibers, named by Galen. It mainly interconnects corresponding areas of the neopallial cortex but does contain some projection fibers. It consists of the following parts:

> **ros´trum** [rostrum corporis callosi, NA] [L. *rostrum* beak]   part of the corpus callosum between the genu and the lamina rostralis.

> **genu** [genu corporis callosi, NA] [L. *genu* knee]   most anterior part of the corpus callosum.

> **body** [truncus corporis callosi, NA] [L. *truncus* stem, trunk]   the large middle part of the corpus callosum between the genu and the splenium.

> **sple´nium** [splenium corporis callosi, NA] [Gr. *splenion* bandage]   the thick, posterior part of the corpus callosum.

corpus cerebel´li [NA], CEREBELLUM   that part of the cerebellum which develops from the cerebellar plates and not from the rhombic lips. It consists of all the cerebellum except the flocculonodular lobe.

corpus medullare /med-u-lar´l/ [NA], CEREBELLUM   deep mass of white matter in the cerebellum.

corpus neuroni [NA]   *See* body, cell.

corpus restiforme   *See* body, restiform.

corpus stria´tum [NA], CEREBRUM, [L. *striatus* striped]   collective term for the caudate nucleus, putamen, and globus pallidus. *See also* striatum *and* ganglia, basal.

cor´puscle, Pacinian [corpusculum lamellosum, NA]   *See* Pacini.

corpuscle, tactile [corpusculum tactus, NA]   peanut-shaped nerve ending, for fine tactile sensibility, located in the dermal papillae. These endings have a thin capsule, stacked, flattened connective tissue cells, and usually at least two myelinated nerve fibers. They are most numerous in the finger and toe tips, palm and sole, lips, and tongue tip. *Syn:* Meissner's tactile corpuscle.

corpus´culum chromati´ni sexual´is [NA]   *See* satellite, nucleolar.

corpusculum lamellosum [NA]   *See* Pacini for the corpuscles of Vater-Pacini.

cortec´tomy   removal of the cortex of a cerebral hemisphere.

cortex /kor´teks/ [*pl.* cortices /kor´tĭ-sēs/; *adj.* cortical] [L. outer layer, bark]   outer layer of gray matter on the surface of the cerebral hemispheres and of the cerebellum. It consists of a laminated mantle of nerve cells and fine, mostly nonmyelinated, nerve fibers and including, most superficially, a synaptic (molecular) layer, composed largely of axonic and dendritic terminals. *See also* area; cortex, cerebral; cortex, cerebellar.

cortex, agranular /a-gran´u-lar/, CEREBRUM   neopallial cortex in which the granular layers are reduced, e.g., motor cortex.

cortex, association (general), CEREBRUM   cerebral cortex which is specifically neither sensory nor motor in function but appears to be concerned with thinking, the processing of information, and the most complex of cortical functioning.

cortex, association, sensory, CEREBRUM   *See* cortex, secondary sensory.

cortex, aud´itory, CEREBRUM   cortex of the transverse temporal gyri on the opercular surface of the temporal lobe. Area 41 is primary auditory cortex and area 42 is secondary auditory cortex.

cortex, cal´carine, CEREBRUM   cortex adjoining the calcarine sulcus in the occipital lobe (Brodmann's area 17); visual cortex.

cortex, cerebel´lar [cortex cerebelli, NA], CEREBELLUM   superficial mantle of gray matter of the cerebellum. The layers of the cerebellar cortex (Figs. C-8, C-9) are as follows:

> **molec´ular (plex´iform) layer** [stratum moleculare (plexiforme), NA]   most superficial layer. It is a synaptic layer containing the dendrites of Purkinje cells, climbing and parallel fibers, basket cells, and certain other cells and fibers.

> **Purkinje cell layer** [stratum neuronorum piriformium, NA]   layer of large cell bodies arranged singly between the molecular and granular layers of the cerebellar cortex.

> **gran´ular layer** [stratum granulosum, NA]   innermost layer of the cerebellar cortex, composed largely of the closely packed granule cells and related fibers. *See also* glomerulus, cerebellar; island, cerebellar; *and* cells, stellate, *def.* 2.

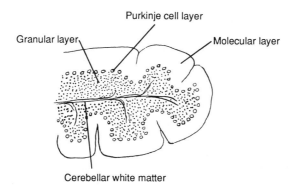

Fig. C-8.   Diagram to show the layers of the cerebellar cortex.

cortex, cer´ebral [cortex cerebri, NA]   superficial mantle of gray matter of the cerebral hemispheres. *See also* Brodmann *and* Fig. B-1. According to the cytoarchitectonic patterns established by Brodmann, Campbell, and Cajal and the myeloarchitectonic pattern of the Vogts, the layers of the neopallial cerebral cortex (Fig. C-10) are as follows:

> **molec´ular (plex´iform) layer, layer I** [lamina molecularis or plexiformis (stratum moleculare or plexiforme), NA]   most superficial layer of the cerebral cortex, a synaptic zone that includes the terminal portions of the apical dendrites of pyramidal cells, the axons of granule cells, and the horizontal cells of Cajal. *Syn:* zonal layer; lamina tangentialis (Vogt).

> **external gran´ular layer, layer II** [lamina granularis externa (stratum granulare

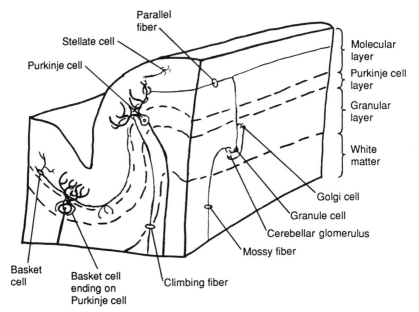

Fig. C-9.   Diagram to show the major connections within the cerebellar cortex. The mossy fibers, parallel fibers, and climbing fibers are excitatory; the axons of the basket cells, Golgi cells, stellate cells, and Purkinje cells are inhibitory.

externum), NA]   layer of small pyramidal cells and many small stellate cells, and containing the stripe of Kaes. This layer appears to be concerned mainly with intracortical connections and to receive its input from other cortical regions. *Syn:* lamina dysfibrosa (Vogt).

external pyram´idal layer, layer III [lamina pyramidalis externa (stratum neuronorum pyramidalium externum), NA]   layer of medium-sized and large pyramidal cells and some small stellate cells. This layer appears to be concerned mainly with intracortical connections and to send its efferent fibers to other cortical regions. *Syn:* lamina suprastriata (Vogt). Layers I, II, and III constitute the supragranular layers.

internal granular layer, layer IV [lamina granularis interna, NA]   layer mainly of small stellate or granule cells and containing the outer stripe of Baillarger. Afferent fibers from subcortical regions end largely in this layer. In the visual cortex, area 17, this layer contains the macroscopic stripe of Gennari. *Syn:* stria Baillarger externa (Vogt).

internal pyramidal (ganglionic) layer, layer V [lamina pyramidalis interna (ganglionaris), NA]   layer of large and medium-sized pyramidal cells with intermingled stellate cells, and, in the motor area, giant pyramidal (Betz) cells. The inner stripe of Baillarger runs through this layer.   Efferent fibers to subcortical regions arise largely from this layer. *Syn:* stratum neuronorum pyramidalium internum; lamina interstriata superficialis and stria Baillarger interna (Vogt).

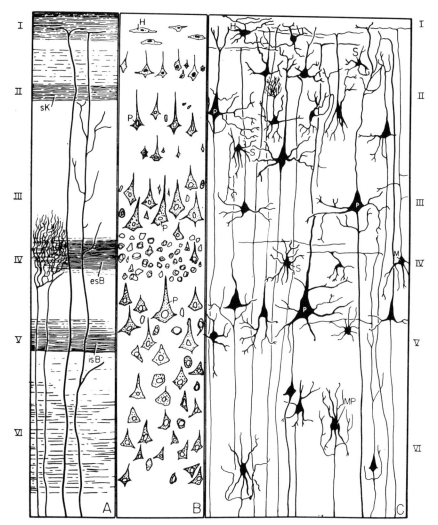

Fig. C-10. Drawing to illustrate the characteristic cell and fiber layers of the six-layered neopallial cortex. A. fiber stain, with (sK) the stripe of Kaes, and the outer (esB) and inner (isB) stripes of Baillarger. B. cell stain. C. Golgi silver stain with H-horizontal, M-Martinotti, MP-modified pyramidal, P-pyramidal, and S-stellate cells. I-molecular layer, II-external granular layer, III-external pyramidal layer, IV-internal granular layer, V-internal pyramidal layer, VI-multiform layer. From E.C. Crosby, T. Humphrey, and E. Lauer, *Correlative Anatomy of the Nervous System,* Copyright (c) 1962, Macmillan Publishing Company. Reprinted with permission of Macmillan Publishing Company.

multiform layer, layer VI [lamina multiformis (stratum neuronorum fusiformium), NA]   layer containing cells of different shapes, including many fusiform and modified pyramidal cells. From this layer fibers enter the white matter for various destinations, including subcortical nuclei projecting to the same cortical area. *Syn:* lamina infrastriata (Vogt). Cajal divided this innermost layer into two layers, a layer of medium-sized pyramidal and triangular cells and a layer of fusiform cells, his layer VII. Layers V and VI constitute the infragranular layers.

cortex, entorhi´nal, CEREBRUM   *See* area, entorhinal.

cortex, eulam´inate, CEREBRUM   *See* cortex, homotypic.

cortex, gran´ular, CEREBRUM   neopallial cortex in which the granular layers predominate and the pyramidal cell layers are reduced, as in the sensory cortex of the parietal lobe and the prefrontal regions of the frontal lobes.

cortex, heterogenet´ic, CEREBRUM   allocortex, the cortex of the archipallium and paleopallium. Brodmann included additional areas of the rhinencephalon and subdivided this cortex into: cortex primativus, cortex rudimentarius, and cortex striatus.

cortex, heterotyp´ic, CEREBRUM   neopallial cortex in which the six layers are obscure, e.g., motor cortex.

cortex, homogenet´ic, CEREBRUM   six-layered cortex of the neopallium. *Syn:* isocortex; neocortex.

cortex, homotyp´ic, CEREBRUM   neopallial cortex in which the six layers are clearly evident, e.g., sensory cortex. *Syn:* eulaminate cortex.

cortex, limitro´phic, CEREBRUM   *See* cortex, transitional.

cortex, motor, CEREBRUM   Brodmann's area 4 (Fig. B-1), in the precentral gyrus and the anterior part of the paracentral lobule, containing giant pyramidal cells, and concerned with skilled voluntary movements.

cortex, perirhi´nal, CEREBRUM   Brodmann's area 28 (Fig. B-1), along the rhinal fissure, a transitional area between the entorhinal cortex of the parahippocampal gyrus and the adjoining neopallial cortex. Brodmann considered it a part of his cortex striata subdivision of heterogenetic cortex.

cortex, prefron´tal, CEREBRUM   cortex in the anterior part of the frontal lobe. It is the general association (non-motor) area of the frontal lobe.

cortex, premo´tor, CEREBRUM   Brodmann's area 6 (Fig. B-1), in the frontal lobe, anterior to the motor cortex. It contributes fibers to the pyramidal tract and to the corticostriate and other systems.

cortex, preoccip´ital, CEREBRUM   *See* area, peristriate.

cortex, primary sensory, CEREBRUM   any area of the cerebral cortex which receives the thalamocortical fibers of a sensory system and is a part of the sensory perception system for that modality.

cortex primativ´us, CEREBRUM   division of Brodmann's heterogenetic cortex, consisting of olfactory bulb, anterior perforated substance, and amygdaloid nucleus, and which he considered as showing no layering.

cortex, projec´tion, CEREBRUM   cerebral cortex which receives fibers from, or sends fibers to, subcortical regions.

cortex, prorhi´nal, CEREBRUM   the lateral part of the entorhinal area.

cortex rudimentar´ius, CEREBRUM   division of Brodmann's heterogenetic cortex, consisting of the dentate gyrus, cornu ammonis, subiculum, indusium griseum, and septum pellucidum, and which he considered as having only incipient layering.

cortex (area), secondary sensory, CEREBRUM   cortical area adjacent to a primary sensory area, especially that next to the postcentral gyrus, and involved in processing information relayed to it from the adjoining sensory area.

cortex, somesthet´ic, CEREBRUM   Brodmann's areas 3, 1, and 2 (Fig. B-1), sensory cortex in the postcentral gyrus, concerned with the perception of discriminatory pain, touch, and kinesthetic sensibility.

cortex, stri´ate, CEREBRUM   occipital lobe cortex (Brodmann's area 17, Fig. B-1) containing in layer IV the macroscopic stripe of Gennari. These fibers are the terminal portions of the optic fibers which end in this region. *Syn:* area striata; visual cortex; calcarine cortex. *See also* cortex, visual.

cortex stria´tus, CEREBRUM   division of Brodmann's heterogenetic cortex, consisting of the cortex of the entorhinal (Brodmann's area 28), perirhinal (Brodmann's area 35), prepiriform, presubicular (Brodmann's area 27), and retrosubicular (Brodmann's area 48) areas.

cortex, transitional, CEREBRUM   cortex in a region where one type borders on another. *Syn:* limitrophic cortex; mesocortex.

cortex, visual, CEREBRUM   occipital lobe cortex adjoining the calcarine fissure and concerned with the perception of visual stimuli (Brodmann's area 17, Fig. B-1). *Syn:* striate cortex; calcarine cortex; area striata.

cortex, visual association, CEREBRUM   cortical area 18 (also called parastriate area) adjacent to area 17 in the occipital lobe, and area 19 (also called peristriate area) next to area 18 in the adjoining parietal and temporal lobes. These areas lack the stripe of Gennari. They are concerned with visual memory and the significance of the remembered images, also with optokinetic (following) eye movements. Area 18 also plays a part in color vision.

Corti, Marchese Alfonso (1822-1888)   Italian histologist born in Sardinia, active in Germany. He was noted for his investigations of the mammalian cochlea, published in 1851. The *organ of Corti* is the spiral organ of the cochlea, the end organ for hearing. Several other cochlear structures have also been named for him, including the *tunnel of Corti* (inner tunnel) and the *ganglion of Corti* (the spiral ganglion).

cortices   plural of *cortex.*

corticifugal /kor-tĭ-sif´u-gal/   carrying impulses away from the cerebral cortex.

corticipetal /kor-tĭ-sip´et-al/   carrying impulses toward the cerebral cortex.

corticopontocerebel´lar   pertaining to a two-neuron chain (corticopontine and pontocerebellar tracts) by which the cerebral cortex of one side is able to modify the functioning of the cerebellum, mainly of the other side. The pontine gray, where the synapses of this system are located, is one region where transneuronal degeneration occurs after destruction of the primary neurons.

Cotugno (Cotunnius), Domenico Felice Antonio (1736-1822)   Italian anatomist, professor of anatomy at Naples, noted for his studies of the ear, including a description of the labyrinthine system and its fluids (1761). He also published the first description of the cerebrospinal fluid (1764). Named for him were the *aqueduct of Cotunnius* (the vestibular aqueduct), the *liquor cotunnii* (perilymph), and the *nerve of Cotunnius* (the nasopalatine nerve).

crest   *See also* crista.

crest, ganglion´ic   *See* crest, neural.

crest, neural [crista neuralis, NA]   cells of ectodermal origin, adjacent to the dorsal part of the neural tube, which become segmentally clustered. From the crest develop the sensory and autonomic ganglion cells, the leptomeninges, the satellite and (at least in part) the sheath cells of PNS neurons, as well as cells of the adrenal medulla and of the paraganglia. Also derived from neural crest are certain amine precursor uptake and decarboxylation (APUD) cells, including: C-cells of the thyroid gland and of the ultimobranchial body, certain cells of the carotid body, pigment cells, and small intensely fluorescent (SIF) cells regarded as interneurons (Pearse, '77). Also thought to be of neural crest origin is the head mesenchyme from which develop the cranial dura mater and certain other connective tissues, some head muscles, and most of the cartilage and bones of the head. There is also some evidence that the islet cells of the pancreas may be of neural crest origin and perhaps even some pituitary cells. *For a review of this subject, see* Johnston *et al.* ('73).

crest, supraoptic /soo-prah-op´tik/, CEREBRUM   ventricular organ of the lamina terminalis.

Creutzfeldt, Hans-Gerhard (1885-1964)   distinguished German neuropathologist and neuropsychiatrist. *Creutzfeldt-Jakob disease,* which both he (1920) and A. Jakob (1921) described, is a degenerative disease of the CNS inherited as an autosomal dominant, or which may be caused by a transmissible virus. It appears to be related to kuru and to two animal diseases, scrapie and transmissible mink encephalopathy (TME). It is characterized by spongiform encephalopathy. There is rapidly progressive dementia and some motor disability, such as myoclonus, as well as pyramidal, extrapyramidal, and cerebellar signs. It is usually fatal within a few months or a few years.

cris´ta [L. crest]   *See also* crest.

crista acus´tica, EAR   *See* crista ampullaris.

cristae al´vei, CEREBRUM   projections of the alveus of the hippocampus into the digitations of the dentate gyrus.

crista ampullar´is [NA], EAR   ridge which projects into the lumen of each membranous ampulla at right angles to the plane of the semicircular duct and which constitutes a sensory end organ for kinetic equilibrium. *Syn:* crista acustica.

crista gal´li [NA] [L. *gallus* cock, hence cock's comb]   bony ridge projecting into the cranial cavity from the ethmoid bone. It lies between the two olfactory bulbs.

crook, shepherd's, MIDBRAIN   axon which arises from the dendrite of a nerve cell in the superior colliculus and forms a loop before entering the stratum album profundum to leave the superior colliculus.

Crosby, Elizabeth Caroline (1888-1983)   American neuroanatomist of the University of Michigan for many years, later also at the University of Alabama, noted for her expertise in correlating lesions in the CNS with the clinical neurologic syndromes which they cause. She was also pre-eminent in the field of comparative neuroanatomy, and beloved as a teacher.

cross section   *See* section, cross.

crown   *See also* corona.

crown, ciliary /sil´T-ar-T/ [corona ciliaris, NA], EYE   sum of the ciliary processes on the posterior surface of the ciliary body.

cru´ra   plural of *crus.*

crus [L. *crus* leg]   *See also* brachium; peduncle.

crus cer´ebri [NA], MIDBRAIN   ventral part of the cerebral peduncle, consisting of a cellular portion, the substantia nigra, dorsally, and a fibrous portion, the pes pedunculi, ventrally. Sometimes this term is used for just the pes pedunculi. *Syn:* basis pedunculi. *See also* peduncle, cerebral.

crus, common [crus membranaceum commune, NA], EAR   channel of the membranous labyrinth, by which the superior and posterior semicircular ducts communicate with the utricle.

crus for´nicis [NA], cerebrum   *See* fornix, crus.

Cruveilhier, Jean (1791-1874)   French physician, anatomist and pathologist of Paris. *Cruveilhier's nerve* is the vertebral nerve. *Cruveilhier's plexus* is the posterior cervical plexus, formed by the dorsal rami of the first three cervical spinal nerves.

CSF   cerebrospinal fluid.

CT   computed tomography. *See* tomography.

cul´men [NA], cerebellum   subdivision of the anterior lobe of the cerebellar vermis between the central lobule and the declive (Figs. C-2, V-6). *See* vermis cerebelli.

cu´neus [NA], cerebrum, [L. wedge]   wedge-shaped segment of the occipital lobe on the medial surface of the cerebrum between the calcarine and parieto-occipital sulci (Fig. C-3B). *Syn:* abrupt convolution.

cu´pula [NA], ear   dome- or cup-shaped structure surmounting the crista ampullaris in each membranous ampulla, into which the hairs from the crista project.

Cushing, Harvey Williams (1869-1939)   pioneer American neurosurgeon of Johns Hopkins, Harvard, and Yale Universities, whose contributions covered many neurological areas, including pituitary gland function and brain tumors of various kinds. *Cushing's loop* is the temporal loop of the optic radiation, more often called Meyer's loop. *See* Fulton ('46) for Cushing's biography.

cybernetics /si-ber-net´iks/ [*n. pl.* but used as a *sing.*] [Gr. *kybernetes* helmsman]   comparative study of electronic calculators and the human nervous system, for the purpose of increasing the knowledge of the functioning of the brain.

cyclopia /si-klo´pī-ah/ [Gr. *kyklos* circle; *ops* eye]   developmental defect named for a mythical race of one-eyed giants. There is only one median orbit in which the eyeball may be normal, double, malformed, or absent. The nose, if present, is located above the orbit.

Cyon, Elie de (1843-1912)   Russian physiologist. The *nerve of Cyon* is the aortic depressor nerve, derived from the superior laryngeal nerve, a branch of the vagus nerve.

cytoarchitecton´ics [*adj.* **cytoarchitectonic**]   cytoarchitecture.

cytoar´chitecture   architecture of the CNS according to the pattern of its cells.

cy´ton (cytone)   *See* body, cell.

d

DA dopamine.

Dandy, Walter Edward (1886-1946) pioneer American neurosurgeon, a skillful and innovative surgeon who devised many neurosurgical procedures, and introduced ventriculography and pneumoencephalography as diagnostic tools.

Darkschewitsch, Liverij Osipovich (1858-1925) Russian neurologist of St. Petersburg. The *nucleus of Darkschewitsch,* also called the ventral nucleus of the posterior commissure, is a small nucleus located in the ventrolateral part of the periaqueductal gray in the rostral part of the midbrain. Its main afferent connections are the lenticular fasciculus from the globus pallidus via connections in the nucleus of the field of Forel, and ascending fibers of the medial longitudinal fasciculus from the vestibular nuclei. Its efferent connections enter the medial longitudinal fasciculus for discharge to motor nuclei of the brain stem and perhaps the spinal cord (Fig. F-2). The *tract of Darkschewitsch,* considered by Darkschewitsch to pass from the optic tract to the habenula, then through the posterior commissure to the oculomotor nucleus for pupillary impulses, is doubtful. *Syn:* ventral nucleus of the posterior commissure.

dB or **db** decibel.

decerebration /de-ser-ĕ-bra´shun/ section of the brain stem low in the midbrain.

decibel (dB or **db)** /des´ĭ-bel/ smallest change of sound intensity detectable by the human ear.

declive /de-klīv´/ [NA], CEREBELLUM, [L. *declivis* sloping] most rostral segment of the vermis posterior lobe (Figs. C-2, V-6). *Syn:* clivus; declivus. *See* vermis cerebelli.

decomposition of movement motor disability in which movements normally carried out simultaneously are performed in succession. It occurs with lesions of a cerebellar hemisphere or superior cerebellar peduncle.

decortica´tion removal of all or part of the cerebral cortex.

decoupling, ciliary /de-kup´ling, sil´ĭ-ar-ĭ/ separation of the stereocilia of the outer hair cells of the spiral organ of the cochlea from the overlying tectorial membrane, with consequent auditory impairment.

decussa´tion [decussatio, NA] [L. *decussare* to intersect, from *decussis* ten, X] place where nerve fibers cross the median plane, or the nerve fibers which take part in the crossing. *See also* commissure.

decussation, fountain, MIDBRAIN   *See* decussation, tegmental, dorsal.

decussation, hypothalamic, anterior, HYPOTHALAMUS   old term for the dorsal supraoptic decussation.

decussation, hypothalamic, inferior, HYPOTHALAMUS   old term for either the ventral supraoptic decussation alone or the ventral supraoptic and intrachiasmatic decussations taken together.

decussation, hypothalamic, posterior, HYPOTHALAMUS   *See* decussation, supramamillary.

decussation, hypothalamic, superior, HYPOTHALAMUS   old term for the dorsal supraoptic decussation.

decussation, intrachiasmat´ic, HYPOTHALAMUS   place where fibers which cross the median plane within the optic chiasm in subprimates. It is the most ventral of the supraoptic decussations, and is said to connect the medial geniculate nuclei in some species. When the dorsal and ventral supraoptic decussations are considered subdivisions of the dorsal supraoptic commissure, this one is called the ventral supraoptic commissure or Gudden's commissure. It is also sometimes called the ventral division of the inferior hypothalamic decussation in the older literature.

decussation (of the) lemnisci, medial /lem-nis ´l/ [decussatio lemniscorum medialium, NA], MEDULLA   *See* decussation, sensory.

decussation, motor [decussatio motoria, NA], MAINLY MEDULLA   *See* decussation, pyramidal.

decussation, postmam´illary, HYPOTHALAMUS   *See* decussation, supramamillary.

decussation, pyram´idal (motor) [decussatio pyramidum (motoria), NA], MAINLY MEDULLA   decussation in the region of the medulla-spinal cord junction, where 70% to 90% of the pyramidal tract fibers cross the median plane from the pyramid to enter the lateral funiculus of the spinal cord as the lateral corticospinal tract. *See also* tract, corticonuclear *and* corticospinal.

decussation, sen´sory [decussatio sensoria (lemniscorum medialium), NA], MEDULLA   decussation in the closed medulla, rostral to the pyramidal decussation. The fibers arise from the nucleus gracilis and the nucleus cuneatus of each side, and after crossing the median plane, ascend in the medial lemnisci. They are secondary sensory fibers carrying impulses for sense of position, vibratory sensibility, and tactile discrimination to the ventral posterolateral nucleus of the dorsal thalamus. *Syn:* superior pyramidal decussation.

decussation (of the) superior cerebel´lar pe´duncles [decussatio pedunculorum cerebellarium superiorum (rostralium), NA], MIDBRAIN   decussation in the caudal part of the midbrain tegmentum. Most of the fibers belong to the dentorubral or dentothalamic tract. A lesion of this structure causes extreme hypotonicity and a marked bilateral cerebellar tremor. *Syn:* decussation of Werekinck.

decussation, superioer pyramidal, MEDULLA   old term for the sensory decussation.

decussation, suprachiasmatic /soo-prah-ki-az-mat´ik/, HYPOTHALAMUS   old term for the ventral supraoptic decussation.

decussation (commissure), supramam´illary, HYPOTHALAMUS   place where fibers which cross the median plane, dorsal to the mamillary bodies, at the junction of the hypothalamus and the midbrain tegmentum. It consists of fibers connecting various diencephalic and mesencephalic nuclei, including hypothalamotegmental bundles, connections between the two subthalamic nuclei, some fornix longus fibers from the anterior column of the fornix, and others. *Syn:* commissure of Forel; posterior hypothalamic decussation; postmamillary decussation.

decussation, supraop´tic, HYPOTHALAMUS   either of two fiber bundles, dorsal and ventral, which cross the median plane in the floor of the third ventricle dorsal to the optic chiasm and, in subprimates, also including the intrachiasmatic decussation. They are said to connect parts of the basal ganglia, diencephalon, and midbrain with parts of such areas on the contralateral side, but the precise terminations and functions of these fibers have not all been established. There are many overlapping synonyms for these bundles, including various supraoptic commissures and hypothalamic decussations. *For a discussion of this subject, see* Mettler ('48, pp. 357-359).

decussation, supraoptic, dorsal, HYPOTHALAMUS   most dorsal of the supraoptic decussations. From the midbrain, fibers ascend to a point medial to the globus pallidus and internal capsule, then arch over the fornix and cross the median plane in the floor of the third ventricle, to end in the contralateral globus pallidus. In addition to some mesencephalic connections, it may contain pallidohypothalamic fibers from the medial segment of the globus pallidus to the ventromedial nucleus of the hypothalamus, but the connections and functions have not been verified. *Syn:* commissure of Ganser; anterior (or superior) hypothalamic decussation (or commissure); commissure of the fibrae ansulatae; dorsal division of the dorsal supraoptic commissure. *See also* Meynert.

decussation, supraoptic, ventral, HYPOTHALAMUS   largest of the supraoptic decussations, on the dorsal surface of the optic chiasm and tracts. It presumably contains fibers which arise from the subthalamic nucleus, pass through the internal capsule, and end in the contralateral globus pallidus. Some fibers may extend into the midbrain but their exact connections have not been firmly established. *Syn:* formerly also called the ventral division of the dorsal supraoptic commissure. *See also* decussation, intrachiasmatic.

decussation, tegmen´tal [decussationes tegmenti, NA], MIDBRAIN   either of two decussations, ventral and dorsal, which cross the median plane in the rostral part of the mesencephalic tegmentum.

decussation, tegmental, dorsal (of Meynert), MIDBRAIN   fibers of the tectorubral, medial tectobulbar, and tectospinal tracts which cross the median plane in the dorsal part of the tegmentum at upper midbrain levels. *Syn:* fountain decussation.

decussation, tegmental, ventral, MIDBRAIN   decussation of the rubrospinal tracts in the upper midbrain tegmentum, ventromedial to the red nucleus. *Syn:* decussation of Forel; commissura ansulata.

decussation, trochlear /trok´le-ar/ [decussatio trochlearis (nervorum trochlearium), NA], MIDBRAIN, PONS   decussation of the trochlear nerve fibers in the anterior medullary velum, at the junction of the pons and midbrain.

degenera´tion, ascending   degeneration of axons and myelin sheaths of ascending tracts, progressing rostrally from the site of injury.

degeneration, descending   degeneration of axons and myelin sheaths of descending tracts, progressing caudally from the site of injury.

degeneration, ret´rograde   degeneration back toward the cell body of a neuron after injury to its axon.

degeneration, sec´ondary   complete degeneration of the axis cylinder, myelin sheath, and nerve endings of nerve fibers after injury to or separation from their cell bodies. *Syn:* Wallerian degeneration.

degeneration, transneuro´nal   degeneration of neurons after destruction of the neurons from which they receive their stimulation. *Syn:* transsynaptic degeneration.

degeneration, transsynap´tic   *See* degeneration, transneuronal.

Deiters, Otto Friedrich Carl (1834-1863)   German anatomist of Bonn, a pupil of Virchow's, noted for his studies of the ear and related parts of the nervous system. The *cells of Deiters* are the outer phalangeal cells of the spiral organ of the cochlea. The *nucleus of Deiters* (1865) is the lateral vestibular nucleus or the lateral and the inferior vestibular nuclei taken together. The (ventrolateral) vestibulospinal tract is sometimes called the *Deiterospinal tract* and the reticular formation, *Deiter's formation.*

Dejerine, Joseph Jules (1849-1917)   French neurologist, a pupil of Charcot's, and later professor of neurology and clinical chief at the Salpêtrière. Several neurologic disorders bear his name: *Landouzy-Dejerine dystrophy* is facio-scapulo-humeral muscular dystrophy; *see also* dystrophy, muscular. *Dejerine-Sottas disease* is hypertrophic interstitial neuritis; *Dejerine-Thomas atrophy* is olivopontocerebellar atrophy; *Dejerine-Klumpke paralysis* is paralysis of the hand muscles with a lower brachial plexus injury. The thalamic syndrome is also called *Dejerine-Roussy syndrome.* The *tract of Dejerine* is the ventral spinothalamic tract.

DeJong, Russell Nelson (1907-1990)   American neurologist of the University of Michigan. He served as president of the American Academy of Neurology and was a founding editor of *Neurology,* its official journal. Among other publications were his textbook, *The Neurologic Examination,* the last edition published in 1979, and *A History of American Neurology,* published in 1982.

Del Rio Hortega   *See* Hortega.

demarche de coq   high-stepping walk characteristic of certain cerebellar disorders.

dementia [L. *de* down, away; *mens* mind]   an acquired impairment of intellectual capacity that includes disorders of such functions as language, memory, visual-spatial ability, cognitive ability, and personality (Benson, '79).

dementia praecox [L. *praecox* precocious]   old term for schizophrenia.

Demours, Pierre (1702-1795)   French ophthalmologist. The *membrane of Demours* is the posterior limiting membrane of the cornea, also named for Descemet.

demyelina´tion   pathologic process whereby myelinated nerve fibers lose their myelin sheaths.

dendrax´on   single process of a unipolar neuron, which divides into two branches, one of which conducts impulses from the periphery toward the cell body and the other of which conducts centrally, toward the CNS.

den´drite [dendritum, NA], [Gr. *dendron* tree]   process of a neuron which conducts impulses to the cell body. Dendrites were so named by Golgi in the late 19th century. The large peripheral processes of some afferent neurons are histologically indistinguishable from the axons of motor neurons and are sometimes also called axons. *Syn:* dendron.

dendrite, a´pical, CEREBRUM   process extending from the apex of a cortical pyramidal cell toward the surface of the cerebral cortex.

dendrite, bas´ilar, CEREBRUM   process extending horizontally from the base of a pyramidal cell of the cerebral cortex.

den´dron   *See* dendrite.

den´tate [L. *dentatus* toothed]   having a scalloped edge. *For* dentate gyrus, ligament, *and* nucleus, *see the nouns.*

dentes acustici [NA], ᴇᴀʀ   *See* teeth, auditory (of Huschka).

depolariza´tion   sudden rise of sodium ions in a nerve fiber, changing the membrane potential from negative to positive during the initial phase of an action potential.

der´matome   cutaneous area innervated by the afferent fibers of a particular spinal nerve.

Descemet, Jean (1732-1810)   French physician, professor of anatomy and surgery at Paris. He described the posterior limiting membrane of the cornea *(Descemet's membrane)* in 1758, although it is said to have been described earlier by Duddell, an English oculist.

descen´dens cervical´is [ansa cervicalis, radix inferior, NA]   bundle of nerve fibers which arises from spinal cord segments C2 and C3. It joins the descendens hypoglossi to form the ansa cervicalis of the cervical plexus, branches of which supply certain muscles of the neck. *See also* plexus, cervical.

descendens hypoglos´si [ansa cervicalis, radix superior, NA]   bundle of nerve fibers not from the hypoglossal nerve as the name implies but from cervical spinal cord segment C1. It joins the descendens cervicalis to form the ansa cervicalis of the cervical plexus to supply certain muscles of the neck. *See also* plexus, cervical.

detachment, ret´inal   disorder in which the sensory layers of the retina are separated from the pigment layer. The term *detachment* is a misnomer because the separation occurs *within* the retina, between derivatives of the inner and outer layers of the embryonic optic cup and not between the retina and the choroid.

diagonal´is te´nia, ᴄᴇʀᴇʙʀᴜᴍ   *See* band, diagonal (of Broca).

Diamidino Yellow   trademark for a fluorescent tracer used to mark the nuclei of nerve cell bodies. *See also* tracer, fluorescent.

diaphragma sellae /di-ah-frag´mah sel´i/ [NA]   ring of dura mater around the pituitary stalk, separating the pituitary gland from the hypothalamus.

diastematomye´lia   abnormality in which the spinal cord is doubled. It is frequently associated with other spinal cord malformations.

diencephalon /di-en-sef´al-on/ [NA], ꜰᴏʀᴇʙʀᴀɪɴ, [Gr. *dia* or *di* through; *enkephalos* brain]   most caudal subdivision of the forebrain, derived from the prosencephalon. It consists of the dorsal thalamus and metathalamus, ventral thalamus, hypothalamus, and epithalamus. *Syn:* 'tweenbrain; interbrain.

dimyelia /di-mi-e´ll-ah/   abnormality in which there is a complete duplication of the spinal cord. Each cord has a complete set of roots. *See also* diplomyelia.

diplegia /di-ple´ji-ah/   paralysis of two corresponding limbs or both sides of the face.

diplomyelia /dip-lo-mi-e´ll-ah/   abnormality in which there is an accessory spinal cord lying either dorsal or ventral to the normal cord. The accessory cord lacks nerve roots. *See also* dimyelia.

diplo´pia   double vision.

disc   *See* disk.

disinhibition /dis-in-hib-ish´un/   inhibition of an inhibitory neuron.

disk, optic [discus nervi optici, NA], ᴇʏᴇ   pale circular area of the fundus of the eye where the optic nerve fibers leave the retina; the blind spot of the retina.

disk, tac´tile (Merkel's) [epithelioidocytus tactus, NA]   specialized intraepithelial nerve ending located mainly in the margins of the tongue. Such endings consist of small, cuplike nerve fiber terminations and the modified epithelial cells on which they end.

disynap´tic   having two synapses.

DLF   dorsal longitudinal fasciculus.

DMD   Duchenne's muscular dystrophy. *See* Duchenne.

doc´trine, neu´ron   tenet formulated in the last century (1886-1890) which holds that the nervous system is not a syncytial net but is composed of discrete units, neurons, which contact one another at what are now called synapses, but do not fuse with with one another. The concept, affirmed by Forel, His, Waldeyer, and others, was widely debated in the early years but clearly established by Cajal and is now universally accepted.

Dogiel, Alexander Stanislavovic (1852-1922)   Russian neurologist and histologist, noted for his studies of nerve endings, especially the terminal end bulbs.

do´pa [dihydroxyphenylalanine]   an intermediary compound in the catabolism of tyrosine. It is the precursor of dopamine and an intermediate product in the biosynthesis of norepinephrine, epinephrine, and melanin. L-dopa (levodopa), the biologically active form of this agent, is used in the treatment of Parkinson's disease.

do´pamine [DA, 3-hydroxytyramine]   a catecholamine formed during the metabolism of tyrosine. It is a precursor of norepinephrine and epinephrine and also an important neurotransmitter in its own right. It occurs in various parts of the CNS and PNS, including the retina, olfactory bulb, fibers arising from the hypothalamus and zona incerta, and a periventricular system, but is mainly known for its role as an inhibitory neurotransmitter synthesized by the large pigmented cells of the substantia nigra (pars compacta) and carried by fibers of the nigrostriate tract for release in the caudate nucleus and putamen. *See also* neurotransmitters.

dors´al   1. pertaining to the back.
2. sometimes used as a synonym for *thoracic*. This use of the term can be misleading if confused with *def.* 1.

Down, John Langdon Haydon (1828-1896)   English physician who devoted his career to the study and care of the mentally retarded. *Down's syndrome,* formerly called *mongolism,* is a genetically transmitted mental disorder. Most patients have a total of 47 chromosomes with trisomy of chromosome 21.

Doyère, Louis (1811-1863)   Russian physiologist and zoologist. *Doyère's eminence* or *hillock* is the slight elevation of muscle tissue at the termination of a motor neuron.

Duchenne (de Boulogne), Guillaume Benjamin Amand (1806-1875)   French neurologist noted for his studies of muscular disorders. *Duchenne's muscular* or *pseudomuscular dystrophy* (DMD) is a severe, progressive, childhood muscular disease, inherited almost always by boys, and carried on the X-chromosome. *Duchenne's paralysis* is a progressive bulbar paralysis, and *Duchenne-Erb paralysis* is an upper arm paralysis following injury of spinal nerve roots C5 and C6.

duct, coch´lear [ductus cochlearis, NA], ᴇᴀʀ   spiral tube of the membranous labyrinth, separated from the scala vestibuli by the vestibular membrane and from the scala tympani by the spiral membrane (basilar membrane and osseous spiral lamina). *Syn:* scala media.

duct, endolymphat´ic [ductus endolymphaticus, NA], ᴇᴀʀ   narrow channel in the vestibular aqueduct, between the utriculosaccular duct and the endolymphatic sac of the membranous labyrinth. *Syn:* otic duct.

duct, o´tic, EAR   *See* duct, endolymphatic.

duct, perilymphat´ic [ductus perilymphaticus, NA], EAR   *See* aqueduct, cochlear.

duct, perio´tic, EAR   *See* aqueduct, cochlear.

duct, sac´cular, EAR   narrow channel connecting the saccule and the endolymphatic duct.

duct, semicir´cular [ductus semicircularis, NA], EAR   any of three membranous tubes (superior, posterior, and lateral) contained within the semicircular canals of the bony labyrinth. Oriented at right angles to one another, they connect by five openings with the utricle of the membranous labyrinth.

duct, utricular /u-trik´u-lar/, EAR   narrow channel which connects the utricle and the endolymphatic duct.

duct, utric´ulosac´cular [ductus utriculosaccularis, NA], EAR   narrow channel which connects the utricle and saccule of the membranous labyrinth of the internal ear with the endolymphatic duct.

ductus reuniens /re-u´nĭ-enz/ [NA], EAR   short, small channel that connects the cochlear duct and the saccule of the membranous labyrinth.

Duddell, Benedict (18th century)   English oculist. *Duddell's membrane* is the posterior limiting membrane of the cornea, later described by and named for Descemet.

Duke-Elder, Sir William Stewart (1898-1978)   world-renowned Scottish ophthalmologist, later of London. Throughout his life he received numerous honors for his many accomplishments. His monumental *Textbook of Ophthalmology* was later expanded to a 15-volume *System of Ophthalmology.*

Duncan, Daniel (1649-1735)   French physician. *Duncan's ventricle* is the cavum septi pellucidi.

du´ra ma´ter [NA] [L. *dura* hard or strong; *mater* mother]   outermost and heaviest layer of the meninges covering the brain and spinal cord. *Syn:* pachymeninx. *See also* mater.

Duret, Henri (1849-1921)   French neurosurgeon. In Charcot's laboratory he studied the blood supply of the brain and the associated vascular pathology. *Duret's lesion* is a cerebral hemorrhage in the region of the fourth ventricle. *Duret's arteries* are the anterolateral central arteries of the cerebrum (Fig. C-5).

Dusser de Barenne, Joannes Gregorius (1885-1940)   Dutch neurophysiologist, active at Utrecht University and later at Yale University in the United States. He was noted for his studies of cortical function and for the use of strychnine as an investigative tool.

dust, ear, EAR   *See* statoconia.

dynor´phin [Gr. *dynamis* power + *morphine*]   an endorphin, an endogenous opioid peptide, occurring widely throughout both the CNS and the PNS. One form of this neurotransmitter, Dyn-A, has been found to have powerful analgesic properties (Goldstein, '87). *See also* neurotransmitters.

dysarth´ria [Gr. *dys* difficult or faulty; *arthroun* to articulate]   faulty articulation of consonant and vowel sounds.

dysdiadochokine´sia   *See* adiadochokinesia.

dyskine´sia [Gr. *dys-*; *kinesis* movement]   motor disability in which there are purposeless, involuntary movements.

dyslex´ia   [Gr. *dys-*; *lexis* diction] learning disability in children of normal intelligence, more frequently boys than girls. They have difficulty in learning to read and to spell and in mastering the interpretation of visual symbols.

dysme´tria [Gr. *dys-*; *metron* measure]   disorder in the control of the range of movement, characteristic of certain cerebellar lesions.

dyspha´gia [Gr. *dys-*; *phagein* to eat]   difficulty in swallowing.

dyspho´nia [Gr. *dys-*; *phone* voice]   impaired vocalization.

dysto´nia [Gr. *dys-*; *tonus* tension]   muscular disorder, a postural abnormality in which there is extreme and sustained contraction usually of the limb and trunk muscles. *Syn:* torsion spasm.

dystonia musculorum deformans   most severe form of dystonia.

dystrophy, muscular   any of several types of degenerative muscular disease, transmitted by inheritance, and affecting different muscle groups in different forms of the disease. *See also* Dejerine; Duchenne; Hoffmann; Landouzy; Werdnig.

e

ear dust, ᴇᴀʀ   statoconia.

ear, external [auris externa, NA], ᴇᴀʀ   the pinna (auricle) and the external acoustic meatus.

ear, internal [auris interna, NA], ᴇᴀʀ   fluid-filled part of the ear within the petrous bone, comprising a bony labyrinth (scala vestibuli and scala tympani of the cochlea, vestibule, and semicircular canals and related channels) and, suspended within it, the membranous labyrinth (cochlear duct, saccule and utricle, and semicircular ducts, and their connections). *Syn:* labyrinth.

ear, middle [auris media, NA], ᴇᴀʀ   irregular, air-filled chamber consisting of the tympanic antrum and cavity, mastoid air cells, and auditory tube. The tympanic cavity contains three ossicles (malleus, incus, and stapes), connected in series from the tympanic membrane to the oval window, as well as two muscles (tensor tympani and stapedius) and their associated nerves. It is also traversed by the chorda tympani. The auditory tube connects the tympanic cavity and the pharynx.

ecchondrosis physaliphora /ek-kon-dro´sis fiz-al-if´or-ah/   remnant of the rostral end of the notochord, from which an intracranial chordoma may arise.

Eccles, Sir John Carew (b. 1903)   Australian neurophysiologist. He, Sir Alan Lloyd Hodgkin, and Sir Andrew Huxley received the Nobel Prize in medicine and physiology in 1963 for their discoveries concerning the physiology of nervous impulses.

Economo, Constantin von (1876-1931)   neurologist, born in Romania, of Greek descent. He studied in Austria, France, and Germany then practiced in Vienna the rest of his life. *Von Economo's disease* (1917) is lethargic encephalitis.

ec´toderm [Gr. *ektos* outside; *derma* skin]   outer layer of the embryo from which the nervous system and certain other tissues develop.

Edinger, Ludwig (1855-1918)   German anatomist of Frankfurt-am-Main, a pioneer of modern comparative neuroanatomy. The *Edinger-Westphal nucleus* of the oculomotor nerve (1885) is the accessory oculomotor nucleus, the parasympathetic nucleus of the oculomotor nerve, the rostral part for pupillary constriction and the caudal part for accommodation of the lens for near vision (Figs. R-2, R-4; Table C-3). *Edinger's tract* is the lateral spinothalamic tract. The *predorsal bundle of Edinger* is the medial tectospinal tract.

EEG   electroencephalogram or electroencephalographic.

ef´ferent [L. *effere* to carry out from; from *ex* out from, *ferre* to carry]   conducting away. *See* neuron, efferent.

Ehrenritter, Johann (d. 1790)   Austrian anatomist. *Ehrenritter's ganglion* is the superior ganglion of the glossopharyngeal nerve.

Ehrlich, Paul (1854-1915)   neurohistologist, born in Silesia, later of Berlin, Germany. He introduced *intra vitam* staining of nervous tissue with methylene blue and was a pioneer in neurocytochemistry.

electroenceph´alogram (EEG) [*adj.* **electroencephalographic**]   recording of electrical impulses arising from the activity of neurons within the brain.

electroencephalog´raphy   procedure for the recording of electrical activity of neurons within the brain, by the use of electrodes attached to the scalp.

electromy´ogram (EMG)   recording of the electrical activity of motor units (action potentials) of skeletal muscles.

electromyog´raphy   procedure used to study the viability and functioning of skeletal muscle fibers, by the use of needle electrodes inserted into the muscle.

electroret´inogram (ERG)   recording of the sequence of electrical changes that occur when light strikes the retina.

Elliot Smith, Sir Grafton (1871-1937)   British neuroanatomist and ethnologist, born in Australia, later of London, also with many years in Cairo. His work, especially on the comparative morphology of cortical patterns and his analyses of anatomical specimens from the tombs of Egypt, brought him widespread recognition.

ellip´soid, EYE   highly refractile body containing mitochondria, located in the outer half of the inner segment of rods and cones.

EMG   electromyogram.

em´inence, ar´cuate [eminentia arcuata, NA], EAR   elevation on the surface of the petrous part of the temporal bone, overlying the anterior semicircular canal.

eminence, collat´eral [eminentia collateralis, NA], CEREBRUM   eminence on the medial wall of the posterior part of the inferior horn of the lateral ventricle, overlying the collateral sulcus.

eminence, medial [eminentia medialis, NA], PONS, MEDULLA   elevation on the floor of the fourth ventricle, on each side of the median plane, between the median sulcus and the sulcus limitans, and extending the length of the pons and open medulla (Fig. V-4). It includes the facial colliculus in the caudal part of the pons and the vagal and hypoglossal trigones in the medulla. *Syn:* funiculus teres; eminentia teres.

eminence, median, HYPOTHALAMUS   hypothalamic part of the neurohypophysis, a small funnel-shaped extension of the tuber cinereum on the ventral surface of the diencephalon, from which the infundibular stalk extends to the pars nervosa (Fig. N-4).

eminen´tia postre´ma, MEDULLA   old term for the area postrema.

eminentia ter´es, PONS, MEDULLA   medial eminence, particularly its caudal part comprising the facial colliculus and the rostral part of the hypoglossal trigone. *See also* nuclei, parahypoglossal.

eminentia trigem´ini, MEDULLA   *See* tubercle, trigeminal.

encephalocele /en-sef´al-o-sĕl/   abnormality in which the brain is herniated through an opening in the cranium.

enceph´alon [NA] [Gr. *enkephalos* brain; from *en* in, *kephale* head]   brain.

end brain   cerebrum; telencephalon.

end bulb (foot)   *See* bulb, terminal.

end plate, motor   *See* plate, motor end.

ending, an´ulospi´ral   a stretch receptor, the primary nerve ending around the central portion of the intrafusal fibers in a neuromuscular spindle (Fig. S-2).

ending, flower spray   a stretch receptor, the secondary nerve ending around the terminal portions of nuclear chain fibers in a neuromuscular spindle (Fig. S-2).

ending, nerve   specialized termination at the end of a nerve fiber, composed of a branching or otherwise modified axis cylinder and often including components of other tissues, such as connective tissue or muscle. *See also* corpuscle; spindle; plate, motor end.

endolymph /en´do-limf/ [endolympha, NA], ᴇᴀʀ, [Gr. *endon* within; *lympha* clear fluid] fluid secreted by the stria vascularis of the cochlear duct, which fills the cavities of the membranous labyrinth. *Syn:* otic fluid; Scarpa's fluid.

endoneurium /en-do-nu´rĭ-um/ [NA] [Gr. *endon-*; *neuron* nerve]   delicate, interstitial, mesodermal, connective tissue investment of individual nerve fibers within a nerve fascicle or ganglion. *Syn:* epilemma; sheath of Henle; sheath of Key and Retzius; Ruffini's subsidiary sheath.

endor´phin [from a contraction of *endogenous* and *morphine*]   any neurotransmitter which is an endogenous peptide with an opioid action, such as the enkephalins and dynorphin. *See also* neurotransmitters.

engram [Gr. *en* in; *gramma* mark]   a latent memory picture, the lasting trace left by a stimulus or experience.

enkeph´alin   an endorphin, either of two pentapeptides, met-enkephalin (with methionine in its formula) and leu-enkephalin (with leucine), which inhibit pain transmission. It occurs in periaqueductal gray, in Rexed's laminae I and II of the spinal cord, and in the subnucleus caudalis of the spinal nucleus of V. It may inhibit the release of substance P from presynaptic endings in these areas. Enkephalin-labeled cells also occur to some extent in other brain regions. *See also* neurotransmitters.

enlargement, cervical [intumescentia cervicalis, NA], ᴄᴏʀᴅ   enlarged portion of the spinal cord consisting of cord segments C5-T1, associated with the brachial plexus and the innervation of the upper extremities.

enlargement, lumbosacral [intumescentia lumbosacralis, NA], ᴄᴏʀᴅ   enlarged portion of the spinal cord, consisting of cord segments L2-S3, associated with the lumbosacral plexus and the innervation of the lower extremities.

ependyma /ep-en´dĭ-mah/ [NA] [*adj.* **ependymal**] [Gr. *epi* upon; *endyma* garment] cellular lining of the ventricular spaces of the CNS. In the embryo there are multiple layers of nuclei in the ependyma. The processes of these cells extend through the thickness of the neural tube. In the adult the ependyma is a single layer of cells and in most areas their processes do not reach the external surface. In both the embryo and the adult, in man as well as in subhuman forms, ependymal cells have cilia which appear to beat in the direction of the foramina of the fourth ventricle (Worthington and Cathcart, '63).

eph´ase   site of contact of two or more nerve cell processes but without the formation of a true synapse. The possibility that some form of neural transmission takes place at such places has been suggested.

epichoroid /ep-ĭ-kor´oid/, EYE, [Gr. *epi* upon]   suprachoroid layer of the choroid.

epico´nus, CORD   part of the spinal cord just rostral to the conus medullaris, and comprising, approximately, cord segments L4-S2.

epicrit´ic [Gr. *epikritikos* judgment or determination]   pertaining to fine intensity and spatial discriminatory ability or the cutaneous nerve fibers necessary for fine tactile and temperature discrimination.   Epicritic sensibility was named and described by Head in 1908.

epidu´ral   overlying or outside the dura mater.

epilem´ma [Gr. *epi-*; *lemma* husk]   endoneurium.

epilep´sy   neurologic disorder characterized by periodic episodes of motor, sensory, or psychic dysfunction.

epiloia /ep-ĭ-loi´ah/   *See* sclerosis, tuberous.

epineph´rine   a catecholamine, the chief neurohormone of the adrenal medulla, where it is derived from norepinephrine.   In the CNS it is formed in cells in the caudal part of the brain stem for release in the hypothalamus, spinal cord, and elsewhere.   *Syn:* adrenaline.   *See also* norepinephrine; neurotransmitters.

epineur´ium [NA]   loose connective tissue which binds together two or more fascicles of a peripheral nerve or which supports a ganglion.

epiph´ysis cer´ebri, EPITHALAMUS   *See* body, pineal.

epithal´amus [NA], DIENCEPHALON   dorsal, posterior part of the diencephalon, composed of the habenula and its fiber bundles, the pineal body, part of the posterior commissure, and the tela choroidea of the third ventricle.

epithe´lioidocy´tus tac´tus [NA]   *See* disk, tactile.

epithe´lium, cil´iary, EYE   two-layered cuboidal epithelium covering the ciliary body, including its processes.   It is derived from the optic cup and is continuous anteriorly with the posterior epithelium of the iris and posteriorly with the retina. The layer on its free surface secretes aqueous humor.   The deep layer is pigmented.   *Syn:* ciliary retina.

EPSP   excitatory postsynaptic potential.

Erb, Wilhelm Heinrich (1840-1921)   German neurologist.   He introduced the use of the reflex hammer and the testing of tendon reflexes as a part of the neurologic examination.   He was also responsible for the introduction of neurology as a part of the curriculum at Heidelberg.   *Erb's phenomenon* is increased electrical irritability of motor neurons in tetany.   *Duchenne-Erb paralysis* is an upper arm paralysis following a birth injury to the upper part of the brachial plexus (C5 and C6).

ERG   electroretinogram.

Erlanger, Joseph (1874-1965)   American neurophysiologist, noted for his skill in instrumentation and for his studies of autonomic function.   He and his former student, H. Gasser, received the Nobel Prize for medicine and physiology in 1944 for their discoveries of the highly differentiated functions of individual nerve fibers.

Euler, Ulf Svante von (b. 1905)   Swedish neurophysiologist, who discovered that the neurotransmitter at sympathetic postganglionic nerve endings is noradrenaline, and not adrenaline, and for which he, with J. Axelrod and B. Katz, received the Nobel Prize for physiology and medicine in 1970.

Eustachius, Bartolommeo (ca. 1510/1520-1574)   Italian physician and anatomist of Rome.   He discovered and described many structures, including parts of the ear. The *Eustachian tube* is the auditory tube.

exencephaly /eks-en-sef´ah-lī/   abnormality in which the brain projects through the cranial roof.

Exner, Siegmund (1846-1926)   Viennese physiologist. *Exner's writing center* is located in the posterior part of the middle frontal gyrus. *Exner's plexus* is a layer of nerve fibers in the outer part of the cerebral cortex (1881). *Exner's nerve* is the middle laryngeal nerve.

exteroception /eks-ter-o-sep´shun/ [*adj.* **exteroceptive**] [L. *exterus* outside; *capere* to take]   that class of impulses arising from sensory end organs at or near the surface of the body and which relate the individual to the outside world. The term was introduced by Sherrington about 1906. Exteroceptive nerve endings, exteroceptors, include cutaneous nerve endings for pain, temperature, and touch, the photoreceptors of the retina, and the spiral organ of the cochlea.

extinc´tion, sensory   failure to recognize or localize correctly a stimulus on one side when both sides are stimulated simultaneously. The side ignored is contralateral to a lesion in the appropriate sensory association area.

extor´sion   outward rotation of the eyeball, on its anatomical axis as in a trochlear nerve paralysis.

extra-ax´ial   outside the central nervous system.

extrafusal /eks-trah-fu´zal/   outside a muscle spindle, particularly pertaining to the muscle fibers supplied by the alpha motor neurons (Fig. L-1).

extramed´ullary   outside the central nervous system.

extrapyram´idal system   *See* system, extrapyramidal.

eye fields   portions of the cerebral cortex which, when stimulated, produce eye movements. *See* fields, eye, frontal *and* occipital, *also* fields, visual *and* retinal.

f

facial /fa´shal/   *For* facial colliculus, nerve, *and* nucleus, *see the nouns.*

facilita´tion [L. *facilitas*; from *facilis* easy]   process by which the excitability of a subliminally bombarded motor neuron is increased. The nerve cell membrane is partially depolarized by a subliminal stimulus, then a subsequent subliminal stimulus further depolarizes the membrane until it reaches the threshold of impulse initiation.

factors, releasing   hormones produced in the median eminence and tuberal region of the hypothalamus. They are released from nerve fibers into the hypophysial portal sinusoids for activation of anterior pituitary hormones. *See also* hormones, neurosecretory.

Falloppio (Fallopius), Gabrielle (1523-1562)   Italian anatomist, pupil of Vesalius, later professor at Padua. The *Fallopian canal* or *aqueduct* is the facial canal in the temporal bone.

falx cerebel´li /falks/ [NA] [L. *falx* sickle]   narrow, sickle-shaped dural fold between the two cerebellar hemispheres.

falx cer´ebri [NA]   sickle-shaped dural fold located in the longitudinal fissure, between the two cerebral hemispheres (Fig. F-1).

Fañanás, J.   Spanish physician. *Fañanás cells* are neuroglial cells, also called feather cells, in the molecular layer of the cerebellar cortex.

Farabeuf, Louis Hubert (1841-1910)   surgeon of Paris. *Farabeuf's triangle* is the triangular space outlined by the internal jugular vein, the common facial vein, and the hypoglossal nerve.

fascia bulbi /fash´yah bul´bī/, EYE, [L. *fascia* ribbon or band]   thin, fibrous membrane that encloses the eyeball. It is firmly attached to the eyeball anteriorly near the margin of the cornea and posteriorly at the optic nerve and by fine trabeculae to the sclera. It is pierced by the extraocular muscles and by various small blood vessels and nerves. *Syn:* capsule of Tenon.

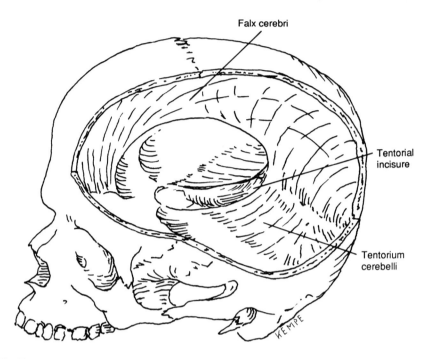

Falx cerebri

Tentorial incisure

Tentorium cerebelli

KEMPE

Fig F-1.   The dural folds within the cranial cavity.   Drawing courtesy of Dr. L.G. Kempe.

fascia dentata /den-tah´tah/ (dentate fascia), CEREBRUM   the dentate gyrus. Sometimes this term is limited to the molecular and granular layers of the dentate gyrus.

fascicula´tion   spontaneous discharges of a motor unit (amplitude of 2 to 6 mV and duration of 5 to 8 milliseconds), indicative of dysfunction of a lower motor neuron. All the muscle fibers of the motor unit contract and the contraction is visible through the skin. *See also* fibrillation.

fascic´ulus [*pl.* **fasciculi**] [L. dim. of *fascis* bundle]   a small bundle of nerve fibers. In the PNS a fascicle is one of the constituent parts of a nerve and is enclosed by perineurium. In the CNS *fasciculus* is sometimes used as a synonym for tract but often refers to a bundle of nerve fibers with diverse origins and terminations, such as the medial longitudinal fasciculus. *See also* tract; bundle; column; fibers.

fasciculus, anterolateral, CORD   ascending fibers in the ventral and lateral funiculi of the spinal cord, concerned with the transmission of pain, temperature, and general (nondiscriminatory) tactile sensibility, and comprising the lateral and ventral spinothalamic tracts. *Syn:* spinal lemniscus.

fasciculus, anterolateral, superficial, CORD   *See* tract, spinocerebellar, ventral.

fasciculus, anulo-ol´ivary, BRAIN STEM   *See* tract, central tegmental.

fasciculus, ar´cuate, CEREBRUM   *See* fasciculus, longitudinal, superior.

fasciculus arcuatocerebellar MEDULLA   *See* striae medullares (of the fourth ventricle).

fasciculus cuneatus /ku-ne-a´tus/ [NA], MEDULLA, CORD [L. *cuneus* wedge]   tract in the lateral part of the posterior funiculus of the cervical (Fig. B-2) and thoracic spinal cord, and in the closed medulla. These fibers, with cell bodies in dorsal root ganglia, conduct impulses from tactile and proprioceptive endings (Fig. T-3) in the upper half of the body primarily to the cuneate and accessory cuneate nuclei of the medulla, but also to the nucleus proprius of the spinal cord. *Syn:* Burdach's tract; funiculus cuneatus. *See also* fasciculus, interfascicular.

fasciculus, dorsal longitudinal, BRAIN STEM   *See* fasciculus, longitudinal, dorsal.

fasciculus, dorsolateral, CORD   *See* tract, dorsolateral.

fasciculus, fronto-occip´ital, CEREBRUM   *See* fasciculus, occipitofrontal.

fasciculus gracilis /gras´il-is/ [NA], MEDULLA, CORD, [L. *gracilis* graceful or slender] tract occupying most of each half of the posterior funiculus in the lower spinal cord and the medial part in the upper spinal cord and closed medulla (Fig. B-2). These fibers, with cell bodies in dorsal root ganglia, conduct impulses from tactile and proprioceptive nerve endings (Fig. T-3) in the lower half of the body, primarily to the nucleus gracilis of the medulla, and to the thoracic nucleus and nucleus proprius of the spinal cord. *Syn:* funiculus gracilis; tract of Goll. *See also* fasciculus, septomarginal.

fasciculus hippocampi /hip-o-kam´pī/, CEREBRUM   *See* band, diagonal (of Broca).

fasciculus, interfascic´ular [fasciculus interfascicularis (semilunaris), NA], CORD tract located in the rostral half of the spinal cord between the fasciculus gracilis and the fasciculus cuneatus. It is composed of short, descending collaterals of tactile and proprioceptive fibers in the fasciculus cuneatus. *Syn:* comma tract; tract of Schultze.

fasciculus, interstitiospi´nal (of Muskens), BRAIN STEM   extrapyramidal or conditioning component of the medial longitudinal fasciculus. Its fibers arise from cells in the nucleus of Darkschewitsch and the interstitial nucleus and end in motor nuclei of the brain stem and cervical spinal cord (Fig. F-2).

fasciculus, lentic´ular, MAINLY FOREBRAIN   fiber tract arising in the lentiform nucleus and, to some extent, from the cerebral cortex. It crosses the posterior limb of the internal capsule, and passes dorsal to the subthalamic nucleus through the H_2 field of Forel. Some fibers end in the nucleus of the field of Forel, the nucleus of the posterior commissure, the interstitial nucleus of the medial longitudinal fasciculus, and/or the red nucleus for relay to the motor nuclei of the brain stem and spinal cord. Other fibers enter the thalamic fasciculus (H_1 field of Forel) for termination in the ventral anterior nucleus and, to a lesser extent, in the ventral lateral nucleus of the dorsal thalamus. Some fibers enter the hypothalamus and terminate in the ventromedial nucleus. *Syn:* dorsal division of the ansa lenticularis, *def.* 2.

fasciculus, longitudinal, dorsal (DLF) [fasciculus longitudinalis dorsalis, NA], BRAIN STEM bundle located in the ventral part of the periaqueductal gray and in the floor of the fourth ventricle, just dorsal to the hypoglossal nucleus. It is composed of fibers mainly from the hypothalamus and dorsal tegmental nucleus, and some from the habenula (Fig. H-1), with endings in all cranial preganglionic parasympathetic nuclei and brain stem motor nuclei other than those innervating the ocular muscles. *Syn:* fasciculus or tract of Schütz; periependymal fasciculus.

fasciculus, longitudinal, (of the) fornicate gyrus, CEREBRUM   *See* cingulum.

fasciculus, longitudinal, inferior [fasciculus longitudinalis inferior, NA], CEREBRUM association bundle of the cerebrum which interconnects occipital lobe cortex and temporal lobe cortex in the inferior and lateral part of the hemisphere. *Syn:* external sagittal stratum.

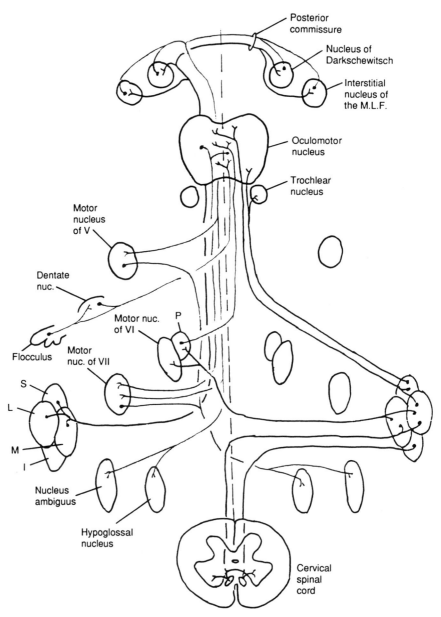

Fig. F-2.   Diagram to show the connections of the medial longitudinal fasciculus, including a vestibular component, an internuclear component, and a conditioning or extrapyramidal component. The descending fibers to the spinal cord constitute the medial vestibulospinal tract. The flocculo-(dento-)oculomotor tract, in the rostral part of the fasciculus, is included. Inhibitory fibers to the nuclei supplying antagonistic muscles are not shown. P-parabducens nucleus. S, L, M, I-superior, lateral, medial, and inferior vestibular nuclei. See the text.

fasciculus, longitudinal, medial (MLF) [fasciculus longitudinalis medialis, NA], BRAIN STEM   fiber tract located close to the median plane just ventral to the gray beneath the ventricular surface, and extending from the midbrain tegmentum into the cervical spinal cord.   It consists mainly of a vestibular component, an internuclear component, and a conditioning or extrapyramidal component. Fibers from the vestibular nuclei end nuclei to supply eye and neck muscles, for compensatory eye and head movements in response to changes in position of the head.   The internuclear component connects brain stem motor nuclei having related functions. The trigeminal, facial, and hypoglossal motor nuclei and the nucleus ambiguus are interconnected for chewing and swallowing and for speech. Other fibers, from the oculomotor to the facial nuclei, coordinate lowering the eyelids with downward movements of the eyes.   From reticular cells in the parabducens nucleus fibers ascend to the oculomotor nucleus, a necessary connection for conjugate deviation of the eyes in the horizontal plane. Striatal modification of the brain stem motor nuclei is possible by way of lenticular fasciculus fibers from the globus pallidus to the nucleus of Darkschewitsch and the interstitial nucleus of the medial longitudinal fasciculus, and the conditioning component of the medial longitudinal fasciculus to the brain stem motor nuclei (Fig. F-2). *Syn:* posterior longitudinal fasciculus or bundle. *See also* nystagmus, vestibular; reflexes, vestibulo-ocular.

fasciculus, longitudinal, posterior, BRAIN STEM   **1.** usually a synonym for the medial longitudinal fasciculus.

2. sometimes for the dorsal longitudinal fasciculus.

fasciculus, longitudinal, superior [fasciculus longitudinalis superior, NA], CEREBRUM association bundle of the cerebrum located along the dorsolateral border of the putamen, lateral to the internal capsule.   It underlies and interconnects the cortices of the frontal, parietal, and occipital lobes, and arches inferiorly and anteriorly with connections in the temporal lobe cortex. *Syn:* arcuate fasciculus.

fasciculus mamillar´is prin´ceps, DIENCEPHALON   fairly substantial bundle of fibers which arises from the medial mamillary nucleus, passes dorsally a short distance, then divides into the mamillothalamic and mamillotegmental tracts.

fasciculus, medial longitudinal, BRAIN STEM   *See* fasciculus, longitudinal, medial.

fasciculus, medial triangular, CORD   sacral part of the septomarginal fasciculus.

fasciculus, occip´ital, lateral, CEREBRUM   association bundle of the cerebrum which passes vertically through the occipital lobe and interconnects the posterior part of the medial occipitotemporal gyrus and the posterior part of the parietal lobe. *Syn:* fasciculus of Wernicke; perpendicular or vertical occipital fasciculus.

fasciculus, occipital, perpendic´ular, CEREBRUM   *See* fasciculus, occipital, lateral.

fasciculi, occipital, transverse, CEREBRUM   two association bundles of the occipital lobe; one connects the upper lip of the calcarine fissure with the superolateral occipital cortex; the other connects the inferior lip of the calcarine fissure with the inferolateral occipital cortex.

fasciculus, occipital, vertical, CEREBRUM   *See* fasciculus, occipital, lateral.

fasciculus, occipitofron´tal, CEREBRUM   either of two association bundles of the cerebral hemispheres (the superior and inferior occipitofrontal fasciculi), which interconnect cortex mainly of the occipital and frontal lobes.

fasciculus, occipitofrontal (fronto-occipital), inferior, CEREBRUM   association bundle of the cerebrum, located along the inferior part of the extreme capsule, dorsal to the uncinate fasciculus.   It interconnects cortex of the lateral or inferolateral part of the frontal lobe and cortex of the occipital lobe, with connections along the way, including the inferior temporal and medial occipitotemporal gyri of the temporal lobe.

fasciculus, occipitofrontal (fronto-occipital), superior, CEREBRUM   association bundle of the cerebrum located along the caudate nucleus medial to the interdigitating fibers of the internal capsule and corpus callosum. Its fibers interconnect the cortex of the occipital and temporal lobes on the one hand with that of the frontal lobe and insula on the other. *Syn:* fasciculus subcallosus.

fasciculus, oval, CORD   lumbar part of the septomarginal fasciculus.

fasciculus, periepend´ymal, BRAIN STEM   *See* fasciculus, longitudinal, dorsal.

fasciculus, predor´sal   *See* tract, tectospinal (medial).

fasciculus pro´prius [fasciculi proprii, NA], MEDULLA, CORD   system of short fibers in the spinal cord and adjoining brain stem, mainly in, but not limited to, the area adjacent to the gray matter, and interconnecting neighboring spinal cord levels. In the spinal animal it provides the necessary connections for many automatic functions, including vasomotor, sudomotor, bowel, and genitourinary functioning, and coordination of the musculature of the trunk and limbs. *Syn:* ground or reflex bundle; propriospinal or spinospinal tract.

fasciculus prosencephal´icus medial´is [NA], FOREBRAIN   *See* bundle, forebrain, medial.

fasciculus pyramidal´is [NA]   *See* tract, pyramidal.

fasciculus retroflex´us   *See* tract, habenulo-interpeduncular.

fasciculus, semilu´nar [fasciculus semilunaris, NA], CORD   *See* fasciculus, interfascicularis.

fasciculus, septomar´ginal [fasciculus septomarginalis, NA], CORD   tract located in the caudal half of the spinal cord between the fasciculus gracilis and the dorsal median septum and composed of short, descending collaterals of tactile and proprioceptive fibers in the fasciculus gracilis. The lumbar part of the septomarginal fasciculus, located along the mid-portion of the septum, is the oval bundle. *Syn:* tract of Flechsig. The sacral portion, located at the dorsal surface, is the triangular fasciculus. *Syn:* medial triangular fasciculus; triangular field of Gombault and Philippe.

fasciculus solitar´ius [tractus solitarius, NA], MAINLY MEDULLA   fiber tract composed of descending visceral afferent fibers of the facial, glossopharyngeal, and vagus nerves. Most fibers terminate in the adjoining nucleus parasolitarius. Some fibers (for taste) descend only a short distance to end in the dorsal visceral gray. *Syn:* Gierke's respiratory bundle. *See also* reflexes, vagal, *and* Fig. R-9.

fasciculus subcallo´sus, CEREBRUM   *See* fasciculus, fronto-occipital, superior.

fasciculus, subthalam´ic [fasciculus subthalamicus, NA], MAINLY FOREBRAIN   fibers which interconnect the globus pallidus mainly with the subthalamic nucleus but also with the zona incerta and the midbrain tegmental gray. It forms the capsule of the subthalamic nucleus. Pallidosubthalamic fibers arise from the outer pallidal segment. Subthalamopallidal fibers end in both outer and inner segments of the globus pallidus. *Syn:* intermediate division of the ansa lenticularis, *def.* 2.

fasciculus, sulcomar´ginal (of Marie) [fasciculus sulcomarginalis, NA], CORD   area adjacent to the ventral median fissure of the spinal cord, containing some combination of descending fiber bundles. The term usually refers to the spinal part of the medial tectospinal and medial reticulospinal tracts but has also been used at times to mean or to include the ventral corticospinal tract.

fasciculus, superior fronto-occip´ital, CEREBRUM   *See* fasciculus, occipitofrontal, superior.

fasciculus, superior longitudinal, CEREBRUM   *See* fasciculus, longitudinal, superior.

fasciculus, thalam´ic [fasciculus thalamicus, NA], DIENCEPHALON   fiber bundle located between the dorsal thalamus and the zona incerta. It consists of fibers from the ansa lenticularis, the lenticular fasciculus, and the dentothalamic and rubrothalamic tracts. Its fibers terminate mainly in the ventral anterior and ventral lateral nuclei of the dorsal thalamus. *Syn:* H_1 field of Forel.

fasciculus, triangular, CORD   sacral part of the septomarginal fasciculus.

fasciculus, uncinate /un´sin-āt/ [L. *uncinatus* hook-shaped]   **1.** BRAIN STEM   fibers which arise in the fastigial nucleus of the cerebellum, cross the median plane, loop over the superior cerebellar peduncle, and enter the juxtarestiform body of the inferior cerebellar peduncle. Most fibers terminate in the vestibular nuclei; some fibers continue caudally and end in the cervical spinal cord. *Syn:* hook bundle; Russell's fasciculus. *See also* tract, cerebellospinal.

2. [fasciculus uncinatus, NA], CEREBRUM   hook-shaped association bundle which interconnects the frontal and the temporal lobe cortices. Its dorsal division joins the cortex in the region of the temporal pole and that of the middle frontal gyrus, whereas its ventral division joins the cortex of the parahippocampal gyrus and the orbital surface of the frontal lobe.

fasciola cinerea /fah-se´o-lah sin-er´e-ah/, CEREBRUM   *See* gyrus, fasciolar.

Fast Blue   trademark for a fluorescent tracer used to mark the cytoplasm of nerve cell bodies. *See also* tracer, fluorescent.

fastigium /fas-tidj´ī-um/ [L. summit]   mid-dorsal apical part of the fourth ventricle (Fig. V-3).

Fechner, Gustav Theodor (1801-1887)   German physicist. *See* Weber *for the* Weber-Fechner law.

feet, sucker   vascular footplates of astrocytes, which form the perivascular glial limiting membrane.

fenes´tra coch´leae [NA], EAR   *See* window, round.

fenestra oval´is [NA], EAR   *See* window, oval.

fenestra rotun´da [NA], EAR   *See* window, round

fenestra vestib´uli [NA], EAR   *See* window, oval.

Ferrier, Sir David (1843-1928)   renowned Scottish neurophysiologist, later of London, noted for his pioneer studies of the cerebral cortex, which established the concept of localization of function in the cerebral hemispheres.

festina´tion [L. *festinare* to hasten]   acceleration of gait with an inability to slow down or stop, characteristic of extrapyramidal dysfunction, as in Parkinson's syndrome.

fi´bers [fibrae, NA]   *See also* bundle; fasciculus; tract.

fibers, A   myelinated, peripheral nerve fibers, as large as 22 μm in diameter, with long internodal segments and a conduction velocity of five to 120 meters per second. Of these the largest and most rapidly conducting carry motor impulses to skeletal muscle or afferent impulses from neuromuscular spindles. Slightly smaller fibers carry impulses for touch or pressure. The smallest of these fibers carry impulses for pain, temperature, or touch.

fibers, ar´cuate   **1.** MEDULLA   any of several fiber bundles in the medulla which take a curved course.

2. [fibrae arcuatae cerebri, NA], CEREBRUM   short association fibers which lie immediately beneath the cerebral cortex adjacent to a cerebral sulcus and which connect adjacent gyri. *Syn:* U-fibers.

fibers, arcuate, dorsal (posterior) external (superficial) [fibrae arcuatae externae dorsales (posteriores), NA], MEDULLA   cuneatocerebellar tract fibers that arise in the accessory cuneate nucleus and turn, almost immediately, into the inferior cerebellar peduncle and terminate in the cerebellar vermis.

fibers, arcuate, external (superficial), MEDULLA   fibers that follow a curved course on the surface of the medulla until they enter the inferior cerebellar peduncle for termination in the cerebellum. *See also* fibers, arcuate, dorsal external *and* ventral external.

fibers, arcuate, internal [fibrae arcuatae internae, NA], MEDULLA   fibers which arise from cells in the gracile and cuneate nuclei and spiral rostrally and ventrally then medially to cross the median plane in the sensory decussation in the rostral part of the closed medulla. They ascend in the medial lemniscus.

fibers, arcuate, ventral (anterior) external (superficial) [fibrae arcuatae externae ventrales (anteriores), NA], MEDULLA   fibers which arise mostly in the arcuate nucleus, adjacent to the pyramid in the medulla oblongata (some from the lateral arcuate and lateral reticular nuclei), and pass dorsolaterally on the surface of the medulla to enter the inferior cerebellar peduncle for distribution in the cerebellum. *Syn:* stratum zonale of Arnold.

fibers, associa´tion (of the cerebral hemispheres), CEREBRUM   nerve fibers which interconnect cortical regions of the same cerebral hemisphere, first described by Meynert. The major ones are: the superior and inferior longitudinal fasciculi, the superior and inferior occipitofrontal fasciculi, the cingulum, and the uncinate fasciculus.

fibers, B   myelinated, peripheral nerve fibers, 3 μm or less in diameter, with a conduction velocity of three to 14 meters per second.   They have shorter internodal segments than type A fibers. Such fibers include all the preganglionic autonomic fibers, the postganglionic sympathetic fibers that supply the arrectores pilorum, and some visceral afferent fibers.

fiber, band   multinucleated syncytial cord formed by the proliferation of neurolemma sheath cells as a part of the regenerative process of peripheral nerve fibers. *Syn:* band of Büngner; Bandfasern.

fibers, bas´ilar, EAR   *See* strings, auditory.

fibers, C   unmyelinated nerve fibers with a slow conduction velocity (0.5 to 2 meters per second). They include most postganglionic autonomic fibers, also some fibers for visceral pain and for poorly localized cutaneous pain and temperature. *Syn:* fibers of Remak.

fibers, cerebellomotor´ius   fibers that are said to arise from cells in the fastigial nuclei of the cerebellum and terminate in motor nuclei of the brain stem.

fibers, climbing [neurofibra ascendens, NA], CEREBELLUM   olivocerebellar and perhaps other nerve fibers which enter the molecular layer of the cerebellar cortex and spiral around the dendritic processes of Purkinje cells, to which they transmit excitatory impulses (Fig. C-9). Collaterals synapsing in the deep cerebellar nuclei are also excitatory.

fibers, commissu´ral (commis´sural) (of the cerebral hemispheres), CEREBRUM   nerve fibers which cross the median plane and interconnect similar cortical regions in the two cerebral hemispheres.

fibers, corticonu´clear (corticobulbar) [fibrae corticonucleares, NA]   pyramidal tract fibers which terminate in motor nuclei of the brain stem.

fibers, corticopon´tine [fibrae corticopontinae, NA]   fibers of the frontal and temporoparieto-occipital corticopontine tracts.

fibers, corticoretic´ular [fibrae corticoreticulares, NA]   fibers which originate in the cerebral cortex and terminate on cells in the reticular formation of the brain stem.

fibers, corticoru´bral [fibrae corticorubrales, NA]   *See* tract, corticorubral.

fibers, corticospi´nal [fibrae corticospinales, NA]   *See* tract, corticospinal.

fibers, dentato-ol´ivary (dento-ol´ivary)   fibers which arise from cells in the dentate nucleus of the cerebellum, ascend through the superior cerebellar peduncle, cross the median plane in caudal part of the midbrain tegmentum, and descend in the central tegmental tract to end in the inferior olivary nucleus (Fig. O-1). *See also* myoclonus, palatal.

fibers, dentatoru´bral (dentoru´bral)   *See* tract, dentatorubral.

fibers, dentatothalam´ic (dentothalam´ic)   *See* tract, dentatothalamic.

fibers, external arcuate, MEDULLA   *See* fibers, arcuate, external.

fibers, gam´ma ef´ferent (motor), CORD   fine axons from small nerve cell bodies in the ventral horn, which terminate on the small, intrafusal muscle fibers within neuromuscular spindles (Figs. L-1, S-2). *See also* loop, gamma.

fibers, internal arcuate, MEDULLA   *See* fibers, arcuate, internal.

fibers, intrafu´sal   thin, modified skeletal muscle fibers within a neuromuscular spindle. Of these, the smaller (nuclear chain) fibers are uniform in diameter. In their central portion the myofibrils are replaced by a chain of large single nuclei. The terminal portions of the larger fibers resemble small extrafusal fibers, but their central, expanded portions, the nuclear bag, contain a cluster of nuclei. Both types have afferent, anulospiral nerve endings around their central portions. The chain fibers also have flower spray endings in their terminal portions (Fig. S-2).

fibers, itin´erant   *See* fibers, projection.

fiber, mossy   1. [neurofibra muscoidea, NA], CEREBELLUM   axon terminal of an excitatory fiber mainly of the pontocerebellar, vestibulocerebellar, and spinocerebellar tracts. Such fibers terminate mostly as rosettes in relation to the claw-shaped dendrites of granule cells in the glomeruli of the granular layer of the cerebellum (Fig. C-9), but also to some extent on the cells in the deep cerebellar nuclei. *See also* glomerulus, cerebellar; island, cerebellar.

2. CEREBRUM   axons of certain cells in the dentate gyrus of the hippocampal formation have also been called mossy fibers.

fiber, nerve   process of a neuron together with its sheaths.

fiber, nuclear bag   small, intrafusal, modified skeletal muscle fiber, usually one to four per neuromuscular spindle. The central, expanded portion of the fiber, the nuclear bag, contains many nuclei and no striations. Wrapped around the nuclear bag is a primary or anulospiral ending of a proprioceptive fiber. Only the terminal, striated portions of the fiber contain motor end plates and are contractile (Fig. S-2).

fiber, nuclear chain   small, intrafusal, modified skeletal muscle fiber, usually one to 10 per neuromuscular spindle. Its central portion, not expanded like that of the larger nuclear bag fibers, contains a line of single nuclei, has no striations, and is not contractile. Wrapped around this part is a primary or anulospiral nerve ending. The terminal, striated parts of the chain fibers have motor end plates and are contractile, and also have secondary afferent or flower spray endings (Fig. S-2).

fibers, orbitofron´tal, CEREBRUM   association fibers of the cerebrum which pass through the anterior part of the extreme capsule and interconnect the posterior part of the orbital gyri and the dorsolateral part of the frontal lobe.

fiber, parallel [neurofibra parallela, NA], CEREBELLUM   axon of a granule cell of the cerebellar cortex. Such fibers course through the molecular layer in a plane parallel to the longitudinal axis of a cerebellar folium. These fibers transmit excitatory impulses to the Purkinje cells and also to the stellate, basket, and Golgi cells of the cerebellar cortex (Fig. C-9).

fibers (of) passage   nerve fibers which pass through a region without synapse.

fibers, pon´tine, transverse [fibrae pontis transversae, NA], PONS   pontocerebellar fibers in the base of the pons. They arise from cells of the pontine gray. Most fibers cross the median plane and enter the middle cerebellar peduncle.

fibers, pontocerebel´lar [fibrae pontocerebellares, NA]   pontine fibers which arise from cells in the pontine gray, cross the base of the pons (transverse pontine fibers), then enter the middle cerebellar peduncle and terminate as mossy fibers in the cerebellar cortex, mainly in the contralateral posterior lobe cerebellar hemisphere.

fibers, postganglion´ic [neurofibrae postganglionares, NA]   nerve fibers of the ANS which have their cells of origin in an autonomic ganglion (sympathetic chain ganglia or prevertebral ganglia of the sympathetic division or terminal ganglia of the parasympathetic division). Such fibers terminate in some visceral organ to activate glandular secretion or to modify the contraction of smooth or cardiac muscle.

fibers, preganglion´ic [neurofibrae preganglionares, NA]   nerve fibers of the ANS which have their cells of origin in the brain stem or spinal cord in a general visceral motor nucleus. Such fibers leave the brain by way of the oculomotor, facial, glossopharyngeal, vagus, and bulbar accessory nerves and the spinal cord by way of spinal nerves T1-L3 and S2-S4. They terminate in autonomic ganglia, synapsing on the cell bodies of postganglionic fibers. *See also* ramus, gray *and* white; trunk, sympathetic; nerves, splanchnic; system, autonomic nervous (Fig. S-3); Tables 1, 2, and 3.

fibers, projec´tion   nerve fibers, ascending or descending, which connect the cerebral cortex and some subcortical region.

fibers, propriospi´nal, CORD   fasciculus proprius fibers that arise and terminate wholly within the spinal cord; intrinsic spinal fibers.

fibers, pyram´idal, aber´rant   fibers which leave the pyramidal tract at brain stem levels to descend with the medial lemniscus and terminate in motor nuclei of the brain stem and the accessory nucleus of the cervical spinal cord (Crosby *et al.*, '62, pp. 262-265).

fibers, superfic´ial ar´cuate, MEDULLA   *See* fibers, arcuate, external.

fibers, transver´sal, CEREBELLUM   axons of the basket cells which course transversely in the molecular layer of the cerebellar cortex just above the Purkinje cell bodies and which synapse with the Purkinje cells.

fibers, trap´ezoid, PONS   transversely running auditory fibers of the trapezoid body, which arise from cells in the cochlear nuclei and, with or without synapses in course, continue into the lateral lemniscus to end in the inferior colliculi and medial geniculate nuclei. *See also* body, trapezoid.

fibers, tun´nel, EAR   terminal portions of olivocochlear fibers as they cross the inner tunnel (of Corti) to end on the hair cells of the spiral organ of the cochlea. *See* *also* bundle, olivocochlear.

fibers, ventral superficial (external) arcuate, MEDULLA   *See* fibers, arcuate, ventral external.

fi´brae ansat´ae, FOREBRAIN   nerve fibers connecting the area in front of the lamina terminalis with the tuber cinereum.

fibrilla´tion   small, irregular, asynchronous potentials in a single muscle fiber (amplitude of 10 to 20 μV, duration of 1 to 2 milliseconds). They can be detected by electromyography but do not produce any shortening of the muscle fiber and cannot be detected visually through the skin. They occur in muscle undergoing denervation, but cease either when reinnervation is established or when denervation is complete. *See also* fasciculation.

fields of Forel   *See* Forel.

field, fron´tal eye, CEREBRUM   area of the frontal lobe cortex (area 8) concerned with voluntary eye movements. *For additional information on the control of eye movements, see* Crosby and Schneider ('82).

field, occip´ital eye, CEREBRUM   area of the occipital lobe cortex concerned with vision (area 17), with optokinetic (following) eye movements, and with visual association (Brodmann's area 18). Area 19 of the adjoining cortex is usually also included.

field, preru´bral, MAINLY MIDBRAIN   area just rostral and dorsolateral to the red nucleus and containing rubrothalamic and dentatothalamic fibers. These fibers continue into the thalamic fasciculus. *Syn:* H or tegmental field of Forel.

field, receptive, EYE   area of the retina, stimulation of which causes a retinal ganglion cell to respond. Stimulation of the inner part of the field, its central zone, may activate the neuron to excitation or to inhibition, whereas that of the area around the central zone, the surround, tends to inhibit such activity. *See also* cells, on-center *and* off-center.

field, ret´inal, EYE   area of the retina which "sees" a part of the visual field.

field, triang´ular (of Gombault and Philippe), CORD   sacral part of the septo-marginal fasciculus.

field, visual   area seen by one or both eyes.

Fielding, George Hunsley (1801-1871)   English anatomist. *Fielding's membrane* is the tapetum of the corpus callosum.

fi´la   plural of *filum.*

fila, lateral, of the pons   one or more strands of fibers which course along the upper surface of the base of the pons next to the cerebral peduncle, then turn down in the groove between the middle and the superior cerebellar peduncles.

fila, olfac´tory   delicate fascicles of olfactory nerve fibers which arise from specialized olfactory cells in the upper part of the nasal mucosa, pass through openings in the cribriform plate, and end in the olfactory bulb.

fillet /fil´et/ [Fr. *filet* a band]   *See* lemniscus.

fi´lum termina´le [NA] [*pl.* fila] [L. *filum* thread]   threadlike filament of pia mater extending caudally from the caudal tip of the spinal cord through the subarachnoid space, acquiring arachnoid and dural investments, and attaching to the dorsal surface of the coccyx.

filum terminale externum [NA]   that part of the filum terminale outside the subarachnoid space, having arachnoid and dural investments. *Syn:* coccygeal ligament.

filum terminale internum [NA]   that part of the filum terminale within the subarachnoid space, extending caudally from the caudal tip of the spinal cord to the caudal end of the arachnoid.

fim´bria hippocam´pi [NA], CEREBRUM, [L. *fimbria* fringe]   the main efferent bundle of nerve fibers arising from the hippocampal formation. It extends posteriorly along the surface of the hippocampus (Fig. C-7). The fibers arise from the large pyramidal cells in the cornu ammonis and subiculum, emerge to enter the alveus, then collect to form the fimbria, and, posterior to the hippocampus, continue into the fornix.

fissu´ra pri´ma [NA], CEREBELLUM   *See* fissure, primary.

fissura secun´da [NA], CEREBELLUM   *See* fissure, secondary.

fis´sure [fissura, NA] [L. *fissura* cleft or slit]   This term has been variously used in the past, sometimes with reference to any major, deep groove on the surface of the brain or spinal cord, or to any groove deep enough to cause an elevation on the ventricular surface of the brain (total fissure or complete sulcus), or to any groove which separates the lobes of the cerebral hemispheres. It is also sometimes used interchangeably with sulcus. Now it is reserved primarily for the large clefts separating the two cerebral hemispheres, the grooves between subdivisions of the cerebellum, and certain other grooves on the surface of the brain stem and spinal cord. *For the grooves on the surface of the cerebral hemispheres, see* sulcus.

fissure, chor´oid   1. [fissura choroidea, NA], CEREBRUM   fissure located between the lamina affixa on the upper surface of the thalamus and the lateral edge of the fornix in the body of the lateral ventricle, and between the stria terminalis and the edge of the fimbria in the inferior horn. It is closed by the choroid plexus of the lateral ventricle, which is attached along the margins of the fissure and projects into the ventricle.

2. EYE   *See* fissure, optic.

fissure, dorsolateral   1. [fissura dorsolateralis (posterolateralis), NA], CEREBELLUM   fissure between the flocculus and the hemisphere of the posterior lobe of the cerebellum.

2. MIDBRAIN   fissure on the lateral surface of the midbrain, between the tectum and the tegmentum.

fissure, great horizontal, CEREBELLUM   *See* fissure, horizontal.

fissure, great longitudinal, CEREBRUM   *See* fissure, longitudinal.

fissure, horizontal (great) [fissura horizontalis, NA], CEREBELLUM   fissure which approximately separates the superior and inferior halves of the cerebellum, between the folium vermis and the superior semilunar lobules above, and the tuber and the inferior semilunar lobules below (Figs. C-2, V-6).

fissure, interhemispher´ic, CEREBRUM   *See* fissure, longitudinal.

fissure, interlo´bar   any fissure which serves as a boundary between lobes.

fissure, intralo´bar   any fissure contained within the boundaries of a lobe.

fissure, longitudinal (great) [fissura longitudinalis cerebri, NA], CEREBRUM   deep vertical fissure between the two cerebral hemispheres. *Syn:* interhemispheric fissure.

fissure, op´tic [fissura optica, NA], DIENCEPHALON   fissure extending along the ventral surface of the optic cup and the optic stalk of the developing eye and optic nerve. Through this fissure branches of the ophthalmic artery and vein communicate with the vessels within the eyeball. *Syn:* choroid fissure of the eye.

fissure, postcen´tral   1. CEREBRUM   *See* sulcus, postcentral.

2. CEREBELLUM   fissure on the superior surface of the cerebellum, separating the central lobule and ala centralis anteriorly from the culmen and anterior quadrangular lobules posteriorly.

fissure, postcli´val, CEREBELLUM   fissure on the superior surface of the cerebellum between the declive of the vermis and the posterior quadrangular lobules of the hemispheres anteriorly and the folium vermis and the superior semilunar lobules posteriorly (Figs. C-2, V-6). It separates the lobulus simplex from the remainder of the posterior lobe.

fissure, posterolateral (dorsolateral) [fissura posterolateralis (dorsolateralis), NA], CEREBELLUM   lateral extension of the postnodular fissure of the cerebellum between the flocculus anteriorly and the tonsil and biventer posteriorly.

fissure, postnod´ular, CEREBELLUM   fissure on the anterior, inferior surface of the vermis between the nodule anteriorly and the uvula posteriorly (Fig. V-6).

fissure, postpyram´idal, CEREBELLUM   fissure on the inferior surface of the cerebellum between the pyramis vermis and biventer anteriorly and the tuber vermis and inferior semilunar (and gracile) lobules posteriorly (Fig. V-6). *See also* fissure, prepyramidal.

fissure, precen´tral   1. CEREBRUM   *See* sulcus, precentral.
    2. CEREBELLUM   fissure on the superior surface of the cerebellum between the lingula and the central lobule of the cerebellar vermis (Fig. V-6).

fissure, precli´val, CEREBELLUM   *See* fissure, primary.

fissure, prepyram´idal [fissura secunda, NA], CEREBELLUM   fissure on the inferior surface of the cerebellum between the uvula and tonsils anteriorly and the pyramis vermis and biventers posteriorly (Fig. V-6). Sometimes the pre- and postpyramidal fissures are named according to their rostro-caudal position in relation to the pyramis vermis, so that their order is reversed from that given here.

fissure, primary [fissura prima, NA], CEREBELLUM   fissure on the superior surface of the cerebellum between the culmen and anterior quadrangular lobules anteriorly and the declive and posterior quadrangular lobules posteriorly. It separates the anterior and posterior lobes of the cerebellum (Figs. C-2, V-6). It is the first fissure to appear in the corpus cerebelli, but the second to develop in the cerebellum as a whole. *Syn:* preclival fissure.

fissure of Rolando, CEREBRUM   *See* sulcus, central, *also* Rolando, Luigi.

fissure, secondary [fissura secunda, NA], CEREBELLUM   fissure on the surface of the cerebellar vermis, between the pyramis and the uvula. *Syn:* prepyramidal fissure (Fig. V-6).

fissure, sim´ian, CEREBRUM   *See* sulcus, lunate.

fissure, superior or´bital [fissura orbitalis superior, NA]   opening between the greater and lesser wings of the sphenoid bone, through which the oculomotor, trochlear, and abducens nerves, the ophthalmic branch of the trigeminal nerve, and the ophthalmic vein pass.

fissure, Sylvian, CEREBRUM   *See* sulcus, lateral, *also* Sylvius, Franciscus.

fissure, total, CEREBRUM   *See* sulcus, complete.

fissure, transverse cerebral [fissura transversa cerebri, NA]   fissure separating the occipital lobes above and the cerebellum below, in which the tentorium cerebelli is located. It continues forward under the splenium of the corpus callosum and over the roof of the third ventricle below.

fissure, ventrolateral, MIDBRAIN   fissure on the lateral surface of the midbrain between the tegmentum and the basis pedunculi.

fissure, ventral (anterior) me´dian [fissura mediana ventralis (anterior), NA] MEDULLA,

CORD   deep groove on the midventral surface between the pyramids of the medulla and between the ventral funiculi of the spinal cord.

fit, uncinate /un´sin-āt/   disorder characterized by olfactory hallucinations, usually of an unpleasant nature, associated with an irritative lesion of the uncus of the temporal lobe.

flaccid /flak´sid/   completely lacking in muscle tone, such as the state of the muscle in a peripheral nerve paralysis.

Flack, Martin W. (1882-1931)   English physiologist. *Flack's node* or the *node of Keith and Flack* is the sinuatrial node.

Flechsig, Paul Emil (1847-1929)   German neuroanatomist and professor of psychiatry in Leipzig, noted for his studies of myelogenesis and of CNS tracts. The *oval area of Flechsig* is the lumbar portion of the septomarginal fasciculus. *Flechsig's tract* is the dorsal spinocerebellar tract. *Flechsig's loop*, more often called Meyer's loop, is the temporal loop of the optic radiation. The *arcuate nucleus of Flechsig* is the ventral posteromedial nucleus of the dorsal thalamus. Flechsig also described and named the pyramidal tract.

flex´or reflex afferents (FRA)   the various afferent inputs that may set off a flexor reflex, such as those resulting in withdrawal from a painful stimulus.

flex´ure, cephal´ic [flexura cephalica, NA]   ventral flexure of the embryonic brain in the region of the midbrain. It occurs in embryos 3 to 4 mm in length. In the adult human brain this bend is located at the junction of the forebrain and the midbrain. *Syn:* mesencephalic flexure.

flexure, cer´vical [flexura cervicalis, NA]   ventral flexure of the embryonic CNS. It occurs at the junction of the brain and the spinal cord in embryos about 4 mm in length, shortly after the formation of the cephalic flexure.

flexure, mesencephal´ic   *See* flexure, cephalic.

flexure, pon´tine [flexura pontina, NA]   dorsal flexure of the embryonic brain that occurs at the junction of the met- and myelencephalon. It begins to gain prominence in the embryo at the 10 mm stage.

floc´culus [NA], CEREBELLUM, [L. little tuft of wool]   most caudal subdivision of the cerebellar hemisphere, on the anterior surface of the cerebellum, just lateral to the attachment of the vestibulocochlear nerve at the pontomedullary junction (Figs. C-2, F-2).

Flourens, Marie Jean Pierre (1794-1867)   French physiologist and anatomist who demonstrated that the cerebrum is concerned with thought and will power, and that the cerebellum has to do with motor coordination.

fluid, cerebrospi´nal (CSF) [liquor cerebrospinalis, NA]   clear, colorless liquid secreted by the choroid plexus of the lateral, third, and fourth ventricles, and contained within the ventricular system of the brain and spinal cord and within the subarachnoid space.

fluid, o´tic, EAR   *See* endolymph.

fluid, perio´tic, EAR   *See* perilymph.

Foerster, Otfrid (1873-1941)   German neurologist and neurosurgeon, noted for many studies, including those on the cytoarchitecture of the cerebral cortex and the dermatomal pattern of spinal nerves. He also introduced tractotomy as a surgical procedure for the relief of pain.

Foix, Charles (1882-1927)   French neurologist, a pupil of Marie's. His main interest was the syndromes resulting from occlusion of various arteries. He and his colleagues also demonstrated that the substantia nigra is particularly involved in Parkinson's disease (1921).

fold, dural   membrane of the dura mater, separating the two cerebral hemispheres (falx cerebri), the two cerebellar hemispheres (falx cerebelli), and the two cerebral hemispheres from the cerebellum (tentorium cerebelli) (Fig. F-1).

fold, neural   each lateral wall of the neural groove.

fo´lia, cerebel´lar [folia cerebelli, NA] [*sing.* **folium**], CEREBELLUM, [L. *folium* leaf] narrow, leaflike gyri on the surface of the cerebellum.

fo´lium ver´mis [NA], CEREBELLUM   subdivision of the cerebellar vermis between the declive and the tuber (Figs. C-2, V-6). *See also* vermis cerebelli.

Fontana, Abbada Felice Gaspar Ferdinand (ca. 1720/1730-1805)   Italian anatomist of Pisa and Florence, whose contributions to neurological knowledge covered a wide range of subjects. The *spaces of Fontana* are the small spaces in the trabecular meshwork of the pectinate ligament at the iridocorneal angle of the eye. They transport aqueous humor from the anterior chamber of the eye to the venous sinus of the sclera (canal of Schlemm).

foot, end   *See* bulb, terminal.

foot, perivas´cular   vascular footplate, the process of an astrocyte, which is applied to the surface of a blood vessel within the CNS. Collectively they form the perivascular glial membrane. *Syn:* sucker foot.

fora´men [NA] [*pl.* **foram´ina**] [L. opening; from *forare* to bore]   any small opening in a bone, a membrane, or the brain.

foramen cecum /se´kum/ [L. *caecus* blind, hence a depression or cul-de-sac], MEDULLA   small depression at the upper end of the ventral median fissure on the ventral surface of the brain stem, between the two pyramids and just below the pons.

foramina cribro´sa [NA]   small openings in the cribriform plate of the ethmoid bone in the floor of the cranial cavity through which the fibers of the olfactory nerve enter the cranial cavity. *Syn:* olfactory foramina.

foramen, hypoglos´sal   *See* canal, hypoglossal.

foramen, interventric´ular [foramen interventriculare, NA], FOREBRAIN   opening between the lateral ventricle and the third ventricle (Fig. V-5). Originally this term was used to mean the opening from one lateral ventricle to the other across the third ventricle, so there was only one foramen. Later usage associated the term with the opening of each lateral ventricle into the third ventricle, so now there are two. *Syn:* foramen of Monro.

foramen, interver´tebral [foramen intervertebrale, NA]   opening between the pedicles of adjacent vertebrae on each side of the vertebral column. Through these spaces pass the spinal nerves, their coverings, and their associated blood vessels.

foramen, jug´ular [foramen jugulare, NA]   opening in the base of the skull between the occipital and temporal bones. The glossopharyngeal, vagal, and accessory nerves pass through its medial part, and the sigmoid sinus empties into the internal jugular vein through its lateral part.

foramen lacerum /las´er-um/ [NA]   gap in the dry bone in the base of the skull, medial to the foramen ovale, normally filled with fibrocartilage. The internal carotid artery passes over its intracranial surface toward the cavernous sinus.

foramen mag´num [NA]   large opening in the occipital bone at the base of the skull, through which the spinal cord is continuous with the brain, and through which also pass the spinal accessory nerves and the vertebral arteries and veins.

foramina nervo´sa [NA], EAR   series of small radial slits along the tympanic lip of the spiral limbus, through which small fascicles of cochlear nerve fibers pass to enter the spiral organ of the cochlea.

foramina, olfac´tory   *See* foramina cribrosa.

foramen, op´tic   *See* canal, optic.

foramen oval´e [NA]   opening in the sphenoid bone, in the base of the skull, for the mandibular division of the trigeminal nerve.

foramen proces´sus transver´si (vertebrarteriale) [NA]   *See* foramen, transverse.

foramen rotun´dum [NA]   opening in the sphenoid bone, in the base of the skull, for the maxillary division of the trigeminal nerve.

foramen singular´e [NA], ear   small opening in the wall of the internal auditory meatus for the nerve to the ampulla of the posterior semicircular duct.

foramen spino´sum [NA]   opening in the sphenoid bone, in the base of the skull, through which the middle meningeal artery enters the cranial cavity.

foramen, stylomas´toid [foramen stylomastoideum, NA]   opening in the temporal bone, just behind the styloid process, through which the facial nerve emerges from the skull.

foramen, transverse [foramen processus transversi (vertebrarteriale), NA]   opening in each of the transverse processes of cervical vertebrae 1-6, through which the vertebral artery, passes along with a plexus of small veins and sympathetic branches from the inferior cervical ganglion. *Syn:* foramen transversarium.

foramen, ver´tebral [foramen vertebrale, NA]   large opening in each of the vertebrae. It is surrounded by the body of the vertebra ventrally and the arches of the vertebra laterally and dorsally. Together the vertebral foramina constitute the vertebral canal.

foramen, vertebroarte´rial [foramen processus transversi, NA]   *See* foramen, transverse.

foram´ina   plural of *foramen.*

for´ceps, anterior, cerebrum, [L. *forceps* a pair of tongs]   *See* forceps minor.

forceps frontal´is [NA], cerebrum   *See* forceps minor.

forceps major (occipital´is) [NA], cerebrum   fibers of the corpus callosum which extend posteriorly into the occipital lobes. *Syn:* forceps posterior; occipital radiation.

forceps minor (frontalis) [NA], cerebrum   fibers of the corpus callosum which extend forward into the frontal lobes. *Syn:* forceps anterior; frontal radiation.

forceps occipitalis [NA], cerebrum   *See* forceps major.

forceps, posterior, cerebrum   *See* forceps major.

forebrain   cerebrum and diencephalon, taken together. It is the part of the brain derived from the prosencephalon, the most rostral subdivision of the embryonic brain.

Forel, August Henri (1848-1931)   Swiss neurologist of Zurich. The *commissure of Forel* is the supramamillary decussation; the *decussation of Forel* is the ventral tegmental decussation. The *fields of Forel* are areas located in the ventral thalamus of the diencephalon. The designation H, H_1, and H_2 for these fields stands for *Haubenregion,* the German word for tegmentum (Forel, 1877). The *H field of Forel* is the prerubral field containing dentatothalamic and rubrothalamic fibers and pallidothalamic fibers before they enter the thalamic fasciculus. The H_1 *field of Forel* is a narrow fiber zone between the dorsal thalamus and the zona incerta containing the thalamic fasciculus. The H_2 *field of Forel* is a narrow zone between the zona incerta and the subthalamic nucleus containing fibers of the lenticular fasciculus and the capsule of the subthalamic nucleus.

forma´tion, Am´mon's, CEREBRUM   *See* formation, hippocampal; hippocampus.

formation, hippocam´pal, CEREBRUM   complex of the hippocampus or cornu ammonis, dentate gyrus, and subiculum; archicortex. *See also* cornu ammonis; hippocampus.

formation, retic´ular [formatio (substantia) reticularis, NA], MAINLY BRAIN STEM, [L. *reticulum* small net, dim. of *rete*]   area in the tegmentum of the midbrain and pons and its continuation into the medulla and upper spinal cord, consisting of small groups of nerve cells interspersed among horizontally and vertically running nerve fibers, and excluding the cranial nerve nuclei and roots and the long fiber tracts.

fornix /for´niks/ [NA] [*pl.* **fornices** /for´nĭ-sēz/], FOREBRAIN, [L. arch]   bundle of fibers continuous with the fimbria, which arches over the diencephalon and downward into the hypothalamus. Most fibers descend posterior to the anterior commissure (postcommissural fornix) to end in the mamillary body. Some end in the anterior nucleus of the dorsal thalamus or join the stria medullaris thalami to end in the habenular nucleus. Others pass anterior to the anterior commissure (precommissural fornix) to end in the septal area and to some extent the anterior hypothalamic area. *See also* indusium griseum; striae, longitudinal; gyrus, fasciolar; nucleus, septohippocampal. The major parts of the fornix, from caudal to rostral, are as follows:

> **crus** [crus fornicis, NA]   the posterior part of the fornix, continuous with the fimbria. From the back of the hippocampus it arches upward and medially almost to meet its counterpart from the other side where some fibers cross the median plane in the hippocampal commissure (Fig. P-2). *Syn:* pillar, posterior pillar, or posterior column of the fornix.

> **body** [corpus fornicis, NA]   segment which passes forward and downward in the free edge of the septum pellucidum from the hippocampal commissure to a point just above the interventricular foramen and the anterior commissure. *Syn:* trunk of the fornix; subcallosal fornix.

> **genu**   segment which arches anterior to the interventricular foramen.

> **column** [columna fornicis, NA]   segment which turns backward and downward behind the anterior commissure into the hypothalamus to end mainly in the mamillary body. This segment divides the hypothalamus into medial and lateral areas. *Syn:* anterior column or anterior pillar of the fornix; postcommissural fornix.

fornix, dorsal, CEREBRUM   slender strands of fibers, arising from cells in the indusium griseum or possibly the cingulate cortex, that pass through the corpus callosum and join the column of the fornix. Sometimes this term is used as a synonym for fornix longus and sometimes to mean a part of it.

fornix long´us, MAINLY FOREBRAIN   slender strands of fibers that arise from cells in the indusium griseum, the cortex of the cingulate gyrus, and possibly other cortical areas. They may run for a variable distance in the longitudinal striae above the corpus callosum then pass through it and join the column of the fornix to enter the hypothalamus. They do not end in the mamillary body but cross, at least in part, in the supramamillary decussation and enter the tegmentum of the midbrain. Their termination in man is not known.

fornix peripher´icus, CEREBRUM   old term for cingulum.

fornix, postcommis´sural (postcommissu´ral) [columna fornicis, NA], FOREBRAIN   segment of the fornix which passes behind the anterior commissure into the hypothalamus.

fornix, precommis´sural (precommissu´ral), FOREBRAIN   fornix fibers which pass anterior to the anterior commissure to end in the septal and anterior hypothalamic areas.

fornix, subcallo´sal, CEREBRUM   *See* fornix, body.

fornix, superior, CEREBRUM   *See* stria, longitudinal, medial *and* lateral.

fornix transver´sus   *See* commissure, hippocampal.

fossa, cra´nial, anterior [fossa cranii anterior, NA] [L. *fossa* ditch]   depression on the floor of the cranial cavity, above the orbit and containing the frontal lobes of the cerebrum.

fossa, cranial, middle [fossa cranii media, NA]   depression on the floor of the cranial cavity, posterior to the greater wing of the sphenoid bone, and containing the temporal lobes of the cerebrum.

fossa, cranial, posterior [fossa cranii posterior, NA]   that part of the cranial cavity caudal to the tentorium cerebelli, and containing the medulla, pons, cerebellum, and part of the midbrain.

fossa, intercru´ral, MIDBRAIN   *See* fossa, interpeduncular.

fossa, interpedun´cular [fossa interpeduncularis, NA], MIDBRAIN   space on the anterior surface of the midbrain between the bases of the two cerebral peduncles (Fig. P-1). *Syn:* fossa of Tarini; intercrural fossa.

fossa, olfac´tory   depression in the anterior fossa of the cranial cavity, on either side of the crista galli. Its floor is the cribriform plate of the ethmoid bone, and it contains the olfactory bulb.

fossa, rhomboid /rom´boid/ [fossa rhomboidea, NA], PONS, MEDULLA   floor of the fourth ventricle (Fig. V-4).

fossa, Syl´vian, CEREBRUM   *See* Sylvius, Franciscus.

fossula /fos´u-lah/ [L. dim. of *fossa* ditch]   small depression.

fossula fenes´trae coch´leae [NA], EAR   small depression in the wall of the tympanic cavity adjacent to the round window.

fossula fenestrae vestib´uli [NA], EAR   relatively deep, narrow niche surrounding the footplate of the stapes in the oval window.

fo´vea central´is [NA], EYE, [L. *fovea* pit]   slight depression in the center of the macula lutea of the retina, containing only cones and no rods, and constituting the area of keenest vision.

fovea, inferior [fovea inferior (caudalis), NA], MEDULLA   shallow, angular depression in the sulcus limitans in the medullar part of the rhomboid fossa, at the junction of the vestibular area and the hypoglossal and vagal trigones (Fig. V-4).

fovea, superior [fovea superior (rostralis), NA], PONS   shallow, angular depression in the sulcus limitans above the facial colliculus, between the medial eminence and the vestibular area in the pontine part of the rhomboid fossa (Fig. V-4).

fove´ola [NA], EYE, [L. small pit, dim. of *fovea*]   small depression in the center of the fovea centralis of the retina.

Foville, Achille Louis (1799-1878)   French neurologist. *Foville's fasciculus* is the stria terminalis.

Foville, Achille Louis François (1831-1887)   French psychiatrist. *Foville's syndrome* consists of an ipsilateral paralysis of the facial muscles, an inability to turn the eyes toward the side of the lesion, and a contralateral hemiplegia, resulting from a unilateral paramedian lesion in the pons involving the genu of the facial nerve, the abducens nucleus, and the medial longitudinal fasciculus dorsally, and the corticospinal tract ventrally.

FRA   flexor reflex afferents.

Frankenhäuser, Ferdinand (1832-1894)   German gynecologist. *Frankenhäuser's ganglion* is a cluster of parasympathetic ganglion cells in the uterovaginal plexus.

fren´ulum ve´li medullar´is rostral´is (superius) [NA], MIDBRAIN, [L. *frenulum* small bridle]   narrow median band extending rostrally from the anterior medullary velum into the tectum between the two inferior colliculi.

Freud, Sigmund (1856-1939)   Viennese neurologist and psychiatrist, the founder of psychoanalysis. He stressed the importance of the subconscious and believed that neuroses resulted from the suppression of some psychic trauma, especially of a sexual nature. His views remain controversial.

Friedemann, Max   German neurologist, active at the University of Berlin in 1912. The *semilunar nucleus of Friedemann* is the ventral posteromedial nucleus of the dorsal thalamus.

Friedreich, Nikolaus (1825-1882)   German neurologist and neuropathologist of Würzburg and Heidelberg. *Friedreich's ataxia* (1875) is a familial spinal ataxia, with an associated loss of sense of position, usually inherited as an autosomal recessive. There is progressive degeneration of the fibers of the gracile and cuneate fasciculi and the spinocerebellar tracts and sometimes also the outer fibers of the lateral corticospinal tracts.

Fritsch, Gustav Theodor (1838-1927)   German zoologist who, with Hitzig, used a weak electrical current to explore the cerebral cortex of the dog. They were able to demonstrate discrete movements, the first definitive work on cerebral localization.

fron´tal [L. *frons* forehead]   **1.** CEREBRUM   pertaining to the frontal lobe or its cortex. **2.** *See also* section, frontal.

Froriep, August von (1849-1917)   German anatomist. *Froriep's ganglion* is a small ganglion on the hypoglossal nerve, present in the embryo but absent in the adult.

-fu´gal   suffix denoting efferent conduction from the region indicated.

fun´dus mea´tus acu´stici inter´ni [NA], EAR   thin plate of bone that separates the internal acoustic meatus from the cochlea and vestibule, at which point the facial nerve enters the facial canal.

fundus oc´uli, EYE   retinal surface of the eyeball, visible through the pupil.

funiculus /fu-nik´u-lus/ [NA] [L. dim. of *funis* cord], CORD   one of the large masses of white matter of the spinal cord, set off by the dorsal and ventral horns of the gray matter, the dorsal median septum, and the ventral median fissure.

funiculus, anterior [funiculus ventralis (anterior), NA], CORD   *See* funiculus, ventral.

funiculus cunea´tus, MEDULLA, CORD   *See* fasciculus cuneatus.

funiculus, dorsal [funiculus dorsalis (posterior), NA], MEDULLA, CORD   white matter on each side of the spinal cord, between the dorsal median septum and the dorsal horn and continuing rostrally into the closed medulla. It is composed mainly of the fasciculus gracilis and fasciculus cuneatus (Figs. B-2, T-3). *Syn:* dorsal (posterior) column.

funiculus gracilis /gras´il-is/, MEDULLA, CORD   *See* fasciculus gracilis.

funiculus, lateral [funiculus lateralis, NA], MEDULLA, CORD   white matter on each side of the spinal cord, between the dorsal and ventral horns, and continuing rostrally into the medulla. *Syn:* lateral column.

funiculus, posterior [funiculus dorsalis (posterior), NA], MEDULLA, CORD   *See* funiculus, dorsal.

funiculus sep´arans [NA], MEDULLA   band of thickened ependyma and neuroglial tissue between the vagal trigone and the area postrema in the caudal part of the rhomboid fossa (Fig. V-4).

funiculus ter´es, PONS   *See* eminence, medial.

funiculus, ventral (anterior) [funiculus ventralis (anterior) [NA], CORD   white matter on each side of the spinal cord, between the ventral median fissure and the ventral horn. *Syn:* ventral (anterior) column.

Fuse, G. (20th century)   the *nucleus of Fuse* is the parabducens nucleus.

fusimotor /fu-zī-mo´tor/ [L. *fusus* spindle]   pertaining to the gamma motor neurons which innervate the intrafusal muscle fibers of a neuromuscular spindle.

fu´sus neuromuscular´is [NA]   *See* spindle, neuromuscular.

fusus neurotendine´us [NA]   *See* spindle, neurotendinous.

g

GABA   gamma-aminobutyric acid.

Gabelzellen, CEREBRUM   large, modified pyramidal cells of the auditory cortex. They have a broad base and a relatively short vertical diameter.

GAD   glutamic acid decarboxylase.

Galen, Claudius (ca. 131-201 AD)   Greek physician who practiced in Rome. He was the leading medical authority of the Christian world for 1400 years. He described many parts of the brain. The *vein* (or *great vein) of Galen* is the great cerebral vein. The *lesser* (or *small*) *vein of Galen* is the internal cerebral vein.

Gall, Franz Joseph (1758-1828)   German anatomist. Although he made a number of real contributions to knowledge of the brain, he is best known as the founder of phrenology, which was later discredited as a science.

gamma-aminobutyr´ic acid (GABA)   the most important inhibitory neurotransmitter in the CNS. In particular, it is the neurotransmitter whereby the neurons of the caudate nucleus and putamen inhibit the globus pallidus and pars reticulata of the substantia nigra, and the Purkinje cells inhibit the cerebellar nuclei. *See also* neurotransmitters.

gam´ma ef´ferent   pertaining to the small cells of the ventral horn which supply the intrafusal fibers of neuromuscular spindles. *See also* loop, gamma.

gang´lion [*pl.* **ganglia;** *adj.* **ganglion´ic**] [Gr. swelling]   **1.** [NA] any group of sensory or autonomic nerve cell bodies located outside the CNS.
2. formerly any group of nerve cells, inside or outside the CNS. Sometimes *ganglion cell* is still used as a synonym for any nerve cell body, and the cell masses within the cerebrum are still commonly called *basal ganglia*.

ganglia, aorticore´nal [ganglia aorticorenalia (renalia), NA]   prevertebral, sympathetic ganglia near the origin of each renal artery. They receive preganglionic fibers, mostly from the least splanchnic nerve, and send postganglionic fibers to the kidney and adjoining structures.

ganglion, auric´ular   *See* ganglion, otic.

ganglia, ba´sal [nuclei basales, NA], CEREBRUM   subcortical masses of gray matter of the cerebrum, classically comprising the caudate nucleus, putamen, globus pallidus, amygdala, and claustrum. Sometimes this term is limited to the corpus striatum, i.e., the caudate nucleus, putamen, and globus pallidus, important for their role in the control of movement. *For additional information, see* Alheid and Heimer ('90).

ganglion, basal op´tic, HYPOTHALAMUS   old term for the supraoptic nucleus.

ganglia, car´diac [ganglia cardiaca, NA]   small parasympathetic ganglia in the superficial cardiac plexus below the arch of the aorta. They receive preganglionic fibers from the left inferior cardiac branch of the vagus nerve and supply postganglionic fibers to the heart and coronary arteries. They are concerned with slowing the heart and constricting the coronary arteries. *Syn:* ganglion of Wrisberg.

ganglion, carot´id   small ganglionic swelling in the internal carotid plexus on the underside of the carotid artery in the cavernous sinus. *Syn:* Bock's or Laumonier's ganglion.

ganglion caudal´is [NA]   *See* ganglion, inferior (of the glossopharyngeal and vagus nerves).

ganglia, ce´liac [ganglia celiaca (coeliaca), NA]   relatively large prevertebral, sympathetic ganglia in the celiac plexus on either side of the celiac artery. The cells receive preganglionic fibers from the thoracic splanchnic nerves and send postganglionic fibers to the stomach, duodenum, liver, spleen, and pancreas (Fig. S-3). *Syn:* ganglion solare; Vieussens' ganglion.

ganglion cell   *See* cell, ganglion.

ganglia, central   collective term sometimes used for the dorsal thalamus and basal ganglia combined.

ganglion, cer´vical, inferior   most caudal of the cervical sympathetic ganglia. It is usually fused with the first (and sometimes also the second) thoracic chain ganglion to form the stellate ganglion.

ganglion, cervical, middle [ganglion cervicale medium, NA]   smallest and most variable of the cervical sympathetic ganglia. When present it is usually located in the middle to lower third of the neck, but it is frequently absent.

ganglion, cervical, superior [ganglion cervicale superius, NA]   most rostral ganglion of the sympathetic trunk. It receives preganglionic fibers from the lateral horn of the uppermost thoracic spinal cord segments. Its postganglionic fibers are distributed mainly via: (1) the internal carotid plexus to structures within the orbit, including the lacrimal gland, the dilator muscle of the pupil, and the smooth muscle of the upper eyelid (Fig. R-3); (2) the external carotid plexus to the salivary glands (Fig. C-4); (3) the upper cervical nerves for the sweat glands, cutaneous blood vessels, and smooth muscle of the hair follicles of the face, neck, and upper shoulder; and (4) a small cervical cardiac nerve to the heart (Fig. S-3).

ganglion, cervicodor´sal   *See* ganglion, stellate.

ganglion, cervicothorac´ic [ganglion cervicothoracicum (stellatum), NA]   *See* ganglion, stellate.

ganglia, chain   *See* ganglia (of the) sympathetic trunk.

ganglion, ciliary /sil´ī-ar-ī/ [ganglion ciliare, NA]   parasympathetic ganglion of the oculomotor nerve (Fig. S-3), located in the posterior part of the orbit between the lateral rectus muscle and the optic nerve. It receives preganglionic fibers from the

Edinger-Westphal (accessory oculomotor) nucleus of the oculomotor nerve and supplies postganglionic fibers for the ciliary muscle (Fig. R-2) and for the constrictor muscle of the iris (Fig. R-7). *See also* Table C-3.

ganglion, coccygeal /kok-sĭ-je´al/ *See* ganglion impar.

ganglion, coch´lear, EAR *See* ganglion, spiral.

ganglia, coeliac /se´lĭ-ak/ *See* ganglia, celiac.

ganglia, collat´eral *See* ganglia, prevertebral.

ganglia, cranial parasympathetic terminal ganglia located in the head (Fig. S-3), including the ciliary and episcleral ganglia of nerve III (Figs. R-2, R-7), the pterygopalatine (Fig. R-6), submandibular, and Langley's ganglia of nerve VII (Fig. C-4), and the otic ganglion of nerve IX. *See also* Tables C-1, C-2, C-3.

ganglion, dorsal root *See* ganglion, spinal.

ganglion, episcler´al parasympathetic ganglion of the oculomotor nerve, located on the sclera of each eye. It receives preganglionic fibers from the Edinger-Westphal (accessory oculomotor) nucleus and sends postganglionic fibers to the constrictor muscle of the iris. It is said to be concerned with pupillary constriction in accommodation (Fig. R-2). *See also* Table C-3.

ganglion, genic´ulate [ganglion geniculi (geniculatum), NA] sensory ganglion of the facial nerve. It is located at the bend of the facial nerve in the facial canal and consists of unipolar cell bodies. *See* Table C-2.

ganglion, haben´ular, EPITHALAMUS *See* habenula.

ganglion im´par [NA] [L. *impar* unequal, having no fellow, hence single] inconstant, unpaired sympathetic ganglion located in the pelvis at the junction of the two sympathetic trunks, anterior to the coccyx. *Syn:* coccygeal ganglion.

ganglion, inferior [ganglion inferius (caudalis), NA] **1.** visceral afferent ganglion of the glossopharyngeal nerve, located in the lower part of the jugular foramen, in a notch on the underside of the petrous part of the temporal bone. It contains the unipolar cell bodies of fibers from the carotid body and sinus, and taste fibers from the posterior third of the tongue. It is larger than the superior ganglion of nerve IX, which may be fused with it. *Syn:* petrosal ganglion; ganglion of Andersch. *See also* Table C-1.
2. visceral afferent ganglion of the vagus nerve, located in the jugular foramen below the superior ganglion of the vagus. It contains the unipolar cell bodies of fibers from the pharynx, larynx, trachea, and esophagus and all the organs in the thorax and abdomen which receive vagal autonomic fibers. It also contains the cell bodies of some taste fibers from the region of the epiglottis. *Syn:* nodose ganglion. *See also* reflexes, vagal, Fig. R-9 *and* Table C-1.

ganglion intercarot´icum *See* body, carotid.

ganglion, jug´ular somatic afferent ganglion of the vagus nerve. *See* ganglion, superior, *def.* 2.

ganglion, juxtava´gal nonchromaffin paraganglion next to the inferior ganglion of the vagus nerve. *Syn:* intravagal paraganglion.

ganglion, Langley's *See* Langley.

ganglion, mesenter´ic, inferior [ganglion mesentericum inferius, NA] prevertebral sympathetic ganglion near the origin of the inferior mesenteric artery. It receives preganglionic fibers from cord segments L1-L3 by way of the lumbar splanchnic nerves and sends postganglionic fibers to the descending and sigmoid colon and some pelvic organs (Fig. S-3).

ganglion, mesenteric, superior [ganglion mesentericum superius, NA] prevertebral sympathetic ganglion near the origin of the superior mesenteric artery. It receives preganglionic fibers from the more caudal segments of the thoracic cord, by way of the thoracic splanchnic nerves, and sends postganglionic fibers to the small intestine and to the ascending and the transverse colon (Fig. S-3).

ganglion, nodose /no-dōs/ [L. *nodus* a knot]   visceral afferent ganglion of the vagus nerve. *See* ganglion, inferior, *def.* 2.

ganglion, o´tic [ganglion oticum, NA]   parasympathetic ganglion of the glosso-pharyngeal nerve, located just outside the skull medial to the mandibular nerve. It receives preganglionic fibers from the lesser petrosal nerve and provides postganglionic fibers for the parotid gland by way of the auriculotemporal nerve. *Syn:* Arnold's ganglion; auricular ganglion. *See also* Table C-1.

ganglia, paraver´tebral   *See* ganglia (of the) sympathetic trunk.

ganglia, pel´vic [ganglia pelvica, NA]   terminal ganglia near or in the walls of the pelvic organs. For the most part they receive preganglionic parasympathetic fibers from spinal cord segments S2-S4 by way of the pelvic splanchnic nerves, but may also receive some sympathetic preganglionic fibers. Postganglionic fibers from these ganglia distribute to the organs of the pelvis (Fig. S-3).

ganglion, petro´sal (petrous) [Gr. *petra* rock]   visceral afferent ganglion of the glossopharyngeal nerve. *See* ganglion, inferior, *def.* 1.

ganglion, petrosal, superior   somatic afferent ganglion of the glossopharyngeal nerve. *See* ganglion, superior, *def.* 1.

ganglia, prever´tebral   sympathetic ganglia located near the origin of one of the major abdominal arteries, *viz.* the celiac, superior mesenteric, inferior mesenteric, and aorticorenal ganglia. To reach these ganglia, preganglionic fibers arise from the thoracic and lumbar spinal cord, pass through the sympathetic trunk without synapse, then pass through one of the splanchnic nerves. Postganglionic sympathetic fibers supply organs of the abdomen and pelvis (Fig. S-3). *Syn:* collateral ganglia. *See also* trunk, sympathetic; system, nervous, autonomic.

ganglion, pterygopalatine /ter-ig-o-pal´at-ĕn/ [ganglion pterygopalatinum, NA] parasympathetic ganglion of the facial nerve, located in the pterygopalatine fossa. Although it is attached to the maxillary nerve by way of its pterygopalatine branches, its preganglionic fibers come from the greater petrosal branch of the facial nerve. It supplies postganglionic fibers for the lacrimal (Fig. R-6), nasal, and palatine glands by way of branches of the maxillary nerve. *Syn:* sphenopalatine ganglion; Meckel's ganglion. *See also* Table C-2.

ganglia, re´nal [ganglia renalia, NA]   *See* ganglia, aorticorenal.

ganglion rostral´is [NA]   *See* ganglion, superior.

ganglion, semilunar /sem-ĭ-loo´nar/   sensory ganglion of the trigeminal nerve. *See* ganglion, trigeminal.

ganglion, so´lar [ganglion solare]   *See* ganglion, celiac.

ganglion, sphenopalatine /sfe-no-pal´at-ĕn/   *See* ganglion, pterygopalatine.

ganglia, spinal [ganglia spinalia, NA]   ganglia on the dorsal roots of spinal nerves, containing unipolar cells of origin for sensory neurons of spinal nerves. *Syn:* dorsal root ganglia.

ganglion, spiral [ganglion spirale, NA]   somatic afferent (exteroceptive) ganglion of the cochlear nerve (Fig. R-8), located in the modiolus of the cochlea and composed of bipolar cell bodies. *Syn:* ganglion of Corti; cochlear ganglion. *See* Table C-2.

ganglion, stel´late (cervicothoracic) [ganglion stellatum (cervicothoracicum), NA] fused inferior cervical, first thoracic, and occasionally second thoracic ganglia of the sympathetic trunk, or the inferior cervical ganglion alone. *Syn:* cervicodorsal ganglion.

ganglion, subling´ual [ganglion sublinguale, NA]   small cluster of parasympathetic ganglion cells, sometimes located just anterior to the submandibular ganglion and apparently a displaced part of it. Like the submandibular ganglion, it supplies the sublingual gland.

ganglion, submandib´ular [ganglion submandibulare, NA]   parasympathetic ganglion of the facial nerve. It is located on the hypoglossus muscle near the posterior border of the mylohyoid muscle and is suspended from the lingual nerve by two short roots. It receives preganglionic fibers from the chorda tympani branch of the facial nerve and supplies postganglionic fibers for the sublingual gland (Fig. C-4). *Syn:* submaxillary ganglion. *See also* Langley for Langley's ganglion; nerve, facial; chorda tympani; Table C-2.

ganglion, submax´illary   *See* ganglion, submandibular.

ganglion, superior [ganglion superius (rostralis), NA]   **1.** somatic afferent ganglion of the glossopharyngeal nerve, located in the upper part of the jugular foramen, just above and sometimes fused with the inferior ganglion. It contains the unipolar cell bodies of afferent fibers from the posterior third of the tongue, the posterior part of the soft palate, the tonsil and faucial pillars, and the pharynx from the auditory tube to the epiglottis (Fig. O-2). *Syn:* superior petrosal ganglion; ganglion of Ehrenritter. *See* Table C-1.
2. small, somatic afferent ganglion of the vagus nerve, located in the jugular foramen posterior to the glossopharyngeal nerve. It contains the unipolar cell bodies of afferent fibers from part of the external ear and from part of the tympanic membrane (Fig. O-2). *Syn:* jugular ganglion. *See* Table C-1.

ganglia, sympathetic chain   *See* ganglia (of the) sympathetic trunk.

ganglia (of the) sympathetic trunk [ganglia trunci sympathici, NA]   series of ganglia in the sympathetic trunk, located along the sides of the vertebral column and belonging to the sympathetic division of the ANS. They contain the cell bodies of the postganglionic sympathetic fibers to skin viscera and to visceral structures in the head and in the thorax. (Fig. S-3.) *Syn:* paravertebral ganglia; chain ganglia. *See also* ganglia, prevertebral.

ganglion, ter´minal [ganglion terminale, NA]   any parasympathetic ganglion located in or near the organ innervated. The most important are: the cranial parasympathetic ganglia *viz.* the ciliary (III nerve), pterygopalatine and submandibular (VII nerve), and otic (IX nerve) ganglia; and the ganglia on or within the walls of the thoracic and abdominal viscera (X nerve and sacral 2-4) (Fig. S-3).

ganglion, trigem´inal [ganglion trigeminale, NA]   somatic afferent ganglion of the trigeminal nerve, located in a pocket of the dura mater, cavum trigeminale, in the lower part of the lateral wall of the cavernous sinus. It is the only ganglion located within the cranial cavity. It contains the unipolar cell bodies of somatic sensory (exteroceptive) fibers from the face (except the angle of the jaw) and from most of the oral cavity (Figs. O-2, R-3, R-4, R-6). *Syn:* semilunar ganglion; Gasserian ganglion. *See also* reflexes, vagal, Fig. R-9 *and* Table C-2.

ganglia trunci sympathici [NA]   *See* ganglia (of the) sympathetic trunk.

ganglion, ver´tebral [ganglion vertebrale, NA]   small sympathetic ganglion on or near the vertebral artery as it begins its ascent through the transverse foramina of the cervical vertebrae. Usually regarded as a detached part of the middle cervical or stellate ganglion, it supplies postganglionic fibers for the vertebral artery and its branches.

ganglion, vestib´ular [ganglion vestibulare, NA]   somatic afferent (proprioceptive) ganglion of the vestibular nerve, located in the internal auditory meatus of the temporal bone. It contains bipolar cell bodies and consists of two parts, a superior part for innervation of the horizontal and superior semicircular ducts, the utricle and, part of the saccule, and an inferior part for innervation of the posterior semicircular duct and most of the saccule. *Syn:* Scarpa's ganglion. *See also* Table C-2.

Ganser, Siebert J.M. (1853-1931)   German psychiatrist. The *commissure of Ganser* is the dorsal supraoptic decussation. The *nucleus of Ganser* is the basal nucleus of the substantia innominata, usually called the basal nucleus of Meynert.

gap, synap´tic   *See* cleft, synaptic.

Gasser, Herbert Spencer (1888-1963)   American neurophysiologist, pupil and later a colleague of J. Erlanger's, with whom he shared the Nobel Prize in medicine and physiology in 1944 for their work on individual nerve fibers.

Gasser, Johann Laurentius (1702-1777)   Austrian anatomist of Vienna. The trigeminal ganglion, the sensory ganglion of the trigeminal nerve, was originally named the *Gasserian ganglion* in his honor (1765) by Antonius Hirsch, one of his students.

gate-control theory of pain   according to this theory, activation of the small myelinated (A-delta) and unmyelinated (C) fibers of the dorsal root causes depolarization of the T-cells (transmission cells) of the dorsal horn, whereas activation of the larger afferent fibers, both dorsal root fibers and descending fibers from higher centers, causes presynaptic inhibition of these neurons. The T-cells are concerned with the onward transmission of impulses. The substantia gelatinosa, an intermediary between the afferent fibers and the T-cells, serves as a gate-control system which tends to determine the input from the periphery. When the input from the periphery is great enough, pain occurs. Spontaneous activity of the small afferent fibers, according to this theory, underlies spontaneous pain when it occurs, and also serves to "keep the gate open" (Melzack and Wall, '65). *For a review of this subject, see* Nathan ('76).

Gehrig, Lou (1903-1941)   American baseball player who became afflicted with amyotrophic lateral sclerosis. After his death the disease became popularly known as Lou Gehrig's disease.

gemmules, dendrit´ic /jem´ūlz/ [gemmula (spinula) dendritica, NA] [L. *gemmula* small bud]   *See* spines, dendritic.

general somat´ic af´ferent (sensory) (GSA, GSS)   *See* component, nerve.

general somatic ef´ferent (motor) (GSE, GSM)   *See* component, nerve, somatic efferent.

general visceral afferent (sensory) (GVA, GVS)   *See* component, nerve.

general visceral efferent (motor) (GVE, GVM)   *See* component, nerve.

geniculate /jen-ik´u-lāt/ [L. *geniculare* to bend the knee]   *For* geniculate ganglion *and* the lateral and medial geniculate body and nucleus, *see the nouns.*

geniculum (of the) facial nerve /jen-ik´u-lum/ [geniculum nervi facialis, NA] [L. dim. of *genu* knee]   sharp bend of the facial nerve within the facial canal at the point where the facial canal bends sharply backward. *Syn:* external genu of the facial nerve.

Gennari, Francisco (1752-1797)   Italian physician of Parma who recognized the macroscopic stripe in the occipital lobe cortex, the *line* or *stripe of Gennari*, or visual stria, as early as 1776 and described it in 1782. These fibers, in layer IV of area 17, constitute a well-developed outer stripe of Baillarger in the visual cortex and are mostly the terminal parts of optic radiation fibers with, perhaps, some additional association fibers.

genu /je ´nu/ [*pl.* **genus, genua**; *adj.* **geniculate**] [L. knee]   term used with respect to any of several structures which exhibit a bend, as the genus of the corpus callosum, the internal capsule, and the facial nerve. *See also* knee.

genu, internal (of the facial nerve), PONS   sharp bend of the motor root of the nerve over the rostral end of the abducens nucleus in the facial colliculus of the pons.

genu, external (of the facial nerve)   *See* geniculum.

Gerstmann, Josef (1887-1969)   Viennese neurologist, later a resident of the United States. *Gerstmann's syndrome* is a neurologic disorder consisting of: finger agnosia (difficulty in naming or identifying the fingers), dysgraphia (inability to write), dyscalculia (loss of ability to perform arithmetical calculations), and right-left confusion. It is attributed to a lesion of the left angular gyrus. *For additional information, see* Critchley ('66).

Giacomini, Carlo (1840-1898)   Italian anatomist. *Giacomini's band* or *frenulum* (1878) is a gray band at the anterior end of the dentate gyrus next to the inferior surface of the uncus.

Gibbs, Erna Lenhardt (b. 1904) and **Frederic Andrews Gibbs** (b. 1903)   American neuropathologists. The *sinus of Gibbs* is the tentorial sinus.

Gierke, Hans Paul Bernard (1847-1886)   German anatomist. *Gierke's respiratory bundle* is the fasciculus solitarius.

gland, pine ´al [glandula pinealis, NA]   *See* body, pineal.

gland, pitu ´itary [glandula pituitaria, NA]   *See* hypophysis.

glaucoma /glaw-ko ´mah/   eye disorder characterized by excessive intraocular pressure.

glia /gle ´ah/ [Gr. glue]   shortened form used as a synonym for neuroglia.

glia limitans /lim ´it-anz/ [membrana limitans, NA]   *See* membrane, limiting.

glia, ra ´dial   elongated, cylindrical glial cells which span the full thickness of the developing cerebral wall. They are thought to provide guide lines along which young nerve cells migrate from the ventricular or subventricular zone to a more superficial position in the cerebral plate (Rakic, '72).

gliosomes /gle ´o-sōmz/ [Gr. *glia; soma* body]   granules present in the cytoplasm of astrocytes.

glo ´bus pal ´lidus [NA] [L. *globus* ball or globe; *pallidus* pale], CEREBRUM   one of the basal ganglia, the medial part of the lentiform nucleus (Fig. C-1), separated from the putamen by an external medullary lamina. It is subdivided by an internal medullary lamina into an outer segment (globus pallidus lateralis, NA; pallidus II) and an inner segment (globus pallidus medialis, NA; pallidus I). The inner segment, in turn, is partially subdivided by an accessory medullary lamina. Ansa lenticularis fibers arise from the outer part of the inner segment, lateral to the accessory medullary lamina. Lenticular fasciculus fibers arise from the inner part of the inner segment, medial to the accessory medullary lamina. Efferent fibers in the subthalamic fasciculus arise from the outer segment of the globus pallidus and afferent fibers terminate in both the outer and inner segments. Although it is regarded as a part of the cerebrum, there is now evidence that suggests that the globus pallidus is derived from the embryonic diencephalon, rather than the telencephalon, as formerly thought (Richter, '65). *Syn:* pallidum or dorsal pallidum; paleostriatum.

glomer´ulus [NA] [L. *glomerulus* little ball]   synaptic complex consisting of one or more axon terminals and the dendritic terminals with which they synapse. Such structures are found in a number of places in the CNS, including the olfactory bulbs and the cerebellar cortex.

glomerulus, cerebel´lar, CEREBELLUM   synaptic formation in a cerebellar island in the granular layer of the cerebellar cortex. Such structures consist of axon terminals of mossy fibers and Golgi cells, and the claw-like dendritic terminals of the granule cells with which they synapse (Fig. C-9).

glomeruli, olfac´tory, CEREBRUM   spherical structures in the superficial part of the olfactory bulb. They are composed of the terminal parts of olfactory nerve axons and the mitral cell dendrites with which they synapse.

glo´mus [NA] [L. *glomus* ball]   *See also* paraganglion.

glomus aor´ticum [NA]   *See* body, aortic.

glomus carot´icum [NA]   *See* body, carotid.

glomus choroideum /kor-oid´e-um/ [NA]   expanded portion of the choroid plexus in the collateral trigone of the lateral ventricle.

glomus jugular´e   nonchromaffin paraganglion, located in the wall of the jugular bulb. The most common tumors of the middle ear arise from this tissue.

glu´tamate (glutamic acid) (Glu)   neurotransmitter abundant throughout the CNS. It is synthesized from glutamine and has many metabolic functions, including that of precursor to the inhibitory neurotransmitter, GABA. However, Glu and the closely related compound, aspartate, are the leading excitatory transmitters of the CNS, especially for corticostriate fibers, parallel and climbing fibers of the cerebellum, and various hippocampal connections. *See also* neurotransmitters.

glutamic acid decarboxylase (GAD)   enzyme that synthesizes GABA and is localized mainly in inhibitory neurons that release GABA. *See also* neurotransmitters.

gly´cine (Gly)   inhibitory neurotransmitter, occurring mainly in the spinal cord as the transmitter for interneurons. *See also* neurotransmitters.

Golgi, Camillo (1843-1926)   Italian anatomist and pathologist. He introduced the silver chromate technique for nerve cells (1873) and described many features of silver-stained material, including the neurotendinous spindle *(Golgi tendon organ,* 1880), the reticular apparatus *(Golgi apparatus,* 1898) and *Golgi type I* and *type II cells* (1886). A *Golgi type I cell* (neuronum multipolare longiaxonicum, NA) is a neuron having a large cell body and a long axon which leaves the area of which the cell body is a part. A *Golgi type II cell* (neuronum multipolare breviaxonicum, NA) is a neuron having a small cell body and a short axon which terminates in the nearby gray matter. Internuncial neurons present throughout the CNS, stellate cells of the cerebral and cerebellar cortices, and the granule cells of the cerebellum are examples of this kind of cell. The so-called *Golgi cell* (neuronum stellatum magnum, NA) of the cerebellum is a neuron with a small cell body in the outer part of the granular layer. The dendrites of such cells branch profusely in the molecular layer; the axons branch in the underlying granular layer immediately beneath the spread of the dendrites and terminate in the cerebellar glomeruli, where they are inhibitory in function (Fig. C-9). The *Golgi-Mazzoni corpuscle* is a small, somewhat spherical nerve ending with a relatively thin capsule containing a coiled nerve fiber and thought to be a pressure receptor. In 1906 Golgi shared the Nobel Prize in medicine and physiology with

Ramón y Cajal. *See also* cells, stellate.

Goll, Friedrich (1829-1903)   Swiss anatomist. The *column of Goll* (1860) is the fasciculus gracilis. The *nucleus of Goll* is the nucleus gracilis.

Gombault, François Alexis Albert (1844-1904)   French physician who described the sacral part of the septomarginal fasciculus, which was also described by Philippe and then known as the *triangle of Gombault-Philippe*.

Gordon, Alfred (1874-1953)   American neurologist. *Gordon's sign* is dorsiflexion of the great toe in response to squeezing the muscles of the leg and is indicative of injury to the corticospinal tract. *See also* Babinski.

Gowers, Sir William Richard (1845-1915)   English physician who published notable descriptions of many neurologic disorders. He was one of the first to recognize the usefulness of the ophthalmoscope and to describe retinal findings in a number of diseases. *Gowers' tract* usually refers to the ventral spinocerebellar tract, which he described in 1880, but the term has also been applied to the spinothalamic fibers and sometimes to the entire complex of ascending tracts in the anterolateral quadrant of the spinal cord.

gracilis /gras´il-is/ [L. slender]   *See* fasciculus gracilis; nucleus gracilis.

Granit, Ragnar Arthur (b. 1900)   Finnish neurophysiologist, noted especially for his work on the visual system, including the excitatory and inhibitory processes of the retina and its "on/off" cells. In 1967 he was awarded the Nobel Prize in medicine and physiology with H.K. Hartline and G. Wald.

granula´tions, arachnoid /ar-ak´noid/ [granulationes arachnoideales, NA]   clusters of arachnoid villi, located mainly in lacunae of the superior longitudinal sinus, through which cerebrospinal fluid enters the venous system.

granules, chromatophil´ic   *See* substance, chromatophilic.

granules, ti´groid   *See* substance, chromatophilic.

Gratiolet, Louis Pierre (1815-1865)   French anatomist and zoologist. *Gratiolet's optic radiation* is the optic radiation, sometimes also including the ansa pedunculaaris. The *convolutions of Gratiolet* are small convolutions buried beneath the lateral surface of the occipital lobe. The *canal of Gratiolet* is the channel in the brain which contains the anterior commissure.

gray   pertaining to CNS tissue composed mostly of nerve cells and few myelinated fibers. In the United States and Canada *gray* is usually the preferred spelling. In Great Britain *grey* is usually preferred. *See also* nucleus; matter, gray.

gray, central   cellular area around the cerebral aqueduct (periaqueductal gray) of the midbrain, or around the central canal, especially that of the closed medulla.

gray, dorsal funicular, cord   *See* nucleus proprius.

gray, dorsal visceral, mainly medulla   subdivision of the nucleus solitarius located just dorsomedial to the fasciculus solitarius and best developed at the level of the entering glossopharyngeal nerve fibers. It is a receptive nucleus for incoming gustatory fibers of the facial, glossopharyngeal, and vagal nerves. From it secondary fibers cross the median plane, join the medial lemniscus, and terminate partly in the dorsal thalamus. *Syn:* dorsal nucleus of the fasciculus solitarius; gustatory nucleus; dorsal sensory nucleus. *See* Table C-1.

gray, parahypoglos´sal, mainly medulla   *See* nuclei, parahypoglossal.

gray, parasol´itary, mainly medulla   *See* nucleus parasolitarius.

gray, periaqueductal /per-ĭ-ak-wĕ-duk´tal/, midbrain   cellular area surrounding the cerebral aqueduct of the midbrain. This area, rich in enkephalins and opiate receptors, is concerned with pain inhibition. Lesions are known to result in akinetic mutism. In cats, stimulation of this area has been shown to produce defense reactions and aggressive behavior, and lesions have been shown either to eliminate or attenuate these reactions. *Syn:* anulus of the aqueduct.

gray, perihypoglos´sal, MEDULLA   *See* nuclei, parahypoglossal.

gray, periventric´ular, HYPOTHALAMUS   *See* nucleus, periventricular, posterior.

gray, retic´ular, lateral, MEDULLA   *See* nucleus, reticular, lateral.

gray, reticular, medial, MEDULLA   diffusely arranged cells in the medial part of the reticular formation of the medulla oblongata. Among its connections are fibers to and from the cerebellum and descending fibers to the spinal cord via the medial, lateral, and ventrolateral reticulospinal tracts. *Syn:* medial reticular nucleus.

gray, pon´tine   *See* nuclei, pontine.

gray, sec´ondary visc´eral, CORD   *See* substance, visceral, secondary.

gray, sublenticular, CEREBRUM   cellular area ventral to the lentiform nucleus, the dorsal portion of the substantia innominata. The medial part underlying the globus pallidus is the ventral pallidum; the lateral part underlying the putamen is the ventral striatum. *Syn:* substriatal gray.

gray, subru´bral, MIDBRAIN   tegmental gray of the midbrain, located caudal and ventral to the red nucleus.

gray, substriatal, CEREBRUM   *See* gray, sublenticular.

gray, tegmen´tal, deep, MIDBRAIN   *See* nucleus, mesencephalic, deep.

gray, trap´ezoid, PONS   cells of the trapezoid body, in the ventral and caudal part of the pontine tegmentum. They receive fibers from the ventral cochlear nucleus and their axons (trapezoid fibers) enter the lateral lemniscus.

Greenfield, Joseph Godwin (1884-1958)   British neuropathologist, born in Scotland, for many years at the National Hospital at Queen Square in London. His interests covered a wide range of disorders, including encephalitis, spinocerebellar degeneration, and diffuse sclerosis. The textbook, *Neuropathology,* of which he was the senior author, was published in 1958, after his death.

grey   *See* gray.

groove, neur´al   groove formed by the buckling of the neural plate. When the neural folds on either side thicken and their dorsal parts fuse, the neural groove becomes the neural tube.

ground bundle, CORD   *See* fasciculus proprius.

GSA   general somatic afferent.

GSE   general somatic efferent.

GSM   general somatic motor.

GSS   general somatic sensory.

Gudden, Johannes Bernhard Aloys von (1824-1886)   German neurologist and psychiatrist, active in Zurich. *Gudden's commissure* is the intrachiasmatic decussation. *Gudden's tract* is the mamillotegmental tract. The *nucleus of Gudden* is the dorsal tegmental nucleus, and *Gudden's ganglion* is the interpeduncular nucleus. *Gudden's atrophy* is retrograde degeneration of the dorsal thalamus after destruction of certain cortical areas.

Guidi, Guido   *See* Vidius, Vidus.

Guillain, Georges (1876-1961)   French neurologist. The *Guillain-Barré syndrome,* also named for Jean Alexandre Barré and sometimes also called the *Landry-Guillain-Barré syndrome,* is an acute idiopathic polyneuritis, characterized by muscle weakness or paralysis without sensory abnormalities. There is usually complete recovery, but if it comes on quickly without respiratory assistance, it can be fatal. The *triangle of Guillain-Mollaret* is a rubro-olivocerebellorubral feedback circuit in which the red nucleus modifies and is modified by the cerebellum and, in turn, modulates motor activity by way of its connections with motor nuclei of the brain stem and spinal cord.

gus´tatory [L. *gustare* to taste]   pertaining to the sense of taste.

GVA   general visceral afferent.

GVE   general visceral efferent.

GVM   general visceral motor.

GVS   general visceral sensory.

gyrencephalic /ji-ren-sĕ-fal´ik/   having a convoluted cerebrum.

gyrus /ji´rus/ [*pl*. **gyri** /ji´rī/] [Gr. *gyros* circle]   elevation or ridge on the surface of the cerebrum, separated from other gyri by sulci. *See also* convolution.

gyrus ambiens /am´bī-enz/, CEREBRUM   lateral prominence on the upper, concealed surface of the uncus, a part of the prepiriform area and the limen insulae.

gyrus, ang´ular [gyrus angularis, NA], CEREBRUM   subdivision of the inferior parietal lobule, Brodmann's area 39. It caps the posterior tip of the superior temporal sulcus just posterior to the supramarginal gyrus (Fig. C-3A). Anomic aphasia, alexia with agraphia, and the Gertsmann syndrome characterize an angular gyrus syndrome.

gyrus, annec´tent [L. *annectere* to join to], CEREBRUM   small gyrus in the depth of some cerebral sulci, hidden beneath the surface of the cerebral hemispheres and connecting two lobes or major gyri. *Syn:* transitional gyrus.

gyri bre´ves in´sulae [NA], CEREBRUM   *See* gyri (of the) insula, short.

gyrus, callo´sal, CEREBRUM   *See* gyrus, cingulate

gyrus, callosomarginal /kal-o-so-mar´jin-al/, CEREBRUM   *See* gyrus, cingulate.

gyrus, central, anterior, CEREBRUM   *See* gyrus, precentral.

gyrus, central, posterior, CEREBRUM   *See* gyrus, postcentral.

gyrus, cingulate /sing´gu-lāt/ [gyrus cinguli (cingulatus), NA], CEREBRUM   gyrus on the medial surface of the cerebral hemisphere between the cingulate sulcus and the sulcus of the corpus callosum. It extends from the subcallosal region beneath the rostrum of the corpus callosum around the genu of the corpus callosum, then posteriorly to pass behind the splenium of the corpus callosum to merge with the isthmus of the cingulate gyrus and continue into the parahippocampal gyrus of the temporal lobe (Fig. C-3B). *Syn:* supracallosal gyrus; callosomarginal gyrus; callosal gyrus.

gyrus, den´tate [gyrus dentatus, NA], CEREBRUM   a subdivision of the hippocampal formation, a narrow, folded, scalloped band of cortex along the dorsal margin of the hippocampal fissure. Its free margins interlock with the edge of the cornu ammonis. It consists of three layers: (1) the stratum moleculare, its outer layer, (2) the stratum granulosum, the conspicuous middle layer, composed of deeply staining, tightly packed granule cells, and (3) the stratum polymorphe, an inner layer, within the hilum of the cellular layer. *Syn:* dentate fascia; fascia dentata; Tarin's fascia. *See also* Fig. C-7.

gyrus, fasc´iolar, CEREBRUM   narrow gyrus posterior to the splenium of the corpus callosum and deep to the isthmus of the cingulate gyrus, a transitional strip of cortex, continuous with the indusium griseum above the corpus callosum and with the dentate gyrus in the temporal lobe. *Syn:* fasciola cinerea; splenial gyrus.

gyrus, for´nicate, CEREBRUM   *See* lobe, fornicate.

gyrus, fron´tal, ascending, CEREBRUM   *See* gyrus, precentral.

gyrus, frontal, inferior [gyrus frontalis inferior, NA], CEREBRUM   gyrus on the lateral surface of the frontal lobe between the inferior frontal sulcus and the lateral sulcus and anterior to the precentral sulcus. It is divided by the anterior horizontal and anterior ascending rami of the lateral sulcus into opercular, triangular, and orbital parts (Fig. C-3A). *See also* Broca's area.

gyrus, frontal, medial [gyrus frontalis medialis, NA], CEREBRUM   gyrus on the medial surface of the frontal lobe, anterior to the paracentral sulcus and between the cingulate sulcus and the superior margin of the frontal lobe (Fig. C-3B).

gyrus, frontal, middle [gyrus frontalis medius, NA], CEREBRUM   gyrus on the lateral surface of the frontal lobe anterior to the precentral sulcus and between the superior and inferior frontal sulci (Fig. C-3A).

gyrus, frontal, superior [gyrus frontalis superior, NA], CEREBRUM   gyrus on the lateral surface of the frontal lobe, anterior to the precentral sulcus and between the superior frontal sulcus and the superior margin of the frontal lobe where it is continuous with the medial frontal gyrus on the medial surface of the hemisphere (Fig. C-3A). *Syn:* marginal gyrus.

gyrus, fusiform /fu´zĪ-form/, CEREBRUM   *See* gyrus, occipitotemporal, medial.

gyrus, hippocamp´al [gyrus hippocampi, NA], CEREBRUM   *See* gyrus, parahippocampal.

gyrus (of the) in´sula [gyri insulae, NA], CEREBRUM   gyrus on the surface of the insula, comprising the short and long gyri of the insula.

gyri (of the) insula, short [gyri breves insulae, NA], CEREBRUM   gyri on the surface of the insula, anterior to the central sulcus of the insula.

gyri (of the) insula, long [gyrus longus insulae, NA], CEREBRUM   gyri on the surface of the insula, posterior to the central sulcus of the insula.

gyrus, intralim´bic, CEREBRUM   semidetached posterior tip of the uncus of the temporal lobe. *Syn:* Retzius' gyrus.

gyrus, ling´ual [gyrus lingualis, NA], CEREBRUM   gyrus on the medial surface of the cerebral hemisphere, located below the calcarine fissure in the occipital lobe and extending forward into the temporal lobe medial to the collateral sulcus to become continuous with the parahippocampal gyrus (Fig. C-3B). *Syn:* lingula.

gyrus long´us in´sulae [NA], CEREBRUM   *See* gyrus (of the) insula, long.

gyrus, mar´ginal, CEREBRUM   *See* gyrus, frontal, superior.

gyrus, occipitotem´poral, CEREBRUM   old term for what is now called the medial occipitotemporal gyrus.

gyrus, occipitotemporal, lateral [gyrus occipitotemporalis lateralis, NA], CEREBRUM   gyrus on the inferior surface of the cerebral hemisphere, lateral to the occipito-temporal sulcus (Fig. C-3B,C). Formerly this was considered a part of the inferior temporal gyrus.

gyrus, occipitotemporal, medial [gyrus occipitotemporalis medialis, NA], CEREBRUM   gyrus on the inferior surface of the cerebral hemisphere between the collateral sulcus and parahippocampal gyrus medially and the occipitotemporal sulcus and lateral occipitotemporal gyrus laterally (Fig. C-3B,C). Formerly this was called the occipitotemporal gyrus. *Syn:* fusiform gyrus.

gyrus, olfac´tory, lateral [gyrus olfactorius lateralis, NA], CEREBRUM   narrow cortical area along the lateral olfactory stria, near the attachment of the olfactory tract on the ventral surface of the frontal lobe, part of the prepiriform area.

gyrus, olfactory, medial [gyrus olfactorius medialis, NA], CEREBRUM   narrow cortical area along the medial olfactory stria, near the attachment of the olfactory tract on the ventral surface of the frontal lobe.

gyri, or'bital [gyri orbitales, NA], CEREBRUM   gyri on the ventral (orbital) surface of the frontal lobe, lateral to the olfactory sulcus, divided into anterior, medial, lateral, and posterior parts by the orbital sulci (Fig. C-3C).

gyrus, paracen'tral, CEREBRUM   *See* lobule, paracentral.

gyrus, parahippocam'pal [gyrus parahippocampalis (hippocampi), NA], CEREBRUM   gyrus on the medial surface of the temporal lobe of the cerebrum, although sometimes it is considered separately as a part of the limbic lobe. It is separated from the medial occipitotemporal gyrus laterally through most of its length by the collateral sulcus and anteriorly by the rhinal sulcus. It is continuous posteriorly with the lingual gyrus of the occipital lobe (Fig. C-3B,C). *Syn:* hippocampal gyrus.

gyrus (area or body), parater'minal [gyrus paraterminalis, NA], CEREBRUM   narrow strip of tissue between the lamina terminalis and the posterior parolfactory gyrus. Sometimes this term is used to include the parolfactory area and even the subcallosal gyrus as well.

gyrus, parolfac'tory, anterior, CEREBRUM   anterior part of the parolfactory area, between the anterior and posterior parolfactory sulci, on the medial surface of the frontal lobe (Fig. C-3B).

gyrus, parolfactory, posterior, CEREBRUM   posterior part of the parolfactory area, between the posterior parolfactory sulcus and the lamina terminalis, on the medial surface of the frontal lobe (Fig. C-3B).

gyrus, postcen'tral [gyrus postcentralis, NA], CEREBRUM   gyrus on the lateral surface of the parietal lobe extending from the lateral sulcus to the superior border of the hemisphere, located between the central and postcentral sulci and containing the somesthetic (sensory) cortex, Brodmann's areas 3, 1, and 2 (Fig. C-3A). *Syn:* ascending parietal convolution; posterior ascending convolution; posterior central gyrus.

gyrus, precen'tral [gyrus precentralis, NA], CEREBRUM   gyrus on the lateral surface of the frontal lobe extending from the lateral sulcus to the superior border of the hemisphere and located between the central and precentral sulci (Fig. C-3A). Brodmann's area 4 is within this gyrus. *Syn:* anterior ascending convolution; anterior central gyrus; ascending frontal convolution.

gyrus rec'tus [NA], CEREBRUM   gyrus on the ventral surface of the frontal lobe, medial to the olfactory sulcus (Fig. C-3C).

gyrus semilunar'is, CEREBRUM   medial prominence on the upper, concealed surface of the uncus. It includes a part of the corticomedial division of the amygdala, in which fibers of the lateral olfactory tract end.

gyrus, sple'nial, CEREBRUM   *See* gyrus, fasciolar.

gyrus, straight, CEREBRUM   *See* gyrus rectus.

gyrus, subcallo'sal, CEREBRUM   small gyrus immediately ventral to the genu and rostrum of the corpus callosum and continuous with the cingulate gyrus (Fig. C-3B). *Syn:* peduncle of the corpus callosum; Zuckerkandl's convolution.

gyrus, subros'tral, CEREBRUM   narrow strip of cortex between the subcallosal gyrus and the overlying rostrum of the corpus callosum.

gyrus, supracallo'sal, CEREBRUM   **1.** old term for the cingulate gyrus.
2. indusium griseum.

gyrus, supramar'ginal [gyrus supramarginalis, NA], CEREBRUM   subdivision of the inferior parietal lobule, Brodmann's area 40. It caps the posterior tip of the lateral sulcus, between the postcentral and angular gyri (Fig. C-3A).

gyrus, tem´poral, first, CEREBRUM   old term for the superior temporal gyrus.

gyrus, temporal, inferior [gyrus temporalis inferior, NA], CEREBRUM   gyrus on the lateral surface of the temporal lobe between the inferior temporal sulcus and the lower margin of the temporal lobe (Fig. C-3A). Formerly it included the lateral occipitotemporal gyrus on the inferior surface of the temporal lobe. *Syn:* third temporal gyrus.

gyrus, temporal, middle [gyrus temporalis medius, NA], CEREBRUM   gyrus on the lateral surface of the temporal lobe between the superior and inferior temporal sulci (Fig. C-3A). *Syn:* second temporal gyrus.

gyrus, temporal, second, CEREBRUM   old term for the middle temporal gyrus.

gyrus, temporal, superior [gyrus temporalis superior, NA], CEREBRUM   gyrus on the lateral surface of the temporal lobe between the superior temporal and the lateral sulci (Fig. C-3A). *Syn:* first temporal gyrus.

gyri, temporal, transverse [gyri temporales transversi, NA], CEREBRUM   two small gyri on the superior surface of the temporal lobe, within the lateral sulcus and comprising the auditory cortex, Brodmann's areas 41 and 42. *Syn:* Heschl's convolutions.

gyrus, temporal, third, CEREBRUM   old term for the inferior temporal gyrus.

gyrus, transitional /tran-zish´un-al/, CEREBRUM   *See* gyrus, annectent.

gyrus, triang´ular, CEREBRUM   triangular part of the inferior frontal gyrus, between the anterior ascending and the anterior horizontal rami of the lateral sulcus; Brodmann's area 45.

gyrus, uncinate /un´sin-āt/, CEREBRUM   *See* uncus.

h

habenula /hah-ben´u-lah/ [NA], EPITHALAMUS, [L. *habena* bridle rein or strap]   small protuberance at the dorsal, posterior corner of the wall of the third ventricle, adjacent to the dorsal thalamus and pineal body. It contains the habenular nuclei and is a major part of the epithalamus (Figs. H-1, V-5).

habenula perforata /per-for-ah´tah/, EAR   row of small openings, the foramina nervosa, along the tympanic lip of the spiral limbus.

Hall, Marshall (1790-1857)   English physiologist whose experiments on spinal cord reflexes established the difference between reflex and voluntary movement.

Haller, Albrecht von (1708-1777)   Swiss anatomist and physiologist. The *commissure of Haller* is the commissura infima. *Haller's layer* is the outer part of the vascular layer of the choroid of the eye. It contains the vorticose veins and branches of the short, posterior ciliary arteries. *Haller's line* is the linea splendens on the midventral surface of the spinal cord. *Haller's ansa* is a loop formed between a branch of the facial nerve and the glossopharyngeal nerve just below the stylomastoid foramen.

Hammond, William Alexander (1828-1900)   American neurologist. *Hammond's disease* is athetosis.

ham´ulus (of the) spiral lamina, EAR   tip of the osseus spiral lamina at the apical end of the cochlea.

harp of David, CEREBRUM   *See* psalterium (Fig. P-2).

Hartline, Haldane Keffer (1903-1983)   American neurophysiologist. He, R. Granit, and G. Wald were awarded the Nobel Prize in physiology and medicine in 1967 for their work on the physiological and chemical activity in the retina.

Head, Sir Henry (1861-1940)   English neurologist who studied cutaneous innervation and the changes in sensibility following section of his own peripheral nerves. During and after World War I his work with brain-injured soldiers greatly advanced knowledge of aphasia and related disorders.

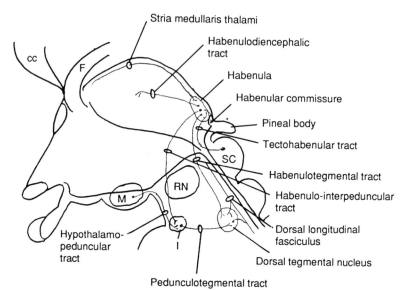

Fig. H-1.   Diagram of a sagittal section showing the wall of the third ventricle, and the midbrain, to illustrate the major connections of the habenula of the epithalamus. CC-corpus callosum; F-fornix; I-interpeduncular nucleus; M-medial mamillary nucleus; RN-red nucleus; SC-superior colliculus.

Held, Hans (1866-1942)   German anatomist. *Held's bundle* is the medial tecto-spinal tract. The *calyces of Held* are pericellular nerve endings in the trapezoid gray. The *commissure of Held* consists of secondary auditory fibers from the ventral cochlear nucleus. They pass through the inferior cerebellar peduncle, cross the median plane dorsal to the trapezoid body, and enter the lateral lemniscus of the opposite side. The *end bulbs of Held* are tiny synaptic terminal bulbs of axons. The *fibers of Held* are fibers that arise from cells in the superior olivary nucleus and were thought at one time to descend and terminate in the dorsal cochlear nucleus. The *marginal glia of Held* constitute the superficial glial limiting membrane at the surface of the brain and spinal cord.

helicotrema /hel-ĭ-ko-tre´mah/ [NA], ᴇᴀʀ, [Gr. *helix* coil; *trema* hole]   the opening at the apex of the cochlea whereby the scala vestibuli communicates with the scala tympani. It was named by Breschet in 1834 but had been described by Cotungo in 1761.

Helmholtz, Hermann Ludwig Ferdinand von (1821-1894)   German physician, physiologist, and physicist who invented the ophthalmoscope (1851) and contributed greatly to knowledge of neurophysiology, particularly in relation to vision and hearing. According to the Helmholtz theory of accommodation, the eye is adapted for near vision when, upon contraction of the ciliary muscle, the suspensory ligament of the lens is relaxed and the lens, because of its elasticity, becomes more globular.

Helweg, Hans Kristian Saxtorph (1847-1901)   Danish physician. *Helweg's tract* is the olivospinal tract.

hemianop´sia (hemiano´pia) [Gr. *hemi* half; *an* not; *opsis* vision]   blindness in one half of the visual field.

hemianopsia (hemianopia), bitem´poral   blindness in the temporal visual field of each eye, after destruction of the crossing fibers in the optic chiasm.

hemianopsia (hemianopia), homon´ymous   blindness in the same half of the visual field for both eyes, after a contralateral, destructive lesion of some part of the visual pathway posterior to the optic chiasm.

hemiballismus /hem-ĭ-bal-liz´mus/ **(hemibal´lism)** [Gr. *hemi-*; *ballismos* jumping] disorder characterized by sudden violent muscular contractions on one side of the body, mainly the proximal limb muscles, and especially the upper extremity, producing flinging movements of the extremity. The movements may occur almost continuously and be interrupted only by sleep. The underlying lesion, usually vascular, involves the subthalamic nucleus on the side opposite the affected limbs.

hemichorea /hem-ĭ-kor-e´ah/ [Gr. *hemi-*; *chorea* dance]   chorea confined to one half the body, resulting from a destructive lesion of the contralateral caudate nucleus.

hemipar´esis [Gr. *hemi-*; *paresis* a letting go, slackening]   weakness of the two extremities on one side of the body.

hemiple´gia [Gr. *hemi-*; *plege* stroke]   paralysis of one half of the body.

hemiplegia, alternate   lower motor neuron paralysis of the muscles supplied by one cranial nerve and an upper motor neuron paralysis of the muscles of the opposite side of the body, resulting from a brain stem lesion on the side of the cranial nerve paralysis. *Syn:* crossed paralysis.

hemiplegia, crossed   1. paralysis of one upper extremity and the opposite lower extremity due to a lesion in the pyramidal decussation on the side of the upper extremity paralysis. *Syn:* crossed paralysis. *See also* paralysis, brachial cruciate. 2. *See* hemiplegia, alternate.

hemisphere, cer´ebral [hemispherium cerebrale, NA]   cerebral cortex, its underlying white matter, and the basal ganglia of one half of the cerebrum. *See also* cerebrum.

hemispherec´tomy   removal of one cerebral hemisphere.

Henle, Friedrich Gustav Jacob (1809-1885)   German anatomist who made many contributions in the field of microscopic anatomy. *Henle's sheath* is the endoneurium, the delicate, mesodermal connective tissue investment of individual peripheral nerve fibers.

Hensen, Victor (1835-1924)   German physiologist and anatomist of Kiel. In addition to making contributions in the field of embryology, he described a number of structures in the internal ear, including: the ductus reuniens (*Hensen's canal,* 1902) and the tall supporting cells of the spiral organ (*Hensen's cells*) between the outer hair and phalangeal cells on one side and the cuboidal epithelium of the cells of Claudius on the other.

Herbst, Ernst Friedrich Gustav (1803-1893)   German anatomist who described a specialized encapsulated nerve ending (*Herbst's corpuscles,* 1848) in the tissue around the bill and in the tongue of birds.

Hering, Heinrich Ewald (1866-1948)   German physiologist of Cologne, noted for his studies of respiratory reflexes. *Hering's nerve* is the carotid sinus branch of the glossopharyngeal nerve. A *Hering-Breuer reflex* is a respiratory reflex that inhibits inspiration and initiates expiration. Afferent fibers, from the lungs, are carried by the vagus nerve. *See also* reflexes, respiratory.

Herophilus (ca. 335-280 BC)   Greek physician of Alexandria. The *torcular Heroph-ili* is the confluence of the dural sinuses at the internal occipital protuberance.

Herrick, Charles Judson (1868-1960)   American neuroanatomist of the University of Chicago, noted for his contributions especially to comparative neuroanatomy.

Herrick, Clarence Luther (1858-1904)   American neuroanatomist, brother of C.J. Herrick. He was the founder of the Journal of Comparative Neurology (1891).

Herring, Percy Theodore (1872-1967)   English physiologist. *Herring bodies* are rather large, often irregularly shaped masses visible at the ends of nerve fibers in the neurohypophysis, which appear to be accumulations of neurosecretory material.

Hertz, Heinrich Rudolph (1857-1894)   German physicist. A *hertz* (Hz), named for him, is a unit of frequency measured in cycles per second.

Heschl, Richard L. (1824-1881)   Austrian anatomist and pathologist of Vienna. *Heschl's convolutions* (1855) are the transverse temporal gyri on the superior surface of the temporal lobe, within the lateral sulcus; auditory cortex.

Hess, Walter Rudolf (1881-1873)   Swiss neurophysiologist, noted for his studies of the diencephalon and of the anatomical relationships of behavior and autonomic nervous system activity. In 1949 he and E. Moniz shared the Nobel Prize for physiology and medicine.

Heubner, Johann Otto Leonhard (1843-1926)   German pediatric neurologist of Leipzig, Berlin, and Dresden. *Heubner's artery* is the recurrent artery, a branch of the anterior cerebral artery.

hic´cup (hiccough)   sudden reflex contraction of the diaphragm and closure of the glottis, dependent on afferent fibers from the lungs, diaphragm, peritoneum, and upper abdominal viscera, and efferent fibers to the diaphragm and glottis, carried by the phrenic and vagus nerves. *Syn:* singultus.

hil´lock, axon [colliculus axonis, NA]   area in the nerve cell body devoid of chromatophilic substance, at the point of origin of the axon.

Hilton, John (1804-1878)   English surgeon. *Hilton's law* states that the nerve which supplies a joint also supplies the muscles that move the joint and the cutaneous area over their articular insertion.

hindbrain   that part of the brain derived from the rhombencephalon, the most caudal subdivision of the embryonic brain, and comprising the medulla, pons, and cerebellum. *Syn:* afterbrain.

hippocamp´us [NA], CEREBRUM, [L. sea horse; from Gr. *hippos* horse; *kampos* sea monster]   **1.** eminence first observed by Achillini but named by Arantius. A gyrus of the limbic system, it projects into the inferior horn of the lateral ventricle. Its anterior part is marked by several shallow grooves, giving it the appearance of an animal's paw, and so this part is called the pes hippocampi. The hippocampus consists mainly of the dentate gyrus and cornu ammonis, and their associated nerve fibers. *See also* formation, hippocampal.
2. This term is also used for the cornu ammonis alone.

hippocampus, dorsal, CEREBRUM   In some mammals (e.g., cat, dog) in which part of the hippocampus is located above the diencephalon, just beneath or posterior to the corpus callosum, that part is called the dorsal hippocampus.

hippocampus major, CEREBRUM   old term for the cornu ammonis.

hippocampus minor, CEREBRUM   old term for the calcar avis.

hip´pus   condition or state of pupillary hyperexcitability.

Hirsch, Anton Balthasar Raymund (b. 1743)   pupil of J.L. Gasser's, in whose honor he named the trigeminal ganglion the *Gasserian ganglion.*

Hirschprung, Harald (1830-1916)   prominent Danish pediatrician of Copenhagen. *Hirschsprung's disease,* a disorder involving megacolon in infancy, results from the failure of neural crest cells to migrate caudally and form the parasympathetic ganglia for innervation of the caudal part of the gastrointestinal tract.

His, Wilhelm, Sr. (1831-1904)   Swiss anatomist in Germany, noted for his studies on the embryologic development of the nervous system. The *spaces of His* are probably shrinkage artifacts, located between the external surface of small blood vessels (less than 100 μm in diameter) and the footplates of the astrocytes in the brain and spinal cord. These spaces surround vessels of smaller caliber than do the Virchow-Robin spaces.

his´tamine   monoamine arising in the CNS from cells in the mamillary nuclei and upper midbrain tegmentum and distributed widely throughout the telencephalon. It probably is involved in the control of sleep and wakefulness and in some neuroendocrine functions (Schwartz and Pollard, '87). *See also* neurotransmitters.

Hitzig, Julius Eduard (1838-1907)   German psychiatrist who, with G. Fritsch, used a weak electrical current to explore the cerebral cortex of the dog, from which they were able to demonstrate discrete movements, the first definitive work on cerebral localization.

Hoffmann, Johann (1857-1919)   professor of neurology at Heidelberg. His description (1893) of infantile spinal muscular atrophy, *Werdnig-Hoffmann disease,* followed by two years that of Werdnig. Inherited as an autosomal recessive, the disorder is usually fatal by four years of age. *See also* dystrophy, muscular. The digital reflex, *Hoffmann's sign,* consists of flexion of the thumb and first two fingers when the volar surface of the finger tips is flicked, and is used as a pyramidal sign.

Hoffmann, Paul (1884-1962)   German physician who, treating German casualties during World War I, perceived that if stimulation of the fibers in the proximal stump of an injured nerve produces sensation in the distal, insensitive cutaneous area, regeneration is taking place, and described it (1915) as a test for peripheral nerve regeneration. This finding was also noted and described later in the same year by Tinel treating French soldiers, and is now known as Tinel's sign.

Holmes, Sir Gordon Morgan (1876-1965)   Anglo-Irish neurologist, for many years at the National Hospital in London. He is noted especially for his studies of the visual system and of the cerebellum.

holoprosenceph´aly   developmental defect in which the prosencephalon remains undivided, in conjunction with other abnormalities of the face and head. *For additional information on this and other prosencephalic defects, see* Müller and O'Rahilly ('89).

hook bundle, BRAIN STEM   *See* fasciculus, uncinate, *def.* 1. It was so named because the bundle hooks over the superior cerebellar peduncle.

hormone, adrenocorticotro´pic (ACTH)   *See* adrenocorticotropic hormone.

hormone, antidiuret´ic (ADH)   *See* antidiuretic hormone.

hormones, neurose´cretory   two neurohypophysial hormones (antidiuretic hormone and oxytocin) produced by cells of the supraoptic and paraventricular nuclei, and transported along fibers of the hypothalamohypophysial tract to the neurohypophysis. *See also* factors, releasing.

hormones, releasing   *See* factors, releasing.

horn, Ammon's, CEREBRUM   *See* cornu ammonis.

horn, anterior   **1.** [cornu anterius (ventrale), NA], cord   *See* horn, ventral.

2. [cornu anterius (frontale), NA], cerebrum   subdivision of the lateral ventricle, anterior to the interventricular foramen and bounded laterally by the head of the caudate nucleus, superiorly by the corpus callosum, and medially by the septum pellucidum (Fig. V-3).

horn, descending, cerebrum   *See* horn, inferior, of the lateral ventricle.

horn, dorsal (posterior) [cornu dorsale (posterius), NA], cord   dorsal gray column, as seen in cross sections of the spinal cord, and containing the following cell groups: substantia gelatinosa, nucleus proprius, thoracic nucleus, and secondary visceral gray (Fig. N-6).

horn, fron´tal [cornu frontale (anterius), NA], cerebrum   *See* horn, anterior, *def.* 2.

horn, inferior (temporal) [cornu inferius (temporale), NA], cerebrum   subdivision of the lateral ventricle within the temporal lobe and containing a part of the choroid plexus (Fig. V-3). *Syn:* descending horn.

horn, intermediate, cord   *See* horn, lateral.

horn, lateral [cornu laterale, NA], cord   lateral gray column of the spinal cord as seen in sections of cord segments T1-L3 and containing the intermediolateral nucleus (Fig. N-6). *Syn:* intermediate horn.

horn, med´ullary dorsal, medulla   term sometimes applied to the subnucleus caudalis, the most caudal subdivision of the spinal nucleus of V, because of its resemblance to the substantia gelatinosa of the spinal cord.

horn, occip´ital [cornu occipitale (posterius), NA], cerebrum   *See* horn, posterior, *def.* 2.

horn, posterior   **1.** [cornu posterius (dorsale), NA], cord   *See* horn, dorsal.

2. [cornu posterius (occipitale), NA], cerebrum   subdivision of the lateral ventricle projecting posteriorly into the occipital lobe from the collateral trigone (Fig. V-3).

horn, tem´poral [cornu temporale (inferius), NA], cerebrum   *See* horn, inferior, of the lateral ventricle.

horn, ventral (anterior) [cornu ventrale (anterius), NA], cord   ventral gray column as seen in cross sections of the spinal cord, and containing such cell groups as the ventromedial, dorsomedial, ventrolateral, dorsolateral, retrodorsolateral, accessory, central, and sacral parasympathetic nuclei (Fig. N-6).

Horner, Johann Friedrich (1831-1886)   Swiss ophthalmologist. *Horner's syndrome* (1869) consists of unilateral ptosis, miosis, and anhidrosis of the face, neck, and shoulder. An enophthalmus may also be noted. The syndrome may occur as a result of a peripheral lesion of the cervical sympathetic trunk or superior cervical ganglion or a central lesion in the medulla or cervical spinal cord involving the lateral tectotegmentospinal tract (eye signs) and the lateral reticulospinal tract (anhidrosis), as in a cervical Brown-Séquard syndrome (Fig. B-2).

horse´rad´ish perox´idase (HRP)   an enzyme used experimentally to determine the location of the cells of origin of selected neurons. After injection at or near the axonal terminals of neurons, the substance is carried by retrograde transport to their cell bodies (Kristensson and Olsson, '71). HRP, injected into selected areas, can also be used as an orthograde transport marker, and also in conjunction with other tracing techniques (Stewart, '81). *See also* tracer, fluorescent.

Horsley, Sir Victor Alexander Haden (1857-1916)   eminent English surgeon and neurologist. Although he also made significant contributions in other medical fields, he is regarded as the father of modern neurosurgery.

Hortega, Pio del Rio (1882-1945)   Spanish histologist, later of Argentina, noted particularly for his studies of neuroglial cells. *Hortega cells* are microglia.

Hounsfield, Godfrey Newbold (b. 1919)   English electronics engineer who extended the discoveries of Cormack to develop computerized axial tomography (the CAT scan) as a non-invasive procedure for the study of the brain. In 1979 he and A.M. Cormack were awarded the Nobel Prize for their contributions.

H-reflex   reflex contraction of the calf muscles in response to electrical stimulation of the tibial nerve in the popliteal fossa. It is thought to be a monosynaptic reflex arc and to correspond to the Achilles reflex. In both cases the response results from stimulation of neuromuscular spindles.

HRP   horseradish peroxidase.

Hubel, David Hunter (b. 1926)   American neurophysiologist, born in Canada. He and T.N. Wiesel are noted for their studies of the visual system, including the synaptic organization of the visual cortex and its ocular dominance columns. They were awarded the Nobel Prize in physiology and medicine in 1981 for discovering the dependence of vision in later life on sight stimulation in infancy.

humor, a´queous [humor aquosus, NA], EYE, [L. *umor* liquid]   thin, watery fluid which fills the anterior and posterior chambers of the eye. It is secreted by the epithelium on the surface of the ciliary body. From the posterior chamber of the eye, it passes through the pupil into the anterior chamber and leaves the interior of the eyeball at the iris angle, entering first the spaces in the trabecular meshwork at the iridocorneal angle (spaces of Fontana), next the venous sinus of the sclera (canal of Schlemm), and then the conjunctival veins.

humor, vit´reous, EYE   1. [humor vitreus, NA] fluid part of the vitreous body. 2. old term for the vitreous body.

Hunt, James Ramsay (1872-1937)   American neurologist. *Hunt's neuralgia* (1907) is glossopharyngeal neuralgia.

Huntington, George Sumner (1850-1916)   American physician. *Huntington's chorea* (1872) is an inherited disorder, carried on chromosome 4, an autosomal dominant with complete penetrance. It is characterized by motor disabilities, such as chorea, followed by severe mental deterioration. The disorder almost always manifests itself in adult or middle life, in women frequently after their child-bearing years. Pathologic changes are mainly in the caudate nucleus and the cerebral cortex.

Huschke, Emil (1797-1858)   German anatomist of Jena. The *auditory teeth of Huschke* are narrow ridges on the surface of the spiral limbus in the cochlear duct, between the vestibular lip and the tympanic lip.

hy´aloid [Gr. *hyalos* glass; *eidos* resembling]   For hyaloid membrane *and* artery, *see the nouns.*

hydrenceph´alocele   abnormality in which the herniated brain forms a tumor composed in part of fluid.

hydrocephalus /hi-dro-sef´al-us/ [Gr. *hydor* water; *kephale* head]   abnormal condition in which the skull, and often the brain, are enlarged because of some disorder or interference with the secretion, circulation, or drainage of cerebrospinal fluid.

hydrocephalus, communicating   hydrocephalus in which the openings between the ventricular spaces and between the fourth ventricle and the subarachnoid space are patent.

hydrocephalus, compensatory   hydrocephalus in which there is no increase in intracranial pressure. Usually the volume of cerebrospinal fluid is increased because of a loss of neurons in cerebral atrophy. *Syn:* hydrocephalus ex vacuo.

hydrocephalus, external   hydrocephalus in which the subarachnoid space is enlarged, usually in addition to the ventricles.

hydrocephalus ex vacuo   *See* hydrocephalus, compensatory.

hydrocephalus, internal   hydrocephalus in which one or more parts of the ventricular system are enlarged.

hydrocephalus, noncommu´nicating   hydrocephalus in which there is obstruction of the flow of cerebrospinal fluid through the ventricular system or from the fourth ventricle into the subarachnoid space.   One or both interventricular foramina, the cerebral aqueduct, or the lateral and median apertures of the fourth ventricle may be blocked.

hydrocephalus, nonobstruc´tive   hydrocephalus which occurs in the absence of any obstruction either within the ventricular system or outside the brain.   It occurs when cerebrospinal fluid is secreted faster than it can be reabsorbed.

hydrocephalus, obstruc´tive   hydrocephalus in which there is a blockage in the circulation of cerebrospinal fluid, either within the ventricular system as in aqueductal stenosis, or in the subarachnoid space as a result of adhesions or a tumor.

hydromeningocele /hi-dro-men-ing´go-sĕl/   abnormality in which a cystic tumor is caused by herniated meninges.

hydromyelia /hi-dro-mi-e´lī-ah/   dilation of the central canal of the spinal cord or closed medulla.

5-hydroxytryptamine   serotonin.

hyperacusis /hi-per-ah-ku´sis/   hypersensitivity to auditory stimuli, as after injury to the stapedial branch of the facial nerve and paralysis of the stapedial muscle.

hypergraph´ia   disorder characterized by a tendency toward extensive and compulsive writing, often involving subject matter of a strongly religious or political nature, suggesting an emotional motivation.   The disorder has been reported in patients with lesions in the midtemporal and frontotemporal regions.

hyperpolariza´tion   an increase in the charge separation across the nerve cell membrane which increases the negative charge of a resting potential and further reduces its capacity to fire.

hyperstriatum /hi-per-stri-a´tum/   large-celled mass in the dorsolateral part of the telencephalon, which serves as "vicarious cortex," mainly in birds, but also in reptiles (C.U. Ariëns Kappers *et al.* '36, p. 1371).

hypesthesia /hip-es-thĕz´ī-ah/ [Gr. *hypo* under; *aisthesis* sensation]   partial loss of sensation.

hypogeusia /hi-po-goo´zī-ah/ [Gr. *hypo-*; *geusis* taste]   diminished taste sensation.

hypoglos´sal [Gr. *hypo-*; *glossa* tongue]   *For* hypoglossal foramen, nerve, *and* nucleus, *see the nouns.*

hypoglos´sus   *See* nerve, hypoglossal.

hypokinesia /hi-po-kin-e´zī-ah/   reduction in the initiation, implementation, and facility of execution of movement.

hypophysial (hypophyseal) /hi-po-fiz´ī-al, hi-pof-ī-ze´al/   pertaining to the hypophysis.   The spelling, *hypophysial* or *hypophyseal*, has been much debated. Both spellings have been used for many years. In Cushing's 1912 monograph, *The Pituitary Body and its Disorders*, as in his earlier papers on the same subject, *hypophyseal* was used.   So great was the acclaim of this paper that, following its publication, *hypophyseal* gained wide acceptance, although after this time Cushing himself always used *hypophysial*.   Corner ('43) pointed out that there is no philological defense for the -*eal* suffix in this connection, but *epiphyseal*, from the same root, appeared in the 1864 edition of Webster's dictionary and does suggest the pronunciation with the accent on the fourth syllable. *See also* Rioch *et al.* ('40, p. 3).

hypoph´ysis, anterior lobe of   pars distalis of the adenohypophysis, sometimes including the pars tuberalis on the anterior surface of the infundibulum. *See also* adenohypophysis; Rathke.

hypophysis cer´ebri [NA]   pituitary gland, located mostly in the sella turcica, on the upper surface of the sphenoid bone (Figs. S-1, V-5), consisting of a neurohypophysis, derived from a ventral evagination of the diencephalon, and an adenohypophysis, derived from an evagination of the roof of the embryonic pharynx, Rathke's pouch. It is divided into an anterior lobe and a posterior lobe and is an endocrine gland of major importance, playing a vital role in the coordination of neurological and endocrine functions. *See also* adenohypophysis; neurohypophysis; Rathke. *For additional information, see* Fawcett ('86, pp. 479-499) *and* Harris and Donovan ('66).

hypophysis, middle lobe of   pars intermedia of the adenohypophysis. *See also* adenohypophysis.

hypophysis, posterior lobe of   pars nervosa of the neurohypophysis, sometimes including the pars intermedia of the adenohypophysis on its anterior surface. *See also* neurohypophysis.

hypothal´amus [NA]   subdivision of the diencephalon located on either side of the third ventricle, just ventral to the hypothalamic sulcus (Figs. N-4, V-5). It is divided into medial and lateral areas by a sagittal plane through the column of the fornix. The hypothalamus is important in the regulation of various visceral functions. *See also* area, hypothalamic, medial *and* lateral; nuclei, hypothalamic. *For additional information, see* Haymaker *et al.* ('69).

hypoto´nia   less than normal muscle tone, indicated by diminished resistance to passive movement. It is characteristic of certain cerebellar lesions.

Hz   hertz.

imprints, ᴇᴀʀ   shallow pits on the underside of the tectorial membrane of the spiral organ of the cochlea, into which the stereocilia of the outer hair cells attach.

impulse, nervous   manifestation of an action potential, the wave of electrical depolarization that is propagated along the inner surface of the cell membrane of a neuron.

inci´sure (notch), cerebel´lar, anterior, ᴄᴇʀᴇʙᴇʟʟᴜᴍ, [L. *incisura* a cutting into; from *in* into, and *caedere* to cut]   relatively broad indentation on the anterior margin of the superior surface of the cerebellum enclosing the superior cerebellar peduncles and the inferior colliculi.

incisure (notch), cerebellar, posterior, ᴄᴇʀᴇʙᴇʟʟᴜᴍ   narrow indentation on the posterior surface of the cerebellum, containing the falx cerebelli.

incisure, my´elin [incisura myelini, NA]   funnel-shaped structure within the myelin sheath of peripheral nerve fibers. Originally believed to be artifacts, such formations are now known to occur in living fibers and are shearing defects in the myelin lamellae, the layers being separated from one another but still continuous across the incisure. *Syn:* Schmidt-Lanterman incisures or clefts.

incisure (notch), preoccip´ital [incisura preoccipitalis, NA], ᴄᴇʀᴇʙʀᴜᴍ   indentation on the underside of the cerebral hemisphere at the border between the occipital and temporal lobes (Fig. C-3A,B).

incisure (notch), tentor´ial [incisura tentorii, NA]   opening anterior to the tentorium cerebelli and enclosing the midbrain (Fig. F-1). *Syn:* Pacchioni's foramen.

incus /ink´us/ [NA], ᴇᴀʀ, [L. anvil]   middle of the three ossicles of the middle ear. Its articulation with the malleus is a fixed joint, but with the stapes it is a moveable joint. It and the malleus were discovered by Achillini in 1503 but were named and illustrated by Vesalius in 1543.

indol´amine (5-hydroxytryptamine)   a biogenic monoamine, such as serotonin or melatonin. *See also* neurotransmitters.

indusium griseum /in-doo´zĭ-um gre´ze-um/ [NA], CEREBRUM   a hippocampal rudiment, consisting of a thin layer of gray matter on the upper surface of the corpus callosum. Anteriorly it is continuous into the septal region with a poorly developed strand of tissue, the anterior continuation of the hippocampus. Posteriorly the fasciolar gyrus connects it with the dentate gyrus. *Syn:* supracallosal gyrus; gray stripe of Lancisi. *See also* nucleus, septohippocampal.

infratentor´ial   caudal to the tentorium cerebelli, within the posterior fossa of the cranial cavity. The infratentorial parts of the brain are the midbrain (in part), pons, medulla oblongata, and cerebellum. The rostral part of the midbrain is within the tentorial incisure.

infundib´ulum [NA], DIENCEPHALON, [L. funnel]   ventral evagination of the wall of the third ventricle of the developing brain from which the neurohypophysis is derived and, in the adult, the slender stalk connecting the median eminence (Fig. N-4) and the pars nervosa.

Ingram, Walter Robinson (1905-1978)   American neuroanatomist, born in England, for many years at the University of Iowa. He was noted for his research into the neurologic bases of behavior, especially the anatomy and physiology of the hypothalamus. The *nucleus intercalatus of Ingram* is the dorsal part of the lateral mamillary nucleus and the *lateral mamillary nucleus of Ingram* is its ventral part.

inhibition, recurrent /in-hib-ish´un/   mechanism whereby collateral branches of a motoneuron synapse with and inhibit a number of neighboring motoneurons, thus stopping their continuous firing.

inhibition, surround (lateral)   principle whereby the firing of a small group of neurons in a central field inhibits the surrounding cells so that definition and localization of the stimulus is made more precise. The mechanism of surround inhibition is used throughout the nervous system as a general principle of reception. In the visual system it is used to separate the receptive fields of retinal ganglion cells, in the auditory system to separate frequencies, and in cutaneous sensitivity to localize a point stimulated on the skin.

inion /in´ī-on/ [NA] [Gr. back of the head]   tip of the external occipital protuberance, a craniometric point used as a landmark in determining, within the intact skull or in X-rays, the location of certain intracranial features.

innerva´tion, recip´rocal   excitatory innervation of one set of muscles so that they contract, together with inhibition of the antagonistic muscles so that they relax.

in´sula [NA] [*adj.* **insular**], CEREBRUM, [L. island]   part of the cerebral cortex overlying the putamen and claustrum. It forms the floor of the lateral sulcus and is covered by the opercula. *Syn:* island of Reil; central lobe.

in´terbrain [L. *inter* between]   diencephalon.

intercala´ted [L. *intercalare* to insert]   placed between. *Syn:* internuncial. *See* neuron, internuncial.

interneu´ron   *See* neuron, internuncial.

in´ternode   segment of a nerve fiber between two nodes of Ranvier.

internun´cial [L. *inter* between; *nuncius* messenger]   serving as a connecting link. *See* neuron, internuncial.

interoception /in-ter-o-sep´shun/ [*adj.* **interoceptive**] [L. *internus* internal; *capere* to take]   general visceral afferent impulses arising from end organs in viscera.

interocep´tor   afferent nerve ending located within viscera.

interol´ivary   between the two inferior olivary nuclei.

interpedun´cular   between the bases of the two cerebral peduncles of the midbrain.

interthalam´ic connexus, DORSAL THALAMUS   *See* adhesion, interthalamic.

in´tima pia /pe´ah/   *See* pia mater.

intorsion /in-tor´zhun/   inward rotation of the eyeball on its anatomical axis.

intra-ax´ial [L. *intra* within]   within the brain.

intracra´nial   within the cranial cavity.

intrafusal /in-trah-fu´zal/   pertaining to the structures within a neuromuscular spindle, particularly the small muscle fibers supplied by gamma motor neurons (Figs. L-1, S-2).

intramed´ullary   within the central nervous system.

intrathecal /in-trah-the´kal/   within a sheath; in relation to the nervous system, within the spinal subarachnoid space.

intumescen´tia cervical´is [NA], CORD   *See* enlargement, cervical.

intumescentia lumbosacral´is [NA], CORD   *See* enlargement, lumbosacral.

involuntary nervous system   *See* system, nervous, autonomic.

iodopsin /i-o-dop´sin/, EYE   visual pigment present in cones of the retina and sensitive to red light.

IPSP   inhibitory postsynaptic potential.

i´ris [NA], EYE, [Gr. rainbow, named for the Greek goddess Iris, represented wearing a robe of variegated colors]   anterior segment of the vascular tunic of the eye. It separates the anterior and posterior chambers of the eye. The smooth muscle of the iris regulates the size of the pupil and controls the amount of light to reach the retina.

island, CEREBRUM   *See* insula.

island, cerebellar, CEREBELLUM   cell-free area bounded by granule cells in the granular layer of the cerebellar cortex. It contains a cerebellar glomerulus, which is a complex synaptic formation of mossy fiber and Golgi cell axon terminals and granule cell dendrites, as well as astroglial processes. *Syn:* plasma island.

island, plasma, CEREBELLUM   *See* island, cerebellar.

isocor´tex, CEREBRUM, [Gr. *isos* equal; L. *cortex* bark, rind]   6-layered cortex of the neopallium. *Syn:* neocortex; homogenetic cortex.

isocortex agranular´is gigantopyramidal´is, CEREBRUM   Brodmann's area 4 of the frontal lobe. *Syn:* motor area.

isocortex agranularis sim´plex, CEREBRUM   Brodmann's area 6 of the frontal lobe. *Syn:* premotor area.

isthmus (of the) cingulate (fornicate) gyrus [isthmus gyri cinguli (cingulatus), NA], CEREBRUM   part of the cerebral cortex posterior to the splenium of the corpus callosum, which connects the cingulate gyrus of the parietal lobe and the parahippocampal gyrus of the temporal lobe (Fig. C-3B).

isthmus (of the) pons, PONS   that part of the pons rostral to the attachments of the cerebellar peduncles.

isthmus, temporal, CEREBRUM   zone between the posterior part of the body of the lateral ventricle and the posterior part of the insula and containing the temporal loop of the optic radiation, the corticotectal tracts, the auditory radiation, and other fiber bundles. *See* Fig. C-1.

i´ter, MIDBRAIN, [L. a way or street]   *See* aqueduct, cerebral.

j

Jackson, John Hughlings (1835-1911)   English physician noted for his pioneering work in neurology. He published many now classic reports on epilepsy and many other neurologic disorders as well as on the structure and function of the nervous system. *Jacksonian epilepsy* consists of focal seizures resulting from sudden, abnormal discharges of neurons in damaged areas of the cerebral cortex.

Jakob, Alfons Maria (1884-1931)   German neuropathologist. His account (1921) and that of Creutzfeldt (1920) led to the identification of *Creutzfeldt-Jakob disease*, spongiform degeneration of the brain. *See also* Creutzfeldt.

Jacobson, Ludwig Levin (1783-1843)   Danish anatomist of Copenhagen. *Jacobson's organ* (1809) is the vomeronasal organ. Both the tympanic branch of the glossopharyngeal nerve and the vomeronasal nerve are called *Jacobson's nerve*. *Jacobson's plexus* (1818) is the tympanic plexus. *Jacobson's foramen* is the opening in the temporal bone, in the ridge between the jugular bulb and the carotid canal, through which the tympanic branch of the glossopharyngeal nerve enters the tympanic cavity.

jerk   *See also* reflex.

jerk, ankle   *See* reflex, Achilles tendon.

jerk, jaw   *See* reflex, jaw-closing.

jerk, knee   *See* reflex, patellar.

jug´ular [L. *jugulum* throat]   pertaining to the jugular veins and ganglia.

Jung, Carl Gustav (1875-1961)   Swiss psychiatrist and pschoanalist and founder of analytic psychology. In his early years a pupil of Freud's, he later broke with him.

juxtarestiform /juk-stah-res´tĭ-form/ [L. *juxta* near to, close by]   pertaining to a subdivision of the inferior cerebellar peduncle. *See* body, juxtarestiform.

k

Kaes, Theodor (1852-1913)   German anatomist. The *stripe of Kaes* or *Kaes-Bechterew* is a layer of nerve fibers in layer II of the cerebral cortex, also called the stripe of Vicq d'Azyr.

Kanner, Leo (b. 1894)   Austrian psychiatrist, active in the United States. *Kanner's syndrome* is infantile autism.

Katz, Sir Bernard (b. 1911)   German-born British neurophysiologist, noted for his studies of neurotransmitters, including the release of acetylcholine from presynaptic vesicles at neuromuscular junctions. In 1970 he, J. Axelrod, and U. von Euler received the Nobel Prize in medicine and physiology for their discoveries.

Keith, Sir Arthur (1866-1955)   London anatomist. The *node of Keith* or *Keith and Flack* (1907) is the sinuatrial node.

kernic´terus [Gr. *kern* kernel, nucleus; *ikteros* jaundice]   pathologic condition in which certain regions of the CNS are stained yellow with bile pigments, particularly the subthalamic nucleus, hippocampus, and globus pallidus.

Kernig, Vladimir Michalovich (1840-1917)   Russian neurologist. *Kernig's sign* (1884) is a limitation of movement on passive extension of the knee because of spasm of the hamstring muscles and is indicative of meningitis.

Kernohan, James Watson (b. 1897)   American physician and pathologist, born in Ireland. *Kernohan's notch* is an indentation of the brain with necrosis, due to pressure on the brain by the free edge of the tentorium cerebelli, often associated with tentorial herniation.

Key, Ernst Axel Henrik (1832-1901)   Swedish physician. The *foramina of Key and Retzius* are the lateral apertures of the fourth ventricle. The *sheath of Key and Retzius* is the endoneurium of peripheral nerve fibers.

kinesthe´sia [*adj.* **kinesthetic**] [Gr. *kinesis* movement; *aisthesis* sensation]   sense of position or movement of a part of the body, the sense of equilibrium, also the sensibility underlying the ability to estimate weight.

kinocil´ium, ᴇᴀʀ   single protoplasmic filament in each hair process of the hair cells in the cupula of the crista ampullaris of each semicircular duct. Bending of the kinocilia stimulates the sensory nerve fibers when the deflection is *toward* the utricle in the horizontal duct, and *away* from the utricle in the vertical ducts (Lowenstein and Wersäll, '59).

Kiss, F. (20th century)   Hungarian anatomist. *Kiss cells* are multipolar cells in the dorsal root ganglia. They resemble autonomic, postganglionic cell bodies and are thought by some observers to be a part of the spinal parasympathetic system (of Ken Kuré) for peripheral vasodilation.

Klimoff, J. (late 19th century)   *Klimoff-Wallenberg fibers* are the fibers of the flocculo-oculomotor tract.

Klüver, Heinrich (1897-1989)   American psychologist. The *Klüver-Bucy syndrome* results from a lesion, usually bilateral, in the temporal lobe, especially the uncus and hippocampus. It is characterized by a serious deficiency of memory and by behavioral changes including excessive responses to all visual stimuli, perversions of appetite, oral tendencies, hypersexuality, and a reduction in emotional responses including a loss of fear and a decrease in aggressive behavior. *For additional information, see* Terzian and Ore ('55).

knee   *See also* genu.

knee, anterior, of the optic chiasm, ᴅɪᴇɴᴄᴇᴘʜᴀʟᴏɴ   optic nerve fibers from the inferior medial quadrant of each retina which cross in the optic chiasm and deviate into the contralateral optic nerve before they enter the optic tract. Injury to these fibers results in blindness in the upper lateral quadrant of the visual field of the contralateral eye.

knee jerk   *See* reflex, patellar.

knee, posterior, of the optic chiasm, ᴅɪᴇɴᴄᴇᴘʜᴀʟᴏɴ   optic nerve fibers from the superior medial quadrant of each retina which deviate into the homolateral optic tract before they cross in the optic chiasm to enter the contralateral optic tract. Injury to these fibers results in blindness in the lower lateral quadrant of the visual field of the homolateral eye.

Koch, Walter (b. 1880)   German physician. *Koch's node* is the sinuatrial node.

Kölliker, Rudolf Albert von (1817-1905)   Swiss anatomist, a student of Remak's, the first to show that nerve fibers are the processes of nerve cells. He also anticipated by nearly fifty years the concept of the neuron doctrine, established by Waldeyer and Cajal.

koniocortex, ᴄᴇʀᴇʙʀᴜᴍ, [Gr. *konis* dust; L. *cortex* bark, rind]   cortex of a sensory projection area, in which the granular layers predominate.

koniocortex, auditory, ᴄᴇʀᴇʙʀᴜᴍ   Brodmann's area 41. *See* Fig. B-1.

Korsakov, Sergei Sergeivich (1853-1900)   Russian psychiatrist. *Korsakov's syndrome* or *psychosis* consists of amnesia, confabulation, and disorientation. It occurs sometimes, but not always, in alcoholics, and is usually associated with bilateral lesions in the mamillary bodies and sometimes also the septal areas and hippocampus. *Syn:* amnesic or amnestic-confabulatory psychosis; psychosis polyneuritica.

Krabbe, Knud (1885-1965)   outstanding Danish neurologist, with many important scientific contributions to his credit. *Krabbe's disease* (1913) is a neurodegenerative disease of infants, inherited as an autosomal recessive and fatal by two years of age.

Krause, Wilhelm Johann Friedrich (1833-1910)   German anatomist. The *end bulbs of Krause* (1860) are small, spherical nerve endings in the dermal papillae. They have a thin capsule and contain a much coiled nerve fiber and are thought to be cold receptors. *Krause's bundle* is the fasciculus solitarius. The *ventricle of Krause* is the terminal ventricle of the spinal cord.

Kühne, Wilhelm (Willy) (1837-1900)   German physiologist and histologist, professor of physiology at Amsterdam and Heidelberg. He wrote the best early description of the neuromuscular spindle, *Kühne's spindle* (1863). His investigations also included the visual purple (rhodopsin) of the retina.

Kuntz, Albert (1879-1957)   American neuroanatomist. The *nerve of Kuntz* is the intrathoracic nerve.

Kuré, Ken G. Saégusa (20th century)   Japanese neuroscientist who demonstrated vasodilator fibers in the dorsal roots as a part of a "spinal parasympathetic system" (Kuré *et al.*, '30).

1

L   lumbar.

L-dopa (levadopa)   the biologically active form of dopa, used in the treatment of parkinsonism.

Labbé, Leon (1832-1916)   French surgeon of Paris. The *vein of Labbé* is the inferior anastomotic vein on the lateral surface of the cerebral hemisphere.

lab´yrinth [labyrinthus, NA], ᴇᴀʀ   *See* ear, internal.

labyrinth, bony [labyrinthus osseus, NA], ᴇᴀʀ   space within the petrous part of the temporal bone, which contains the various parts of the internal ear.

labyrinth, coch´lear [labyrinthus cochlearis, NA], ᴇᴀʀ   the cochlear part of the internal ear comprising the cochlear duct, scala tympani, scala vestibuli, and their related structures.

labyrinth, endolymphat´ic, ᴇᴀʀ   *See* labyrinth, membranous.

labyrinth, mem´branous [labyrinthus membranaceus, NA], ᴇᴀʀ   system of epithelial ducts and chambers of the internal ear which contain endolymph and are suspended within the periotic space of the bony labyrinth. It comprises the three semicircular ducts, the saccule and utricle, the utriculosaccular and endolymphatic ducts and sac, the ductus reuniens, and the cochlear duct. *Syn:* otic labyrinth; endolymphatic labyrinth.

labyrinth, os´seous, ᴇᴀʀ   *See* labyrinth, bony.

labyrinth, o´tic, ᴇᴀʀ   *See* labyrinth, membranous.

labyrinth, perio´tic, ᴇᴀʀ   space containing perilymph, located between the membranous labyrinth of the internal ear and the epithelial lining of the bony labyrinth. These spaces are: the semicircular canals and vestibule of the vestibular labyrinth, the scala tympani and scala vestibuli of the cochlea, and the perilymphatic duct. *Syn:* periotic space.

labyrinth, vestib´ular [labyrinthus vestibularis, NA], ᴇᴀʀ   the vestibular part of the internal ear, comprising the saccule and utricle in the vestibule, the semicircular ducts in the semicircular canals and their related structures.

lacunae (lakes), lateral /lah-koo´ni/ [lacunae laterales, NA]   lacunae extending outward from the superior longitudinal sinus.

lagena /lah-je´nah/, EAR, [L. flask]   **1.** the flask-shaped organ of hearing in lower vertebrates.

2. sometimes also used for the cecum cupulare.

lakes, lateral (of Trolard)   *See* lacunae, lateral.

lambda [NA] [Greek letter Λ]   point of juncture of the occipital and the two parietal bones of the skull, where the lambdoid and sagittal sutures meet in the form of a lambda. In the infant it is the site of the posterior fontanel. In the adult it can be used as a neuroradiologic point of reference to determine the location of certain intracranial structures, such as the venous angle.

lam´ina [*pl.* **laminae**] [L. plate or layer]   *See also* layer; membrane; stratum.

lamina, acces´sory med´ullary, CEREBRUM   layer of nerve fibers partially subdividing the inner segment of the globus pallidus.

lamina affixa /ah-fik´sah/ [NA], DORSAL THALAMUS   ependymal epithelium covering the dorsal surface of the dorsal thalamus between the attachment of the choroid plexus of the lateral ventricle medially and the stria terminalis laterally and forming part of the floor of the body of the lateral ventricle.

lamina basalis /ba-sal´is/ [NA], EYE   *See* choroid, basal layer.

lamina basilaris /bas-ĭ-la´ris/ [NA], EAR   *See* membrane, basilar.

laminae (of the) cer´ebral cor´tex CEREBRUM   *See* cortex, cerebral.

lamina choriocapilla´ris [NA], EYE   *See* choroid, choroidocapillary layer.

lamina cribro´sa [NA] [L. *cribrum* a sieve]   **1.** EYE   perforated area at the back of the eyeball, where the optic nerve fibers pass through the sclera. *Syn:* area cribrosa.

2. thin horizontal plate of the ethmoid bone with perforations (foramina cribrosa) through which the olfactory fila enter the cranial cavity. *Syn:* cribriform plate.

lamina dis´secans, CEREBELLUM   transient cell-poor zone between the Purkinje cell layer and the internal granular layer of the developing primate cerebellar cortex (Rakic and Sidman, '70), first described for the human fetal brain by Hayashi ('24).

lamina dysfibro´sa, CEREBRUM   Vogt's layer II of the cerebral cortex; the external granular layer.

lamina fus´ca [NA], EYE, [L. *fuscus* dusky]   *See* choroid, suprachoroid layer.

lamina infrastria´ta, CEREBRUM   Vogt's layer VI of the cerebral cortex; the multiform layer.

lamina (membrane), limiting, anterior [lamina limitans anterior, NA], EYE   *See* cornea, anterior limiting membrane.

lamina (membrane), limiting, posterior [lamina limitans posterior, NA], EYE   *See* cornea, posterior limiting membrane.

lamina, med´ullary, accessory, CEREBRUM   layer of medullated nerve fibers that partially divides the inner segment of the globus pallidus.

lamina, medullary, external [lamina medullaris externa, NA], DORSAL THALAMUS   layer of medullated nerve fibers in the dorsal thalamus. It separates the ventrolateral nuclei medially from the reticular nucleus laterally, and is continuous ventrally with the thalamic fasciculus (Fig. N-8).

lamina, medullary, internal [lamina medullaris interna, NA], DORSAL THALAMUS   layer of medullated nerve fibers in the dorsal thalamus. It separates the dorsomedial nucleus medially from the ventrolateral nuclear group laterally. Posteriorly it encloses the centromedian nucleus and anteriorly it adjoins the anteroventral nucleus (Fig. N-8). The mamillothalamic tract passes through it to reach the anterior nucleus.

lamina, medullary, lateral [lamina medullaris lateralis, NA], CEREBRUM   layer of medullated nerve fibers between the putamen and globus pallidus.

lamina, medullary, medial [lamina medullaris medialis, NA], CEREBRUM   layer of medullated nerve fibers between the inner and outer segments of the globus pallidus.

lamina quadrigem´ina, MIDBRAIN   tectum.

lamina, retic´ular, EAR   surface of the spiral organ of the cochlea, through which the cilia of the hair cells project. *See* membrane, reticular.

lamina rostral´is, CEREBRUM   membrane extending from the rostrum of the corpus callosum to the anterior commissure, and forming an anteroventral wall for the cavum septi pellucidi. *Syn:* copula. *See also* lamina terminalis.

lamina (of the) sep´tum pellucidum /pel-loo´sĭ-dum/ [lamina septi pellucidi, NA], CEREBRUM   either of two thin plates of tissue of the septum pellucidum separated by a narrow space, the cavum septi pellucidi.

lamina, spiral, mem´branous, EAR   *See* membrane, basilar.

lamina, spiral, os´seous [lamina spiralis ossea, NA], EAR   bony ridge which spirals around the modiolus on which the spiral limbus rests and to which the basilar membrane is attached.

lamina, spiral, secondary [lamina spiralis secundaria, NA], EAR   bony ridge on the outer wall of the first turn of the cochlea.

lamina suprachoroide´a, EYE   *See* choroid, suprachoroid layer.

lamina suprastria´ta, CEREBRUM   Vogt's layer III of the cerebral cortex; the external pyramidal layer.

lamina tangentialis /tan-jen-she-al´is/, CEREBRUM   Vogt's layer I of the cerebral cortex; the molecular layer.

lamina terminal´is [NA]. CEREBRUM   anterior wall of the third ventricle between the anterior commissure and the optic chiasm (Fig. V-5). With the lamina rostralis, it is the most rostral median part of the CNS. *Syn:* velum terminale.

lamina vasculo´sa [NA], EYE   *See* choroid, lamina vasculosa.

lamina vit´rea [NA], EYE, [L. *vitreus* glassy]   *See* choroid, basal layer.

laminec´tomy   surgical removal of the dorsal arches of a vertebra.

Lancisi, Giovanni Maria (1654-1720)   Italian physician and anatomist. The longitudinal striae overlying the corpus callosum are the *medial and lateral white stripes of Lancisi* which accompany the *gray stripe of Lancisi* (indusium griseum) (1711).

Landouzy, Louis Théophile Joseph (1845-1917)   prominent French neurologist. He collaborated with Dejerine on a number of studies. *Landouzy-Dejerine* disease is muscular dystrophy of the facio-scapulo-humeral type, inherited as an autosomal dominant.

Landry de Thézillat, Jean Baptiste Octave (1826-1865)   French physician who distinguished between several varieties of paralysis. *See* Guillain for the Landry-Guillain-Barré syndrome.

Langley, John Newport (1852-1925)   English physiologist noted for his investigations of the autonomic nervous system. *Langley's ganglion* is a parasympathetic ganglion of the facial nerve, located at the hilus of the submandibular gland, from which postganglionic fibers supply the submandibular gland (Fig. C-4, Table C-2).

Lanterman, A.J.   American anatomist active in Strassburg in 1876. The *incisures* or *clefts of Schmidt-Lanterman* are now called myelin incisures.

Larsell, Olaf (1886-1964)   American neuroanatomist, born in Sweden, noted especially for his studies of the comparative neuroanatomy of the cerebellum.

Lasègue, Ernest Charles (1816-1883)   French physician and pathologist. *Lasègue's sign,* indicative of sciatica, was described by his pupil J.J. Frost (1881), and consists of pain that occurs when the lower extremity is raised with the knee extended but not when the leg and thigh are flexed.

Laumonier, Jean Baptiste Phillippe Nicolas René (1749-1818)   French surgeon. *Laumonier's ganglion* is the carotid ganglion.

layers   *For their layers, see* choroid; colliculus, superior; cornea; cornu ammonis; cortex, cerebral *and* cerebellar; gyrus, dentate; retina; *and* Rexed for the layers of the spinal cord. *See also* lamina; stratum.

layer, epen´dymal [stratum ependymale, NA]   inner layer of the neural tube composed of germinal cells which undergo active mitosis.

layer, gran´ular, CEREBRUM, CEREBELLUM   cortical layer composed predominantly of small cells. *See* cortex, cerebellar (Figs. C-8, C-9) *and* cortex, cerebral.

layers, infragran´ular, CEREBRUM   layers V and VI of the cerebral cortex.

layer, mantle [stratum palliale, NA]   middle layer of the neural tube, composed of nuclei of developing nerve cells.

layer, marginal [stratum marginale, NA]   outermost layer of the neural tube composed of the processes of the developing nerve cells.

layer, med´ullary   general term for any layer of the white matter in the CNS.

layer, molec´ular, CEREBRUM, CEREBELLUM, EYE, [L. *molecula* small mass]   a synaptic layer on the surface of the cerebral and cerebellar (Figs. C-8, C-9) cortices and two (plexiform) layers in the retina. It is composed primarily of unmyelinated axon terminals, the dendritic terminals with which they synapse, and few nerve cell bodies. *See also* cortex, cerebral *and* cerebellar; cornu ammonis; gyrus, dentate; *and* retina, (plexiform) layers (3 and 5).

layer, plexiform /plek´sǐ-form/   *See* layer, molecular.

layer, posterior elastic (limiting), EYE   *See* cornea, posterior limiting membrane.

layers, supragran´ular, CEREBRUM   layers I, II, and III of the cerebral cortex.

LD   lateral dorsal nucleus of the dorsal thalamus.

Le Gros Clark, Sir Wilfred Edward (1895-1971)   British anatomist. The *nucleus intercalatus of Le Gros Clark* is the ventral part of the lateral mamillary nucleus; the *lateral mamillary nucleus of Le Gros Clark* is its dorsal part.

lemmocyte /lem´o-sǐt/   *See* cell, neurolemma sheath.

lemniscus /lem-nis´kus/ [Gr. *lemniskos* band or ribbon]   fiber bundle composed of secondary sensory fibers which arise in one or more sensory nuclei and terminate in the dorsal thalamus. *See also* system, lemniscal.

lemniscus, lateral [lemniscus lateralis, NA]   tract composed of fibers from the ventral and dorsal cochlear nuclei, which, with or without synapses in course, carry auditory impulses mainly to the inferior colliculus and to some extent to the medial geniculate nucleus.

lemniscus, medial [lemniscus medialis, NA]   tract composed mostly of fibers from the nucleus gracilis and nucleus cuneatus, which carry impulses for sense of position, vibratory sensibility, and tactile discrimination to the ventral posterolateral nucleus of the dorsal thalamus. Other fibers incorporated in this bundle are secondary gustatory fibers from the nucleus solitarius (dorsal visceral gray) and descending aberrant pyramidal fibers.

lemniscus, spinal [lemniscus spinalis, NA]   lateral and ventral spinothalamic tracts.

lemniscus, trigeminal /tri-jem´in-al/ [lemniscus trigeminalis, NA]   dorsal and ventral secondary ascending trigeminal tracts.

lens [NA], EYE   transparent, biconvex structure within the eyeball, located immediately behind the pupil and adjacent to the posterior surface of the iris.

lentic´ular [L. lens-shaped]   *See* fasciculus *and* nucleus, lenticular.

Lenz   The *nucleus of Lenz* is the Edinger-Westphal nucleus (accessory oculomotor nucleus).

leptomen´inges [NA] [*sing.* **leptomeninx**] [Gr. *leptos* delicate; *meninx* membrane]   thin, membranous coverings of the brain and spinal cord, consisting of the pia mater and the arachnoid. *Syn:* arachnopia; pia-arachnoid. *See also* meninges.

leu-enkephalin   *See* enkephalin.

levartere´nol   *See* norepinephrine.

Lhermitte, Jean (1877-1959)   French neurologist. *Lhermitte's sign* is an electrical sensation indicative of a cervical spinal cord lesion.

lig´ament, coccygeal /cok-sĭ-je´al/   *See* filum terminale externum.

ligament, den´tate (dentic´ulate) [ligamentum denticulatum, NA]   ligament formed by the reflection of the pia-arachnoid, attached medially along the spinal cord midway between the dorsal and ventral roots and laterally to the arachnoid and dura mater at the base of the skull and at intervals between the emerging spinal nerve roots.

ligament, pec´tinate [ligamentum pectinatum, NA], EYE, [L. *pecten* a comb, having projections like the teeth of a comb]   delicate fibers which arise from the posterior elastic membrane of the cornea, and which constitute a trabecular meshwork. The spaces of the meshwork (spaces of Fontana), which communicate with both the anterior chamber of the eye and the venous sinus of the sclera (canal of Schlemm), contain aqueous humor and function in the drainage of aqueous humor from the interior of the eyeball to the conjunctival veins.

ligament, spi´ral [ligamentum spirale (crista spiralis), NA], EAR   thickened periosteal connective tissue layer on the outer wall of the cochlear duct, not a typical ligament, to which the outer margins of the basilar and vestibular membranes are attached. On its free surface is the stria vascularis.

ligament, suspen´sory, EYE   *See* zonule, ciliary.

lig´ula, MEDULLA, [L. strap]   *See* tenia of the fourth ventricle.

lim´bic [L. *limbus* border]   pertaining to certain gyri which surround the rostral part of the brain stem and adjoining forebrain. *See* lobe *and* system, limbic.

lim´bus cor´neae [NA], EYE   transition zone along the rim of the cornea, between the conjunctiva and sclera on the one hand and the cornea on the other.

limbus cortical´is, CEREBRUM   *See* cornu ammonis.

limbus, spi´ral [limbus laminae spiralis osseae, NA], EAR   thickening of the periosteal connective tissue on the upper surface of the osseous spiral lamina in the cochlear duct. On its upper surface the vestibular membrane is attached near its outer margin, and the tectorial membrane is attached to its vestibular lip. Between the two, the surface of the limbus is covered by a layer of columnar epithelium. The surface of the limbus, between the vestibular lip and the tympanic lip, provides the wall of the internal spiral sulcus. The basilar membrane is attached to its tympanic lip and to the osseous spiral lamina.

li´men in´sulae [NA], CEREBRUM, [L. *limen* threshold]   area at the entrance to the lateral sulcus, a transitional area between the anterior perforated substance and the insular cortex. It is a part of the rhinencephalon and includes the gyrus ambiens on the upper lateral surface of the uncus.

Lindau, Arvid (1892-1958)   Swedish pathologist. *Lindau's disease* (1926) consists of a variable number of developmental abnormalities and neoplasms, including cerebellar and retinal hemangioblastomas with cysts and neoplasms of other organs of the body. It appears to be an inherited disorder, of an autosomal dominant type with a moderate degree of penetrance.

line   *See also* stripe.

line, intrape´riod   fine line in the myelin sheath of peripheral nerve fibers, visible in electron micrographs. It is formed by the fusion of the outer layers of the cell membrane as the Schwann cell spirals around the axis cylinder and forms the myelin sheath (Fig. M-1).

line, major dense   line, heavier than the intraperiod line, in the myelin sheath of peripheral nerve fibers, visible in electron micrographs. It is formed by the fusion of the inner layers of the cell membrane as the Schwann cell encircles the axis cylinder and eliminates the intervening Schwann cell cytoplasm. Myelin, formed in the process and laid down between the major dense and intraperiod lines, is derived from the lipid between the inner and outer layers of the Schwann cell membrane (Fig. M-1).

linea splen´dens CORD   thickening of the pia mater along the midventral surface of the spinal cord. It encloses the anterior spinal artery. *Syn:* Haller's line.

ling´ula [L. little tongue]   **1.** [NA], CEREBELLUM   most rostral subdivision of the cerebellar vermis, mainly in the anterior medullary velum (Figs. C-2, V-6).
    2. CEREBRUM   *See* gyrus, lingual.

lip, rhombic /rom´bik/ [labium rhombencephalicum, NA], CEREBELLUM   thickening at the junction of the alar and roof plates on each side of the rhombencephalon, from which the flocculonodular lobe of the cerebellum develops.

lip, tympan´ic, EAR   lower margin of the spiral limbus to which the basilar membrane of the cochlea is attached, on the side adjoining the modiolus.

lip, vestib´ular, EAR   upper margin of the spiral limbus to which the tectorial membrane of the cochlea is attached.

lipofuscin (lipochrome) /lip-o-fu´sin/   a yellowish pigment occurring as granules in the cytoplasm of some nerve cell bodies, particularly those of sensory and autonomic ganglia, and increasing in amount with age. It appears to have no pathologic significance unless it appears at an unusually early age.

liquor cerebrospinal´is /lik´er/ [NA]   *See* fluid, cerebrospinal.

liquor cotun´nii, EAR   perilymph.

Lissauer, Heinrich (1861-1891)   German neurologist. *Lissauer's tract* is the dorsolateral fasciculus of the spinal cord.

lissencephal´ic [Gr. *lissos* smooth; *enkephalos* brain]   having a smooth cerebrum without sulci and gyri; agyric.

Little, William John (1810-1894)   English orthopedic surgeon. *Little's disease* is congenital spastic diplegia.

lobe   *See* cerebrum and cerebellum, for their major subdivisions.

lobe (gyrus), fornicate, CEREBRUM, [L. *fornix* an arch]   part of the cerebral cortex which partially encircles the upper part of the brain stem and which comprises the cingulate gyrus, isthmus, hippocampus, parahippocampal gyrus, and uncus. It constitutes a part of the limbic lobe.

lobe, lim´bic, CEREBRUM   gyri and associated structures on the medial and basal surface of the cerebral hemisphere, which encircle the upper brain stem. Its parts include: the subcallosal gyrus, anterior and posterior parolfactory gyri, olfactory bulb and stalk, medial and lateral olfactory gyri, cingulate gyrus, isthmus, hippocampus, parahippocampal gyrus and uncus, and sometimes the amygdala. It has been thought to play an important role in relation to behavior and emotion. *See also* system, limbic.

lobe (area), pir´iform (pyriform), CEREBRUM   anterior portion of the temporal lobe medial to the rhinal sulcus, an olfactory relay center. It includes the uncus and lateral olfactory stria, and the anterior part of the parahippocampal gyrus, including the entorhinal area.

lobot´omy   operation in which the white matter of a cerebral lobe is incised.

lob´ule [lobulus, NA]   one subdivision of a cerebral or cerebellar lobe.

lobule, an´siform (of Larsell), CEREBELLUM   combination of the superior and inferior semilunar lobules, above and below the horizontal fissure (Fig. C-2).

lobule, ansoparame´dian (of Larsell), CEREBELLUM   combined ansiform and paramedian lobules; the superior and inferior semilunar and the gracile lobules of the cerebellar hemisphere (Fig. C-2).

lobule, central [lobulus centralis, NA], CEREBELLUM   segment of the vermis between the lingula and the culmen of the anterior lobe (Figs. C-2, V-6). *See also* vermis cerebelli.

lobule, crescentic, anterior, CEREBELLUM   *See* lobule, quadrangular, anterior.

lobule, crescentic, posterior, CEREBELLUM   *See* lobule, quadrangular, posterior.

lobule, gracile /gră-sĕl´/ [lobulus gracilis, NA], CEREBELLUM   slender segment some-times identifiable on the inferior surface of the cerebellar hemisphere, between the inferior semilunar lobule and the biventer (Fig. C-2). *Syn:* paramedian lobule of comparative neuroanatomy.

lobule (gyrus), paracen´tral [lobulus paracentralis, NA], CEREBRUM   cortical area on the medial surface of the cerebrum around the dorsomedial tip of the central sulcus and bounded by the paracentral sulcus anteriorly, the cingulate sulcus ventrally, and the marginal sulcus posteriorly. Its anterior part is in the frontal lobe and its posterior portion is in the parietal lobe (Fig. C-3B).

lobule, parame´dian [lobulus paramedianus, NA], CEREBELLUM   *See* lobule, gracile.

lobule, pari´etal, inferior [lobulus parietalis inferior, NA], CEREBRUM   subdivision of the parietal lobe, on the lateral surface of the cerebral hemisphere, posterior to the lower part of the postcentral sulcus, and between the intraparietal and lateral sulci. The angular and supramarginal gyri constitute the inferior part of this lobule (Fig. C-3A).

lobule, parietal, superior [lobulus parietalis superior, NA], CEREBRUM   subdivision of the parietal lobe, on the lateral surface of the cerebral hemisphere, posterior to the superior part of the postcentral sulcus, and above the intraparietal sulcus (Fig. C-3A).

lobule, posterior inferior, CEREBELLUM   *See* lobule, semilunar, inferior.

lobule, posterior superior, CEREBELLUM   *See* lobule, semilunar, superior.

lobule, quadrang´ular (crescentic or semilunar), anterior [lobulus quadrangularis, pars anterior, NA], CEREBELLUM   segment of the anterior lobe, on the superior surface of the cerebellar hemisphere, located between the postcentral fissure anteriorly and the primary fissure posteriorly. It is continuous with the culmen of the vermis (Figs. C-2, V-6).

lobule, quadrangular (crescentic or semilunar), posterior [lobulus quadrangularis, pars posterior, NA], CEREBELLUM segment of the posterior lobe, the hemispheric part of the lobulus simplex, on the upper surface of the cerebellum between the primary and postclival fissures. It is continuous with the declive of the vermis (Figs. C-2, V-6).

lobule, quad´rate, CEREBRUM *See* precuneus.

lobule, semilu´nar, anterior, CEREBELLUM *See* lobule, quadrangular, anterior.

lobule, semilunar, inferior [lobulus semilunaris inferior (caudalis), NA], CEREBELLUM segment of the posterior lobe, mainly on the inferior surface of the cerebellar hemisphere, caudal to the horizontal fissure, and continuous with the tuber vermis (Figs. C-2, V-6). *Syn:* posterior inferior lobule; ansiform lobule, crus II of comparative neuroanatomy.

lobule, semilunar, posterior, CEREBELLUM *See* lobule, quadrangular, posterior.

lobule, semilunar, superior [lobulus semilunaris superior (rostralis), NA], CEREBELLUM segment of the posterior lobe, on the superior surface of the cerebellar hemisphere, between the postclival and the horizontal fissures, and continuous with the folium vermis (Figs. C-2, V-6). *Syn:* posterior superior lobule; ansiform lobule, crus I, of comparative neuroanatomy.

lob´ulus median´us (of Larsell), CEREBELLUM subdivision of the vermis caudal to the lobulus simplex, comprising the folium vermis, tuber, pyramis, and uvula (Fig. V-6).

lobulus me´dius medianus, CEREBELLUM subdivision of the vermis caudal to lobulus simplex, and comprising: **1.** folium vermis and tuber (Ingvar terminology), **2.** folium vermis, tuber, and pyramis (Elliot Smith terminology).

lobulus sim´plex [NA], CEREBELLUM most rostral subdivision of the posterior lobe, on the superior surface of the cerebellum, between the primary and postclival fissures, and comprising the posterior quadrangular lobules of the hemispheres and the declive of the vermis (Figs. C-2, V-6).

lo´cus coeruleus /ser-oo´le-us/ [NA], PONS, [L. *locus* place; *caeruleus* sky-blue] bluish area on the floor of the fourth ventricle in the lateral part of the isthmus of the pons, overlying the nucleus of the locus coeruleus, the cells of which contain pigment (probably melanin) in their cytoplasm (Fig. V-4). These neurons, rich in noradrenaline, have fibers which distribute widely throughout the CNS, from cerebral cortex to spinal cord. A great number of functions have been attributed to this nucleus, including: the control of blood vessels within the CNS, regulation of respiration, micturition, and paradoxical (REM) sleep. It may also play a part in arousal and in the response to stress. *Syn:* nucleus pigmentosus pontis; substantia ferruginia. *For a review of this subject, see* Amaral and Sinnamon ('77).

loop, gamma a 3-neuron chain whereby normal muscle tone is maintained. The first neuron, the gamma motor neuron, is a small ventral horn cell, stimulated by descending spinal cord fibers. It stimulates the small intrafusal fibers of a neuromuscular spindle to contract. The second, an afferent neuron with stretch receptors in the spindle, synapses in the ventral horn with the third, an alpha motor neuron, which causes the extrafusal muscle fibers to contract (Fig. L-1). *See also* reflex, stretch.

loop, tem´poral, of the op´tic radia´tion, CEREBRUM fibers of the optic radiation which arise from the lateral half of the lateral geniculate nucleus and course around the anterior end of the inferior horn of the lateral ventricle before turning back to enter the occipital lobe. Injury to these fibers results in blindness in the superior quadrant of the contralateral visual field. *Syn:* Meyer's loop; occasionally called Archambault's, Cushing's, or Flechsig's loop.

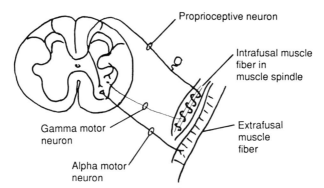

Fig. L-1. Diagram to illustrate the connections of the gamma loop. *See also* Fig. S-2.

Lou Gehrig's disease   *See* sclerosis, amyotrophic lateral. *See also* Gehrig, Lou.

Lorente de Nó, Rafael (1902-1990)   neuroanatomist and neurophysiologist, born in Spain. He studied under Ramón y Cajal and Bárány, and was for many years at the Rockefeller University in New York. He is noted especially for his studies of the cerebral cortex and the electrical and chemical basis of nerve conduction.

LP   lateral posterior nucleus of the dorsal thalamus.

Ludwig, Karl Friedrich Wilhelm (1816-1895)   eminent German physiologist. *Ludwig's ganglion* is a ganglion associated with the cardiac plexus, located near the right atrium of the heart.

Lugaro E. (19th century)   Italian anatomist. The *intermediate cells of Lugaro* are fusiform, horizontal cells in the granular layer of the cerebellar cortex.

lumbar (L), CORD   pertaining to one or more of the five lumbar spinal cord segments, nerves, or vertebrae.

Luschka, Hubert von (1820-1875)   German anatomist of Tübingen. The *foramina of Luschka* (ca. 1863) are the lateral apertures of the fourth ventricle. *Luschka's nerve* sometimes refers to the posterior ethmoidal nerve and sometimes to the sinuvertebral nerves, which are meningeal branches of the spinal nerves that supply structures within the spinal canal.

Luys, Jules Bernard (1828-1897)   French physician. The *body (nucleus) of Luys* or *corpus Luysii* is the subthalamic nucleus, a lesion of which causes hemiballismus.

lyra (of David), CEREBRUM   hippocampal commissure and the adjacent crura (pillars) of the fornix. *Syn:* psalterium (Fig. P-2).

m

macrog´lia [Gr. *makros* large; *glia* glue]   neuroglia of ectodermal origin, comprising the oligodendroglia and astroglia; originally a synonym for just the astroglia.

macroneuron /mak-ro-nu´ron/   neuron with a large cell body and a long axon.

mac´ula [NA], EYE, [L. spot]   *See* macula lutea.

macula acu´stica, EAR   either of two oval thickened areas in the utricle (macula utriculi) and in the saccule (macula sacculi) which constitute the sensory end organs in these vesicles.

macula lu´tea, EYE, [L. *luteus* saffron-yellow]   oval, yellowish area in the posterior part of the retina about 2.5 mm lateral to the optic papilla. It is devoid of all but capillary-size blood vessels but, in its center, the fovea centralis, the area of keenest vision, lacks even capillaries.

macula sac´culi [NA], EAR   sensory end organ of the saccule. It is an oval, thickened area in the anteromedial part of the wall of the saccule, lying in a sagittal plane. From its surface cilia project laterally into an otolithic membrane. It responds to linear acceleration as when the face is displaced forward. It may also respond to slow vibration.

macula utric´uli [NA], EAR   sensory end organ of the utricle. It is an oval, thickened area in the anterolateral part of the wall of the utricle, lying roughly in the plane of the base of the skull. From its surface cilia project vertically upward into an otolithic membrane. It is thought to be concerned with static equilibrium and to be stimulated by the force of gravity as when the head nods.

Magendie, François (1783-1855)   French physiologist of Paris. He described the cerebrospinal fluid and the *foramen of Magendie* (1825), the median aperture of the fourth ventricle. He also confirmed Bell's earlier findings that the ventral roots are motor and determined that the dorsal roots are sensory (about 1820). *See* Bell for the Bell-Magendie law.

magnet´ic res´onance im´aging (MRI)   *See* tomography.

magnetoencephalog´raphy (MEG)   *See* tomography.

magnocel´lular [L. *magnus* large]   composed of large cells.

Magnus, Rudolf (1873-1927)   German pharmacologist noted for his investigations of postural mechanisms (1924). The *Magnus and de Kleijn reflex,* indicative of decerebrate rigidity, consists of extension of one or both limbs and increased muscle tone on the side to which the face is turned when the head is rotated, and flexion of the limbs with loss of tone on the contralateral side.

mal´leus [NA], EAR, [L. hammer]   one of the ossicles of the middle ear. Its long process, the manubrium, is attached to the tympanic membrane. Its head articulates with the incus.

mam´illary, HYPOTHALAMUS, [L. *mamilla* little breast]   pertaining to the mamillary body, its nuclei, or its connections. The term *mamillary* and its various combining forms are used throughout this text, although *mammillary* has been and is still also widely used throughout the neuroscience literature.

manubrium mal´lei /man-oo´brī-um/ [NA], EAR, [L. *manubrium* handle]   the long process of the malleus.

Marchi, Vittorio (1851-1908)   Italian physician and anatomist, a pupil of Golgi's, who developed a technique, the *Marchi method,* for staining degenerating myelin in nerve fibers separated from their cell bodies. Partially degenerated myelin is selectively stained black by osmic acid but normal or completely degenerated myelin is left uncolored. This procedure helped to establish the neuron theory and in more recent years has been used as a research tool to determine the course and direction of conduction of nerve fibers within the CNS.

Marie, Pierre (1853-1940)   French neurologist, a pupil of Charcot's and, after Dejerine, chairman of clinical neurology at the Salpêtrière. Marie was noted for his studies of a number of neurologic disorders, including aphasia. *Marie's ataxia* is hereditary cerebellar ataxia. *Charcot-Marie-Tooth disease* is peroneal muscular atrophy. *See also* Charcot.

Marinescu, Georges (1864-1938)   Romanian neurologist, a pupil of Charcot's. During his long and illustrious career at the University of Bucharest, he and his colleagues reported on many neurologic disorders, including familial diseases, the correlation of a Parkinson tremor with damage to the substantia nigra, and the anatomical basis of the thalamic syndrome.

Martinotti, Giovanni (1857-1928)   Italian physician and anatomist, a student of Golgi's. The *cells of Martinotti* are neurons in the cerebral cortex, intermingled with the pyramidal cells. Their axons, directed toward the surface of the cerebral cortex, give off collaterals to the layers through which they pass, then spread out horizontally in the molecular layer (layer 1) and terminate.

mas´sa interme´dia, DORSAL THALAMUS   *See* adhesion, interthalamic.

mater /mah´ter/ [L. mother]   The term *mater* was applied to the meninges by Haly Abbas, a Persian physician in the tenth century, because it was believed at that time that the meninges gave rise to, or were the *mother* of, all the membranes of the body. *See also* dura mater; pia mater; arachnoid; meninges.

matter, gray [substantia grisea, NA]   that subdivision of the tissue of the CNS composed largely of nerve cell bodies and neuropil.

matter, white [substantia alba, NA]   that subdivision of the tissue of the CNS composed largely of myelinated nerve fibers.

Mauthner, Ludwig (1840-1894)   Austrian ophthalmologist. *Mauthner cells* are giant cells in the medulla oblongata of fishes. *Mauthner's sheath* is the axolemma of peripheral nerve fibers.

Mazzoni, Vittorio (1880-1940)　Italian physician. The *Golgi-Mazzoni corpuscle* is a sensory nerve ending, said to be a pressure ending. It is similar to a Pacinian corpuscle but smaller and simpler in structure.

McCarthy, Daniel J. (1874-1958)　American neurologist. The *McCarthy reflex* is a supraorbital reflex in which tapping of the supraorbital ridge causes contraction of the ipsilateral orbicularis oculi muscle and closure of the eye. Often there is a bilateral response.

meatus, acoustic (auditory), external /me-a´tus, ah-koo´stik/ [meatus acusticus externus, NA], ear, [L. *meatus* channel]　passage in the outer ear from the auricle to the tympanic membrane. It consists of an outer fibrocartilaginous part and an inner osseous part in the tympanic portion of the temporal bone.

meatus, acoustic (auditory), internal [meatus acusticus internus, NA], ear　channel in the petrous part of the temporal bone through which the vestibulocochlear and facial nerves and the internal auditory artery pass from the internal porus acusticus on the surface of the petrous part of the temporal bone, to the fundus of the internal acoustic meatus, where the facial and vestibulocochlear nerves separate to follow different courses.

mechanorecep´tor　superficial nerve ending that responds to mechanical stimulation, i.e. pressure.

Meckel, Johann Friedrich (the elder) (1714-1774)　German anatomist of Berlin. *Meckel's ganglion* (1748) is the pterygopalatine ganglion. *Meckel's lesser ganglion* is the submandibular ganglion and *Meckel's cavity* or *cave* is the space in the dura mater for the trigeminal ganglion, cavum trigeminale.

Meckel, Johann Friedrich (the younger) (1781-1833)　German anatomist and surgeon of Halle, grandson of Meckel the elder. The *cartilage of Meckel* is a cartilaginous bar in the embryo from which the malleus and the incus and certain related ligaments develop.

medul´la [*adj*. medullary, medullar] [L. marrow]　**1.** medulla oblongata. **2.** central core of a brain subdivision.

medulla, cerebel´lar　white matter of the cerebellum, between the cerebellar cortex and the deep cerebellar nuclei.

medulla, closed　caudal part of the medulla oblongata, containing the rostral part of the central canal. It is closed by the rostral parts of the fasciculi gracilis and cuneatus and their related nuclei.

medulla oblongata /ob-long-gah´tah/ [NA] [L. *oblongus* oblong]　caudal subdivision of the hindbrain interposed between the spinal cord and the pons. It is the adult derivative of the myelencephalon, the most caudal subdivision of the developing brain. Its two subdivisions are the open medulla bordering on the fourth ventricle and the closed medulla which surrounds the rostral part of the central canal. *Syn:* bulb; medulla.

medulla, open　rostral part of the medulla oblongata serving as a floor for the caudal part of the fourth ventricle (Fig. V-4).

medulla spinal´is [NA]　*See* cord, spinal.

medul´lar　pertaining to the medulla oblongata.

med´ullary　**1.** pertaining to the myelin sheath of nerve fibers. **2.** medullar.

med´ullate [*n*. medullation]　to have or to acquire a myelin (medullary) sheath. *Syn:* myelinate.

MEG   magnetoencephalography. *See* tomography.

Meissner, Georg (1829-1905)   German anatomist and physiologist of Basle and Göttingen. *Meissner's plexus* (1853) is the submucosal plexus of the gastrointestinal tract. *Meissner's corpuscles* (1853) are the peanut-shaped tactile corpuscles, located in the dermal papillae.

melato´nin   an indolamine, a hormone synthesized by the pineal body which inhibits gonad development and influences estrus in mammals. Its role in humans is unknown.

mem´brane, arachnoid /ar-ak´noid/   *See* arachnoid.

membrane, bas´ilar [lamina basilaris, NA], EAR   membrane suspended between the osseous spiral lamina and the spiral ligament, containing the auditory strings, and on which the spiral organ of the cochlea is located. *See also* membrane, spiral.

membrane, glial /gle´al/   *See* membrane, limiting, *def.* 1.

membrane, glassy, EYE   *See* choroid, basal layer.

membrane, hyaline /hi´a-lin/, EYE, [Gr. *hyalos* glass]   *See* choroid, basal layer.

membrane, hy´aloid, EYE   *See* membrane, vitreous.

membrane, limiting [membrana limitans, NA]   1. any of the glial membranes, composed of the footplates of astrocytes, on the external and ventricular surfaces of the brain and spinal cord and on the surfaces of their blood vessels. *Syn:* glia limitans.
   2. EYE   *See* retina, layers 3 and 10; *also* cornea.

membrane, limiting, anterior, EYE   *See* cornea, anterior limiting membrane.

membrane, limiting, external (outer)   1. *See* membrane, limiting, superficial.
   2. EYE   *See* retina, layer 3.

membrane, limiting, internal (inner)   1. *See* membrane, limiting, periventricular.
   2. EYE   *See* retina, layer 10.

membrane, limiting, outer   *See* membrane, limiting, external.

membrane, limiting, perivas´cular [membrana limitans gliae perivascularis, NA]   membrane composed of the footplates of the processes of astrocytes on capillaries of the CNS. *See also* barrier, blood-brain.

membrane, limiting, periventric´ular [membrana limitans gliae periventricularis, NA]   membrane underlying the ependyma of the ventricular spaces of the CNS. It consists of the footplates of the processes of astrocytes, intermingled with the processes of the ependymal cells. *Syn:* internal glia limitans; internal limiting membrane.

membrane, limiting, posterior, EYE   *See* cornea, posterior limiting membrane.

membrane, limiting, superficial [membrana limitans gliae superficialis, NA]   membrane at the surface of the brain and spinal cord, consisting of the footplates of the processes of astrocytes, attached to the overlying pia mater to form the pia-glial membrane. *Syn:* external (superficial) glia limitans; external limiting membrane; marginal glia (of Held).

membrane, otolith´ic, EAR   *See* membrane, statoconial.

membrane, pia-glial /pe-ah-gle´al/   non-nervous layer on the surface of the brain and spinal cord, composed of the superficial limiting membrane fused with the fibers of the overlying pia mater.

membrane, pu´pillary, EYE   membrane which covers the pupil in the embryo. It is continuous with the substantia propria of the iris. Normally, in man, it disappears before birth.

membrane (lamina), retic´ular [membrana reticularis, NA], EAR   surface of the spiral organ of the cochlea. The intercellular spaces between the hair, pillar, and phalangeal cells and the adjoining border and Hensen cells give the surface of this structure a netlike appearance.

membrane, spi´ral [membrana spiralis (paries tympanicus ductus cochlearis), NA], ᴇᴀʀ the basilar membrane and the osseous spiral lamina which together separate the cochlear duct from the scala tympani in the cochlea.

membrane, stape´dial [membrana stapedis, NA], ᴇᴀʀ delicate membranous layer between the crura and base of the stapes in the middle ear.

membrane, statoco´nial [membrana statoconiorum, NA], ᴇᴀʀ thick, gelatinous structure overlying the maculae of the utricle and saccule of the membranous labyrinth, into which cilia project from the macular surface. It is composed of mucopolysacharides and contains small, tightly packed calcite crystals, the statoconia.

membrane, tector´ial [membrana tectoria, NA], ᴇᴀʀ flexible, gelatinous membrane attached along the vestibular lip of the spiral limbus. It overlies the rest of the spiral organ throughout the length of the cochlear duct.

membrane, tympanic /tim-pan´ik/ [membrana tympani, NA], ᴇᴀʀ membrane that separates the external auditory meatus of the external ear from the tympanic cavity of the middle ear.

membrane, tympanic, secondary [membrana tympani secundaria, NA], ᴇᴀʀ membrane that closes the round window, between the tympanic cavity of the middle ear and the scala tympani of the internal ear. *Syn:* Scarpa's membrane.

membrane, vestib´ular [membrana vestibularis (paries vestibularis ductus cochlearis), NA], ᴇᴀʀ membrane separating the cochlear duct from the scala vestibuli in the cochlea. *Syn:* Reissner's membrane.

membrane, vit´reous [membrana vitrea, NA], ᴇʏᴇ, [L. *vitrum* glass] so-called membrane at the free surface of the vitreous body of the eye. In reality it is a condensation of fibrils at the surface of this structure and not a true capsule. *Syn:* hyaloid membrane.

Menière, Prosper (1799-1862) French otologist. *Menière's syndrome,* a disorder of the internal ear, is characterized by recurrent attacks of vertigo associated with tinnitus and deafness. *Note:* Prosper wrote his name Menière but his son changed it to Ménière.

meninges /men-in´jĕz/ [NA] [Gr. *meninx* membrane] membranous coverings of the brain and spinal cord, *viz.* the dura mater, pia mater, and arachnoid. *See also* mater; leptomeninges; pachymeninx.

meningocele /men-ing´go-sĕl/ saclike protrusion of skin and meninges through a vertebral or cranial defect. *See also* spina bifida cystica.

meningoenceph´alocele abnormality in which both the brain and its meninges are herniated through a defect in the skull. *See also* spina bifida cystica.

meningomy´elocele saclike protrusion of skin, meninges, and spinal cord through a vertebral defect. *See also* spina bifida cystica.

meninx /men´inks/ [*pl.* **meninges**] [Gr. membrane] one of the membranous coverings of the brain and spinal cord. *See also* meninges.

Merkel, Friedrich Siegmund (1845-1919) German anatomist. *Merkel's disks* are specialized nerve endings, tactile disks, in the epidermis.

mesaxon /mez-ak´sŏn/ [NA] [Gr. *mesos* middle] mesentery-like connection of the plasma membrane surrounding the axis cylinder and the innermost coil of the myelin sheath (inner mesaxon) of both central and PNS nerve fibers and a similar connection between the outer coil of the myelin sheath and the neurolemma, the outermost part of the Schwann cell sheath (outer mesaxon) of PNS fibers.

mesencephalon /mez-en-sef´ă-lon/ [NA], MIDBRAIN, [Gr. *mesos-*; *enkephalos* brain] middle segment of the embryonic brain, which unlike the prosencephalon and rhombencephalon, does not further subdivide. In the adult it consists of the tectum and the cerebral peduncles (Fig. P-1).

mesocele /mez´o-sēl/, MIDBRAIN   lumen of the developing mesencephalon.

mesocor´tex [NA], CEREBRUM   transitional cortex in a region where one type borders on another.

mesog´lia [Gr. *glia* glue]   microglia.

met´apore, MYELENCEPHALON, [Gr. *meta* after; *poros* pore]   old term for the median aperture of the fourth ventricle.

metatel´a, MYELENCEPHALON   roof plate of the developing rhombencephalon, from which develop the posterior medullary velum and the choroid plexus in the caudal part of the fourth ventricle.

metathal´amus [NA], DORSAL THALAMUS   those nuclei of the dorsal thalamus located in the caudal and posterior part of the diencephalon, consisting of the lateral and medial geniculate nuclei, the thalamic centers for vision and hearing. *See also* thalamus, dorsal.

metencephalon /met-en-sef´ă-lon/ [NA], HINDBRAIN   that part of the rhombencephalon, from which the pons and cerebellum are derived.

met-enkephalin   *See* enkephalin.

Mettler, Frederick Albert (1907-1984)   American neuroanatomist, for many years a renowned investigator at the College of Physicians and Surgeons of Columbia University, New York.

Meyer, Adolph (1866-1950)   Swiss neuropathologist and psychiatrist, later active in the United States. *Meyer's loop* is the temporal loop of the optic radiation.

Meynert, Theodor Hermann (1833-1892)   Austrian psychiatrist and neurologist of Vienna who made many contributions to the study of the nervous system. He described the association fibers of the cerebrum. Named for him were: *Meynert's decussation* (1869), the dorsal tegmental decussation; *Meynert's bundle* or *fasciculus,* the habenulopeduncular tract or fasciculus retroflexus; and the *ganglion* or *basal nucleus of Meynert* in the substantia innominata. The term *commissure of Meynert* sometimes is used to mean the ventral supraoptic decussation and sometimes is used also to include part of the dorsal supraoptic decussation.

microcephaly /mi-kro-sef´al-ī/ [Gr. *micros* small; *kephale* head]   congenital abnormality in which the cerebrum is underdeveloped, the fontanels close prematurely, and, as a result, the head is small. It was first described by Bartholomaeus Metlinger, a pediatrician, in 1473.

microg´lia [NA] [Gr. *micros-*; *glia* glue]   neuroglial cells of mesodermal origin which, in the resting state, have small elongated, triangular, or kidney-shaped nuclei and scanty cytoplasm, but which enlarge and become phagocytic in many pathologic conditions. *Syn:* Hortega cell; mesoglia; rod cell.

microneuron /mi-kro-nu´ron/   neuron with a small cell body and a short axon.

microtubule /mi-kro-too´būl/   neurotubule.

midbrain   *See* mesencephalon.

Minkowski, Mechyslav (b. 1884)   Polish-born neurologist, active in Switzerland, noted for his studies of cortical function, especially the visual system. He established that the posterior and medial area of the occipital lobe is visual cortex.

miosis /mi-o´sis/ [Gr. *meiosis* lessening]   marked pupillary constriction.

Mitchell, Silas Weir (1829-1914)   leading American neurologist of his time. He is noted for his research on the cerebellum, and for his studies of causalgia and other peripheral nerve disorders during the American Civil War.

mitochondrion /mi-to-kon´drī-on, mit-o-kon´drī-on/ [*pl.* **mitochondria**]   granular or filamentous organoid found in the cell bodies and processes of neurons and in other cells.

MLF   medial longitudinal fasciculus.

modal´ity, sensory   a specific type of sensation, such as touch, pain, vision, or hearing.

modi´olus [NA], ᴇᴀʀ, [L. hub of a wheel]   bony core of the cochlea through which the cochlear nerve passes. It was originally described and named by Eustachius in 1563.

Moebius (Möbius), Paul Julius (1853-1907)   German neurologist who practiced in Leipzig. *Moebius' syndrome* is congenital facial paralysis, sometimes with paralysis of muscles supplied by other cranial nerves. It results from maldevelopment of the motor nuclei and is inherited as an autosomal dominant.

Mollaret, P. (b. 1898)   French neurologist. *See* Guillain for the *triangle of Guillain-Mollaret*.

Monakow, Constantin von (1853-1930)   Russian neurologist, active in Switzerland. Among his other accomplishments he published a monumental work on neuropathology (1897). The *area of Monakow* is the area in the medulla between the spinal nucleus and tract of V dorsolaterally and the inferior olivary nucleus ventromedially, and containing, among others, the lateral spinothalamic tract. The *nucleus of Monakow* is the accessory cuneate nucleus and the *tract of Monakow* is the rubrospinal tract.

Moniz, Egas (1874-1955)   Portuguese physician. His name originally was Antonio Caetano deAbreu Freire. The name of Egas Moniz, a Portuguese national hero, was added at his baptism. He introduced cerebral angiography as a diagnostic procedure in 1927 and in 1949 he shared the Nobel Prize in physiology and medicine, for his introduction of prefrontal leukotomy as a psychosurgery tool.

monoam´ines   group of neurotransmitters comprising the catecholamines dopamine, norepinephrine, and epinephrine and the indolamine, serotonin.

monoplegia /mon-o-ple´jī-ah/   paralysis of one limb.

Monro, Alexander (1733-1817)   the second of three Scottish anatomists of the same name. The *foramen of Monro* (1797) is the interventricular foramen. *Monro's sulcus* is the hypothalamic sulcus. The *cavum Monroi* is the anterior part of the third ventricle, also called the ventriculus impar telencephalicus.

monticulus /mon-tik´u-lus/, ᴄᴇʀᴇʙᴇʟʟᴜᴍ, [L. small eminence]   segment of the cerebellar vermis comprising the culmen, declive, and folium vermis (Fig. V-6).

motoneuron /mo-to-nu´ron/   motor neuron whose cell body is located in a motor nucleus in the CNS, and which conducts impulses to motor end plates in skeletal muscle. *See also* neuron, motor, lower.

MRI   magnetic resonance imaging. *See* tomography.

Müller, Heinrich (1820-1864)   German anatomist noted for his studies of the eye, including the discovery of the visual purple (1851). *Müller's muscle* is the smooth muscle of the eyelid which helps to keep the eye open. The circular fibers of the ciliary muscle are also called *Müller's muscle*. *Müller's cells* are supporting cells, neuroglial in type, located in the retina. Their nuclei are in the inner nuclear layer

(layer 7) of the retina; their delicate processes extend into all retinal layers and also form the inner (layer 10) and outer (layer 3) limiting membranes.

Müller, Johannes (1801-1858)   German neurophysiologist, noted especially for his doctrine of specific nerve energies, according to which each sense organ, regardless of how stimulated, gives rise to its own characteristic sensory modality.

muscarin´ic   pertaining to muscarine, a naturally occurring alkaloid similar to acetylcholine. Muscarinic receptors are activated by ACh and by muscarine and are inhibited by atropine. They are the only receptors at postganglionic parasympathetic endings, where activation results in a slower heart rate and increased glandular secretion. These receptors also occur along with nicotinic receptors on autonomic ganglion cells and in certain CNS areas. *See also* nicotinic.

muscular dystrophy   *See* dystrophy, muscular.

Muskens, L.J.J. (early 20th century)   Dutch neuroanatomist. The *interstitiospinal fasciculus of Muskens* is the extrapyramidal or conditioning component of the medial longitudinal fasciculus (Fig. F-2).

mu´tism, akinet´ic [L. *mutus* silent; Gr. *a* not; *kinesis* movement]   syndrome characterized by a lack of speech and, except when provoked, lack of movement. The patient may retain eye movements and appear to be awake. The disorder is usually associated with lesions involving median or paramedian structures, typically including the periaqueductal gray and upper midbrain tegmentum and the mesodiencephalic junction but sometimes the cerebral hemisphere, especially the septal area and cingulate gyrus. *Syn:* coma vigil. *For additional information on this subject and a review of the literature, see* Alves and Ceballos ('71).

mydri´asis [Gr. *mydros* red hot metal]   dilation of the pupil. Hippocrates is said to have applied the term *mydros* to the instrument he used as a cautery. Because the cautery produced pain and fear with an attendant dilation of the pupils, the term became associated with pupil dilation. *See* reflex, ciliospinal for the connections (Fig. R-3).

myelencephalon /mi-el-en-sef´al-on/ [NA], ʜɪɴᴅʙʀᴀɪɴ, [Gr. *myelos* marrow; *enkephalos* brain]   most caudal subdivision of the rhombencephalon, from which the medulla oblongata is derived.

myelin /mi´el-in/ [Gr. *myelos* marrow]   white, fatty sheath surrounding the axis cylinder of many central and peripheral nerve fibers. The myelin sheath consists of multiple concentric layers of lipid and protein substances around the axis cylinder of many central and peripheral nerve fibers. In the PNS it is continuous with the neurolemma sheath (of Schwann) and formed by the cytoplasm of the sheath cells. Within the CNS it is produced by oligodendroglia (Figs. M-1, R-1).

myelinate /mi´el-in-āt/   to have or to acquire a myelin or medullary sheath. *Syn:* medullate.

myelina´tion   process whereby a nerve fiber acquires its myelin sheath. *Syn:* medullation.

myeli´tis, transverse   transection of the spinal cord.

myeloarchitecton´ic   pertaining to the myeloarchitecture of the CNS.

myeloarchitecton´ics   myeloarchitecture.

myeloarch´itecture   architecture of the CNS according to the pattern of its myelinated nerve fibers. *Syn:* myeloarchitectonics.

myelocele /mi´el-o-sēl/, ᴄᴏʀᴅ   malformation in the region of the developing spinal cord, in which there is incomplete fusion of the neural plate to form the neural tube. Usually the defective spinal cord lies exposed on the surface of the body.

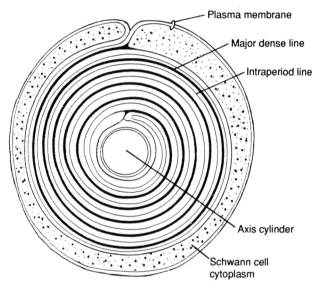

Fig. M-1.   Diagram to show the component layers of the myelin sheath, of a peripheral nerve fiber, and the continuity of the major dense and intraperiod lines with the internal and external layers of the plasma membrane.

my´elogram   roentgenogram of the spinal subarachnoid space following intro-duction of air or radiopaque oil.

my´elomere [Gr. *myelos* marrow; *meros* part]   spinal cord segment.

my´elon   *See* cord, spinal.

myeloschisis /mi-ĕ-lo-ske´sis/, cord   advanced and ultimately fatal form of spina bifida in which the spinal cord is a wideopen, exuding, shiny mass which has protruded entirely through the vertebral defect.

myoclo´nus, pal´atal   rhythmic contractions of the palate after a lesion of the inferior olivary nucleus, or the dento-olivary fibers in the pontine portion of the central tegmental tract (Fig. O-1). *Syn:* palatal nystagmus.

my´oid, eye   part of the inner segment of rods and cones, between the ellipsoid and the outer limiting membrane. This region contains ribosomes, granular endo-plasmic reticulum, and the Golgi apparatus, and may be the site of protein synthesis.

myo´sis   obsolete spelling for miosis.

n

NA   **1.** Nomina Anatomica.

     2. noradrenaline.

naloxone /nal-oks´ōn/   a specific opiate antagonist, used as an antidote to counteract narcotic overdosage.

narcolepsy /nar´ko-lep-sĭ/   disorder characterized by paroxysmal, recurrent, and irresistible diurnal attacks of sleep or drowsiness.

nasion /na´zĭ-on/ [NA]   midpoint of the frontonasal suture at the root of the nose. It is a landmark used in determining, within the intact skull or in X-rays, the location of certain intracranial features.

Nauta, Walle Jetze Harinx   contemporary American neuroanatomist who developed a widely used procedure using silver to stain degenerating nerve fibers.

NE   norepinephrine.

neocerebel´lum [NA], CEREBELLUM, [Gr. *neos* new; cerebellum]   phylogenetically newest part of the cerebellum, comprising the cerebellar hemispheres exclusive of the flocculus. *Syn:* pontocerebellum.

neocor´tex [NA], CEREBRUM, [Gr. *neos-*; L. *cortex* bark]   late-developing 6-layered cortex of the neopallium. It develops primarily through the elaboration of nonolfactory functions and, in man, makes up the major portion of the cerebral cortex. *Syn:* isocortex; homogenetic cortex.

neo-ol´ive, MEDULLA   lateral, late-developing part of the inferior olivary nucleus.

neopal´lium, CEREBRUM   late-developing cerebral cortex (neocortex) and its underlying white matter, exclusive of the piriform area (paleopallium) and of the hippocampal formation (archipallium).

neostria´tum, CEREBRUM   late-developing part of the corpus striatum, comprising the caudate nucleus and putamen. *See also* striatum.

nerve [nervus, NA]   bundle of peripheral nerve fibers bound together into one or more fascicles by connective tissue investments. *See also* nervi; nervus.

nerve, abducens (abducent) (VI) /ab-doo´sens, ab-doo´sent/ [nervus abducens, NA] cranial nerve which arises from cells in the abducens nucleus in the pons. Its fibers emerge from the ventral surface of the brain stem, just lateral to the pyramidal tract, at the junction of the pons and medulla. After leaving the posterior fossa the nerve traverses the cavernous sinus (Fig. S-1) and enters the orbit through the superior orbital fissure to supply the lateral rectus muscle of the eye. *See also* Table C-2.

nerve, accessory (XI) /ak-ses´or-ĭ/ [nervus accessorius, NA] cranial nerve, composed of a spinal part which arises from the cervical spinal cord, and a bulbar part, from the closed medulla. The two parts join the vagus nerve and leave the cranial cavity together through the jugular foramen. *See also* Table C-1.

nerve, accessory, bul´bar (XI) [nervus accessorius pars vagalis, NA] part of cranial nerve XI which arises from visceral motor nuclei in the closed medulla. It joins the vagus nerve and supplements its motor components. Fibers from the caudal part of the nucleus ambiguus become the recurrent laryngeal nerve and innervate laryngeal muscle. Fibers presumably from the caudal part of the dorsal motor nucleus distribute, as part of the vagus nerve, for termination in the ascending and the transverse colon. *See also* Table C-1.

nerve, accessory, spinal (XI) [nervus accessorius pars spinalis, NA] nerve which arises from cells in the accessory nucleus of the cervical spinal cord. The axons of these cells emerge from the lateral surface of the cord between the dorsal roots and the dentate ligament, then collect into a fascicle which turns rostrally and passes through the foramen magnum into the cranial cavity where it joins the bulbar accessory nerve and the vagus nerve. Its fibers supply the sternocleido-mastoid muscle and the upper part of the trapezius muscle. Because of its long course through the subarachnoid space the spinal accessory nerve is especially susceptible to any irritant, such as blood, in the cerebrospinal fluid. Consequently, a stiff neck, caused by contraction of the muscles which this nerve supplies, is used as a sign of subarachnoid hemorrhage. *See also* nucleus, accessory, of the spinal cord; Table C-1. *Syn:* nerve of Willis.

nerve, acoustic (VIII) /ah-koos´tik/ *See* nerve, vestibulocochlear.

nerve, aor´tic depres´sor branch of the vagus nerve with stretch receptors in the aortic arch. It is analogous in function to the carotid sinus nerve. *Syn:* nerve of Cyon.

nerve, auditory (VIII) *See* nerve, vestibulocochlear.

nerve, axillary [nervus axillaris, NA] nerve which arises from the posterior cord of the brachial plexus with fibers from spinal cord segments C5-C6. It supplies mainly the deltoid muscle, which is the chief abductor of the arm at the shoulder joint, and the skin over the same area.

nerve, carot´id si´nus [ramus sinus caroticus glossopharyngei, NA] branch of the glossopharyngeal nerve carrying afferent fibers from the carotid sinus and carotid body. *Syn:* Hering's nerve. *See* reflex, carotid sinus.

nerve cell   1. neuron.

2. *See* body, cell.

nerves, cer´vical [nervi cervicales, NA] any of eight spinal nerves on each side of the spinal cord. They are formed by the fusion of dorsal and ventral roots and emerge from the vertebral column between the skull and the first cervical vertebra (nerve C1), between the cervical vertebrae (nerves C2-C7), and between the seventh cervical and the first thoracic vertebrae (nerve C8).

nerve, cervical sympathet´ic   that part of the sympathetic trunk between the superior cervical ganglion above, and the middle and inferior cervical ganglia below.

nerves, cil´iary [nervi ciliares, NA]   any of certain small nerves in the orbit, composed of autonomic and sensory nerve fibers.

nerves, ciliary, long [nervi ciliares longi, NA]   two or three small branches of the nasociliary nerve within the orbit. They are composed mainly of sensory fibers from the eyeball, and some postganglionic sympathetic fibers for dilation of the pupil and activation of the smooth muscle of the upper eyelid.

nerves, ciliary, short [nervi ciliares breves, NA]   six to 10 small nerves in the orbit, from the ciliary ganglion to the eyeball. They contain postganglionic parasympathetic fibers from the ciliary ganglion for contraction of the pupil and activation of the ciliary muscle and join the long ciliary nerves which also supply the eyeball (Figs. R-2, R-7).

nerve, cochlear (VIII) /kok´le-ar/ [nervus cochlearis, NA]   cochlear division of the vestibulocochlear nerve, composed of fibers from the spiral organ which join the brain stem just lateral to the vestibular nerve and end in the cochlear nuclei of the brain stem. *See also* Table C-2 *and* Fig. R-8.

nerve component   *See* component, nerve.

nerves, cra´nial [nervi craniales, NA]   any of the nerves which attach to the brain. They are: the olfactory (I), optic (II), oculomotor (III), trochlear (IV), trigeminal (V), abducens (VI), facial (VII), vestibulocochlear (VIII), glossopharyngeal (IX), vagus (X), accessory (XI), and hypoglossal (XII) nerves.

nerve, cranial, thirteenth   nerve described by Benedikt and said by him to lie on the floor of the fourth ventricle, to arise from a special nucleus, and to supply the blood vessels and villi of the choroid plexus.

nerve, dorsal   any thoracic nerve.

nerve ending   *See* ending, nerve.

nerve, fa´cial (VII) [nervus facialis, NA]   cranial nerve which arises from the ventrolateral surface of the pons at its junction with the medulla. It enters the petrous bone through the internal auditory meatus and passes through the facial canal. Most of its fibers leave the skull through the stylomastoid foramen. It is composed mostly of motor fibers which supply the muscles of facial expression, including those that close the eye (Fig. R-4) and the stapedial muscle of the middle ear (Fig. R-8), preganglionic parasympathetic fibers for relay to the lacrimal gland in the orbit (Fig. R-6) and to the salivary glands (other than the parotid) (Fig. S-3), taste fibers from the anterior two-thirds of the tongue, and some cutaneous fibers from the external ear (Fig. O-2). Stimulation of the salivatory fibers results in the secretion of a high-volume, low-viscosity saliva (Fig. C-4). *See also* plexus, carotid, external; *and* genu, internal *and* external (of the facial nerve); Fig. T-2 *and* Table C-2.

nerve, fem´oral [nervus femoralis, NA]   largest branch of the lumbar plexus, arising from the ventral primary divisions of nerves L2-L4. It supplies muscles of the anterior compartment of the thigh and the overlying skin, muscles which flex the thigh at the hip joint and extend the leg at the knee joint.

nerve fiber   *See* fiber, nerve.

nerve, fur´cal [L. *furca* fork]   branch, usually of the fourth lumbar nerve but occasionally the third or fifth, which divides and sends one branch to the lumbar plexus and one to the sacral plexus.

nerve, glossopal´atine   *See* nervus intermedius.

nerve, glossopharyngeal (IX) /glos-o-far-in´jī-al/ [nervus glossopharyngeus, NA] cranial nerve which arises by several rootlets from the ventrolateral surface of the medulla just caudal to the attachment of the facial nerve. The rootlets combine into one bundle that leaves the cranial cavity in its own dural sleeve by way of the jugular foramen. It contains visceral afferent nerve fibers important in the regulation of blood pressure and of respiration, taste fibers from the back of the tongue, and sensory fibers from the palate and pharynx (Fig. O-2). It also supplies preganglionic parasympathetic fibers for the parotid gland and the von Ebner glands (small serous glands whose ducts empty into the troughs around the circumvallate papillae at the back of the tongue) (Fig. S-3), and motor fibers for the stylopharyngeus muscle. *See also* nerve, facial; plexus, external carotid; reflex, carotid sinus; reflexes, vagal; Figs. R-9, T-2; Table C-1.

nerve growth factor (NGF)   protein first identified in mouse sarcoma 180 and found to stimulate hypertrophy and hyperplasia of spinal (Bueker, '48), and sympathetic (Levi-Montalcini and Hamburger, '51) ganglion cells. It has since been found in cultures of many cell types, especially in snake venom and male mouse submandibular gland, and is now thought also to help maintain these cells and other types of neurons. *For a review of this subject, see* Mobley *et al.* ('77).

nerve, hypoglos´sal (XII) [nervus hypoglossus, NA]   cranial nerve which arises from cells in the hypoglossal nucleus in the medulla. Its fibers emerge from the medulla between the pyramid and the inferior olive, and collect into a nerve trunk which leaves the posterior fossa through the hypoglossal canal to supply all the muscles of the tongue except the palatoglossus. *See also* Table C-1.

nerve, intermediate   *See* nervus intermedius.

nerves, lum´bar [nervi lumbares (lumbales), NA]   five spinal nerves formed by the fusion of dorsal and ventral roots on each side of the spinal cord. Each nerve emerges from the vertebral column through the intervertebral foramen below the corresponding lumbar vertebra.

nerve, mandib´ular (V₃) [nervus mandibularis, NA]   the inferior division of the trigeminal nerve, which passes through the foramen ovale in the base of the skull. It consists of a small motor root and a large sensory root. Its motor fibers supply the chewing muscles. Its sensory fibers carry impulses for pain, temperature, and tactile sensation from the skin of the lower part of the face (not including the angle of the jaw) and from the floor of the mouth, the tongue, and the lower teeth; it also contains fibers from the temporomandibular joint (Figs. C-4, N-1, T-2). *Syn:* inferior maxillary nerve.

nerve, max´illary (V₂) [nervus maxillaris, NA]   the middle division of the trigeminal nerve, which passes through the lateral wall of the cavernous sinus (Fig. S-1) then the foramen ovale in the base of the skull. It consists exclusively of afferent fibers which carry impulses for pain, temperature, and tactile sensibility from the midportion of the face and the upper part of the oral cavity, including the hard palate and upper teeth (Figs. N-1, T-2). *Syn:* superior maxillary nerve.

nerve, me´dian [nervus medianus, NA]   nerve which arises from the lateral and medial cords of the brachial plexus with fibers mainly from spinal cord segments C6-T1. It supplies all the muscles of the anterior aspect of the forearm except the flexor carpi ulnaris, muscles which flex the wrist and the fingers. It also supplies the muscles of the thenar eminence which act upon the thumb. Its sensory branches supply the lateral part (thumb side) of the palm, the palmar surface and tips of the first three fingers, and the lateral side of the fourth finger.

nerves (of the) medulla oblongata   the glossopharyngeal, vagus, bulbar accessory, and hypoglossal nerves. *See* Table C-1.

nerve, menin´geal, middle [ramus meningeus medius, NA]   branch of the maxillary division of the trigeminal nerve, which passes through the foramen spinosum and provides sensory fibers for the dura mater of the middle cranial fossa.

nerves (of the) midbrain   the oculomotor and trochlear nerves. *See* Table C-3.

nerve, musculocuta´neous [nervus musculocutaneus, NA]   nerve which arises from the lateral cord of the brachial plexus with fibers from spinal cord segments C5-C6. It supplies primarily the muscles of the anterior compartment of the arm, which serve to flex the forearm at the elbow joint. Below the elbow it provides sensory fibers for the skin over the radial (lateral) half of the forearm and a small part of the thenar eminence.

nerve, musculospi´ral   old term for the radial nerve.

nerve, oculomo´tor (III) [nervus oculomotorius, NA]   cranial nerve composed of nerve fibers which arise from the oculomotor and the Edinger-Westphal (accessory oculomotor) nuclei in the midbrain. It emerges from the interpeduncular fossa of the midbrain, passes between the posterior cerebral and superior cerebellar arteries, traverses the cavernous sinus (Fig. S-1), and enters the orbit through the superior orbital fissure to supply most of the extraocular muscles and the parasympathetic innervation for the ciliary muscle and the constrictor muscle of the iris (Figs. R-2, R-7, S-3). *See also* Table C-3.

nerves, olfac´tory (I) [nervi olfactorii, NA]   cranial nerve composed of fascicles of fine unmyelinated nerve fibers which arise from bipolar neurons in the olfactory mucosa, pass through the perforations in the cribriform plate, and terminate in glomeruli of the olfactory bulb. Olfactory neurons are able to regenerate and form new synapses.

nerve, ophthal´mic (V₁) [nervus ophthalmicus, NA]   the superior division of the trigeminal nerve. It passes through the lateral wall of the cavernous sinus (Fig. S-1), then the superior orbital fissure to enter the orbit. It consists exclusively of afferent fibers from the orbit and upper part of the face by way of the lacrimal, frontal, and nasociliary nerves (Figs. N-1, R-4, T-2).

nerve, op´tic (II) [nervus opticus, NA]   cranial nerve composed of nerve fibers from the optic nerve fiber layer (layer 9) of the retina, which are axons of the large cells of the ganglion cell layer (layer 8). Fascicles pass through the perforations in the lamina cribrosa at the back of the sclera. From the back of the orbit the nerve passes through the optic canal in the sphenoid bone into the cranial cavity to reach the optic chiasm where some of its fibers cross the median plane. *See also* Fig. S-1.

nerves, pel´vic   *See* nerves, splanchnic, pelvic.

nerve, phren´ic [nervus phrenicus, NA] [Gr. *phren* diaphragm]   nerve arising primarily from cervical spinal cord segments C3-C6. Its fibers are part of the cervical plexus, and traverse the thorax to supply the diaphragm.

nerve, pneumogastric (X) /nu-mo-gas´trik/ [Gr. *pneumo* lung; *gaster* stomach]   old term for the vagus nerve.

nerves (of the) pons   the trigeminal, abducens, facial, and vestibulocochlear nerves. *See* Table C-2.

nerve, presa´cral   neither a separate nerve nor presacral, it consists of two or three interconnected strands of nerve fibers, which descend anterior to the bifurcation of the aorta, left common iliac vein, last lumbar vertebra, and lumbosacral disk. It is continued caudally as the two hypogastric nerves. *See* plexus, hypogastric, superior.

nerve, ra´dial [nervus radialis, NA] nerve arising from the posterior cord of the brachial plexus with fibers mainly from spinal cord segments C6-C8. It supplies the extensor muscles of the arm and forearm, the overlying skin, and most of the back of the hand and fingers. *Syn:* musculospiral nerve.

nerve root fascicle of nerve fibers of a cranial or spinal nerve, either within the brain or spinal cord or in the subarachnoid space.

nerves, sa´cral [nervi sacrales, NA] five spinal nerves formed by the fusion of dorsal and ventral roots from the sacral spinal cord. Within the sacrum the nerves divide into anterior and posterior primary rami, and the rami then emerge through the anterior and posterior sacral foramina, respectively.

nerve, sciatic (great) /si-at´ik/ [nervus sciaticus (ischiadicus), NA] largest nerve of the body, it arises from the lumbosacral plexus with fibers from spinal cord segments L4-S3. It supplies all the muscles of the leg and foot and those of the posterior part of the thigh and the overlying skin. Its main terminal branches are the tibial and the common peroneal nerves.

nerves, sinuver´tebral [ramus meningeus nervorum spinalium, NA] the meningeal branches of the spinal nerves, which supply structures within the vertebral canal. *Syn:* Luschka's nerve.

nerves, spi´nal [nervi spinales, NA] nerves formed in the intervertebral foramina by the fusion of the dorsal and ventral roots of each spinal cord segment and consisting of the fibers which innervate structures that develop at the corresponding segmental levels.

nerve, spinal acces´sory (XI) *See* nerve, accessory, spinal.

nerves, splanchnic /splank´nik/ [nervi splanchnici, NA] [Gr. *splanchna* viscera] any of the nerves composed primarily of preganglionic sympathetic fibers which arise in the spinal cord, pass through the ganglia of the sympathetic trunk without synapse, and terminate in relation to postganglionic neurons of the prevertebral ganglia (Fig. S-3). Also included are some visceral afferent fibers from the regions innervated.

nerve, splanchnic, greater [nervus splanchnicus thoracicus major, NA] nerve composed primarily of preganglionic sympathetic fibers, usually from spinal cord segments T5-T9, which pass through the ganglia of the sympathetic trunk without synapse. It passes through the diaphragm and ends in the celiac ganglion (Fig. S-3).

nerve, splanchnic, least (lowest) [nervus splanchnicus thoracicus imus, NA] [L. *ima* lowest] smallest splanchnic nerve composed primarily of preganglionic sympathetic fibers, usually from spinal cord segment T12 which pass through the ganglia of the sympathetic trunk without synapse, then through the diaphragm, and end in the aorticorenal ganglion. *Syn:* renal nerve.

nerve, splanchnic, lesser [nervus splanchnicus thoracicus minor, NA] nerve composed primarily of preganglionic sympathetic fibers, usually from spinal cord segments T10-T11. They pass through the ganglia of the sympathetic trunk without synapse, then through the diaphragm, and end in the celiac and superior mesenteric ganglia and in the adrenal medulla (Fig. S-3).

nerves, splanchnic, lum´bar [nervi splanchnici lumbares (lumbales), NA] nerve composed primarily of preganglionic sympathetic fibers, usually from spinal cord segments L1-L3. They pass through the ganglia of the sympathetic trunk without synapse, and end in the inferior mesenteric ganglion for relay to the descending and sigmoid colon, pelvic viscera and genitalia, but excluding the gonads (Fig. S-3).

nerves, splanchnic, pel´vic [nervi splanchnici pelvici (nervi erigentes), NA] preganglionic parasympathetic fibers from spinal cord segments S2-S4 for termination on ganglion cells in the walls of the descending and sigmoid colon, pelvic viscera, and genitalia, but excluding the gonads (Fig. S-3). *Syn:* nervi erigentes; pelvic nerves.

nerve, splanchnic, sa´cral [nervi splanchnici sacrales, NA] small filaments of preganglionic, sympathetic fibers which descend in the sympathetic trunk to sacral levels and terminate in prevertebral ganglia for relay to the pelvic viscera.

nerve, splanchnic, thorac´ic any of the splanchnic nerves (greater, lesser, and least) which arise from spinal cord segments T5-T12 and pass through the diaphragm before reaching the prevertebral ganglia in which they end (Fig. S-3).

nerve, stape´dial [nervus stapedius, NA] small branch which arises from the facial nerve as it descends in the posterior wall of the tympanic cavity. It enters the middle ear and supplies the stapedial muscle. Injury to this nerve, if auditory connections are intact, causes hyperacusis (Fig. R-8).

nerve, statoacoustic (VIII) /stat-o-ah-koo´stik/ old term for the vestibulocochlear nerve.

nerve, terminal *See* nervus terminalis.

nerves, thorac´ic [nervi thoracici, NA] any of 12 spinal nerves formed by the fusion of dorsal and ventral roots from the thoracic spinal cord. Each nerve emerges from the vertebral column through the intervertebral foramen below the corresponding thoracic vertebra.

nerve, trifa´cial (V) old term for the trigeminal nerve.

nerve, trigem´inal (V) [nervus trigeminus, NA] cranial nerve which leaves the lateral surface of the pons. Just peripheral to its ganglion, it divides into three

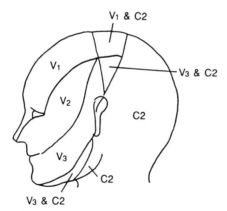

Fig. N-1. Trigeminal nerve, showing the distribution of its branches on the face: the ophthalmic (V_1), maxillary (V_2), and mandibular (V_3) nerves and their overlap with the second cervical nerve, C2. The distribution of the facial, glossopharyngeal, and vagus nerves to the external ear is not included. *See also* Fig. O-2.

branches: the ophthalmic (V_1), maxillary (V_2), and mandibular (V_3) nerves, which leave the cranial cavity by different routes. It is composed primarily of fibers for cutaneous sensibility from the face and oral cavity which end in sensory nuclei in the pons, medulla, and cervical spinal cord, and of motor fibers which arise in the motor nucleus of V in the pons and supply the muscles of mastication (Figs. N-1, O-2, R-3, R-4, R-6). *Syn:* trifacial nerve. *See also* Table C-2; onion-skin pattern; reflexes, vagal *and* Fig. R-9.

nerve, trochlear (IV) /trok´le-ar/ [nervus trochlearis, NA]   cranial nerve which arises as a slender fascicle from cells in the trochlear nucleus of the midbrain. It crosses the median plane in the anterior medullary velum at the junction of the pons and midbrain, and emerges from the dorsal surface of the midbrain (Fig. V-4). It then courses around the midbrain, traverses the cavernous sinus (Fig. S-1), and enters the orbit through the superior orbital fissure to supply the superior oblique muscle. Its action is to depress the eyeball when the eye is turned medially. *Syn:* nervus patheticus. *See also* Table C-3.

nerve, tympanic /tim-pan´ik/ [nervus tympanicus, NA]   parasympathetic and visceral afferent nerve fibers which leave the glossopharyngeal nerve just outside the jugular foramen, pass upward into the middle ear cavity, and join the tympanic plexus.

nerve, ul´nar [nervus ulnaris, NA]   nerve arising from the medial cord of the brachial plexus with fibers from spinal cord segments C8-T1. It supplies muscles on the medial side of the forearm and most of the intrinsic muscles of the hand, the muscles which adduct the hand at the wrist and both adduct and abduct the fingers.

nerve, va´gus (X) [nervus vagus, NA] [L. *vagus* wandering]   cranial nerve which arises by fascicles from the ventrolateral surface of the medulla and passes through the jugular foramen. It provides preganglionic parasympathetic fibers and visceral afferent fibers for thoracic and most abdominal viscera. It also supplies the musculature of the palate, pharynx, and larynx, and carries taste fibers from the epiglottis and some fibers for cutaneous sensibility from the external ear (Figs. O-2, T-2). *Syn:* pneumogastric nerve. *See also* Table C-1; ganglion, inferior *and* superior, *def.* 2; *and* reflexes, vagal (Fig. R-9).

nerve, ver´tebral [nervus vertebralis, NA]   strands of fibers, mostly postganglionic sympathetic, that arise from cells in the vertebral and stellate ganglia. It is located dorsal to the vertebral artery. *Syn:* Cruveilhier's nerve.

nerve, vestib´ular (VIII) [nervus vestibularis, NA]   vestibular division of the vestibulocochlear nerve, consisting of a superior branch composed of fibers from the cristae ampullares of the horizontal and superior semicircular ducts, the macula utriculi, and a small part of the macula sacculi, and an inferior branch from the crista ampullaris of the posterior semicircular duct and the major portion of the macula sacculi. Most fibers end in the vestibular nuclei of the brain stem; some end in the cerebellum. *See* Table C-2.

nerve, vestibulococh´lear (VIII) [nervus vestibulocochlearis, NA]   cranial nerve composed of a cochlear and a vestibular division from the internal ear. It passes through the internal auditory meatus into the middle cranial fossa and joins the brain stem just lateral to the facial nerve at the cerebellopontine angle. *Syn:* auditory nerve; statoacoustic nerve; acoustic nerve. *See also* Table C-2.

nerve, vomerona´sal   nerve composed of unmyelinated fibers arising from specialized epithelium of the nasal septum (vomeronasal organ) and terminating in an accessory olfactory bulb. It is present in many adult mammals and some human embryos, but not in adult man. *Syn:* nerve of Jacobson.

ner´vi plural of *nervus.*

nervi erigen´tes [NA]   *See* nerves, splanchnic, pelvic.

ner´vus im´par filum terminale.

nervus interme´dius [NA]   intermediate nerve; the visceral subdivision of the facial nerve, which leaves the brain between the motor root of VII and the vestibulo-cochlear nerve. It is composed of visceral afferent fibers, including taste, and preganglionic parasympathetic fibers for the innervation of certain glands of the head. *Syn:* glossopalatine nerve; nerve of Sapolini; nerve of Wrisberg; thirteenth cranial nerve.

nervi nervor´um [NA]   small nerve filaments in nerves, presumably for the autonomic supply of the vasa nervorum.

nervus pathet´icus (IV)   old term for the trochlear nerve.

nervus spino´sus branch of the mandibular division of the trigeminal nerve which provides sensory fibers for the dura mater of the middle cranial fossa.

nervus terminal´is [NA]   small nerve, presumably containing autonomic and sensory fibers, which arises from nasal epithelium (but not from olfactory epithelium or the vomeronasal organ) and enters the brain through the lamina terminalis just below the anterior commissure. It is present in many vertebrate forms including man.

nervi vasor´um [NA]   small nerve filaments in the walls of blood vessels.

net, neurokeratin /nu-ro-ker´ah-tin/   *See* neurokeratin.

neural /nu´ral/   pertaining to the nervous system or nervous tissue. *For* neural canal, cavity, crest, fold, groove, plate, *and* tube, *see the nouns.*

neuraxis /nu-rak´sis/   **1.** axial part of the CNS, comprising the brain stem and spinal cord.

2. Sometimes this term is used to include also the diencephalon and cerebellum and sometimes the entire CNS.

3. old term for axon.

neuraxon /nu-rak´son/   old term for axon.

neurilemma /nu-rĭ-lem´ma/   *See* neurolemma.

neurite /nu´rīt/   old term for axon.

neurobiotaxis /nu-ro-bi-o-tak´sis/   tenet which states that nerve cells tend to migrate during their development toward the principal source of their stimulation (C.U. Ariëns Kappers, '14).

neuroblast /nu´ro-blast/ [NA] [Gr. *neuron* nerve; *blastos* germ]   any primitive (embryonic) cell capable of developing into a neuron.

neurocele (neurocoele) /nu´ro-sēl/   *See* canal, neural.

neurocristop´athy any of a group of disorders resulting from maldevelopment of the neural crest.

neurofi´brils [neurofibrilla, NA]   slender filaments within the cell body of a neuron and extending into all its processes. They are visible, after special staining, at the light level. Neurofibrils presumably correspond to the neurotubules and/or neurofilaments visible by electron microscopy.

neurofibromatosis /nu-ro-fi-bro-mah-to´sis/   familial disease inherited as an autosomal dominant trait. It is characterized by skin pigmentation and multiple tumors of the skin and peripheral nerves. There are frequently also congenital abnormalities of the CNS, various endocrine glands, and other organs. *Syn:* von

Recklinghausen's disease.

neurofil´ament [neurofilamentum, NA]   one of the slender, threadlike structures which are constituent parts of neurofibrils. They are 70-100 Å in diameter, and have a dense wall 30 Å thick, and a clear center.

neurog´lia [NA] [Gr. *neuron* nerve; *glia* glue]   connective tissue cells of the CNS, including astrocytes and oligodendroglia of ectodermal origin, and microglia of mesodermal origin. *Syn:* glia.

neurohor´mone   any hormone produced by or acting upon nervous tissue, particularly the neurosecretory substances ADH and oxytocin, produced in the hypothalamus and released in the neurohypophysis.

neurohypophysis /nu-ro-hi-pof´ĭ-sis/ [NA], DIENCEPHALON   that part of the hypophysis derived from a ventral evagination of the diencephalon. It consists of: the median eminence, the infundibular stalk, and the pars nervosa (infundibular process). Axons from hypothalamic cells (supraoptic and paraventricular nuclei) pass through the infundibulum and release neurosecretory material in the pars nervosa. *See also* hypophysis cerebri.

neurokeratin /nu-ro-ker´ah-tin/   network in the myelin sheath of peripheral nerve fibers, visible at the light level under certain conditions after removal of the lipid content of the myelin. It is a fraction of brain proteins first isolated by Ewald and Kühne (1877) and traditionally considered to be associated with the protein network of the myelin sheath.

neurolem´ma [NA] [Gr. *neuron* nerve; *lemma* husk]   outermost part of the ectodermal sheath of myelinated peripheral nerve fibers, including the sheath cell nucleus and its cytoplasm but not the concentric myelin-containing lamellae. Multiple nonmyelinated fibers may be contained within a single neurolemma sheath. The spelling *neurilemma* is frequently used, but it cannot be justified on an etymological basis and may be confusing because originally it was used for the connective tissue investment now called *endoneurium*.   Another spelling, *neurilema,* derived from *neuron* and *eilema* (sheath) is used occasionally but is not recommended. *Syn:* sheath of Schwann; primitive sheath; nucleated sheath. *For discussions of the various spellings and derivations of this word, see* the footnotes in Greenfield *et al.* ('58, p. 15) *and* Beattie *et al.* ('48, p. 1310).

neuromere /nu´ro-mēr/, PONS, MEDULLA   segment of the developing CNS, particularly the segments separated by transverse grooves on the floor of the fourth ventricle of the embryonic hind brain.

neuromod´ulators   substances which act upon the pre- or postsynaptic membrane to increase or decrease the release of a neurotransmitter, or which alter the sensitivity of the target membrane to the neurotransmitter.

neu´ron [neuronum, NA] [Gr. nerve]   the complete nerve cell, including the cell body and all its processes; the structural unit of the nervous system. *See also* cell, nerve.

neuron, af´ferent   one that conducts impulses toward the CNS.

neuron, bipo´lar [neuronum bipolare, NA]   neuron with two processes, one axon and one dendrite. Nerve cells of the spiral and vestibular ganglia of the internal ear and the secondary neurons of the retina (in layer 6) are of this type.

neuron, ef´ferent   one that conducts impulses away from the CNS.

neuron, internun´cial [neuronum internunciale, NA]   small neuron in many parts of the CNS. It has a small cell body and a short axon and acts as a short connecting link between neurons in a neuron chain. *Syn:* interneuron; intercalated or intercalary neuron; Golgi type II cell.

neuron, motor   1. *See* neuron, motor, lower.

2. *See* neuron, motor, upper.

neuron, motor, al´pha   large motor neuron whose axon terminates on large extrafusal muscle fibers (Fig. L-1). *Syn:* alpha motoneuron.

neuron, motor, be´ta   motor neuron with an axon intermediate in size between those of alpha and gamma motor neurons. Such neurons supply both intrafusal and extrafusal muscle fibers. *Syn:* beta motoneuron.

neuron, motor, gam´ma   motor neuron with a small cell body, whose axon, a gamma efferent fiber, terminates on the small intrafusal fibers of a neuromuscular spindle (Fig. L-1).

neuron, motor, lower   large neuron whose cell body is in a motor nucleus of the brain stem or spinal cord ventral horn, and whose axon conducts impulses to motor end plates in skeletal muscle. It provides the last link between the CNS and the muscle fibers it innervates, and so constitutes a final common pathway. *Syn:* motoneuron.

neuron, motor, upper   neuron of the pyramidal tract, whose cell body is in the motor or premotor area of the cerebral cortex and whose axon terminates in a motor nucleus of the brain stem or spinal cord.

neuron, multipo´lar [neuronum multipolare, NA]   neuron having more than two processes, including one axon and more than one dendrite. Most neurons of the CNS and the cells of the autonomic ganglia are of this type. The cell bodies of multipolar neurons are of many different sizes and shapes.

neuron, postganglionic /post-gang-gle-on´ik/   neuron of the ANS whose cell body is located in an autonomic ganglion and which terminates in smooth or cardiac muscle or in glandular tissue.

neuron, preganglionic /pre-gang-gle-on´ik/   neuron of the ANS whose cell body is located in a general visceral motor nucleus within the CNS and which terminates in an autonomic ganglion.

neuron, pseudounipolar /soo-do-u-nī-po´lar/ [neuronum unipolare (pseudounipolare), NA]   *See* neuron, unipolar.

neuron, sen´sory   neuron which conducts impulses in a pathway, characteristically a three-neuron chain, for the perception of some sensory modality.

neuron, sensory, pri´mary   first neuron in a sensory pathway. Its cell body is in a ganglion outside the CNS. Its axon ends, without crossing the median plane, in a CNS nucleus at the level, above the level, or below the level at which the fiber enters the CNS. *See also* pathway, sensory.

neuron, sensory, sec´ondary   sensory neuron having its cell body in a CNS nucleus. Its axon usually crosses the median plane and ends in the dorsal thalamus.

neuron, sensory, ter´tiary   sensory neuron having its cell body in a nucleus in the dorsal thalamus. Its axon, in the sensory radiation, passes through the internal capsule and ends in the homolateral cerebral cortex (Fig. C-1).

neuron, unipo´lar (pseudounipolar) [neuronum unipolare (pseudounipolare), NA]   neuron having a single process which shortly divides into axon and dendrite. Dorsal root ganglion cells and the cells of the sensory ganglia of cranial nerves, except those of the olfactory and vestibulocochlear nerves, are of this type. Cells in the mesencephalic nucleus of V are also unipolar.

neuro´num corbifer´um [NA], CEREBELLUM, [L. *corbis* basket]   *See* cell, basket.

neuronum multipolare breviaxonicum [NA]   neuron having a small cell body and a short axon. *Syn:* Golgi type II cell.

neuronum multipolare longiaxonicum [NA]   neuron having a large cell body and a long axon. *Syn:* Golgi type I cell.

neuropep´tides   several peptides (short chains of amino acids) which are important in neurotransmission, e.g., substance P, the pituitary hormones, hypothalamic releasing factors, and the endorphins (opioid peptides). *See also* neurotransmitters.

neurophysin /nu-ro-fi´sin/   protein formed in the supraoptic and paraventricular nuclei of the hypothalamus, conjugated with the neurohormones, ADH and oxytocin, produced in these nuclei, and transported along the axons of the cells to the neurohypophysis.

neuropil /nu´ro-pil/ [neuropilus, NA] [Gr. *neuron*; *pilos* felt]   feltwork of the terminal processes of axons and dendrites interspersed among the nerve cells in the gray matter of the CNS.

neuroplasm /nu´ro-plazm/   cytoplasm of a neuron.

neuropo´dium [*pl.* **neuropodia**] [Gr. *neuron*; *podion* small foot]   *See* bulb, terminal.

neuropore /nu´ro-por/ [neuroporus, NA] [Gr. *neuron*; *poros* passage]   opening at each end of the neural canal in the developing brain.

neuropore, cau´dal (posterior) [neuroporus caudalis, NA]   opening at the caudal end of the neural canal. It closes at about the 25-somite stage of development.

neuropore, ros´tral (anterior) [neuroporus rostralis (cranialis), NA]   opening at the rostral (anterior) end of the neural canal. It closes at about the 20-somite stage of development.

neuroten´sin (NT)   a tridecapetide present largely in tissues outside the CNS. In the CNS it occurs in many areas, mainly the hypothalamus, amygdala, preoptic area, nucleus accumbens, and olfactory tubercle. It is an important modulator of nociception, body temperature, feeding behavior, and stress responses. *See also* neurotransmitters.

neurotrans´mitters   chemical substances released at the axonal terminations of neurons during the transmission of an impulse across a synapse or at an effector organ. Neurotransmitters either excite or inhibit the target cell and include such substances as acetylcholine, norepinephrine, endorphins, GABA, serotonin, dopamine, glycine, glutamate, histamine, and many others. Techniques to identify neurotransmitters include the use of HRP and fluorescent tracers (Záborszky and Heimer, '89). *Syn:* transmitter substance. *For additional information, see also* Emson ('83).

neurotubules /nu-ro-too´būlz/   extremely fine filamentous structures, apparently tubular in form, visible within the cytoplasm of neurons by electron microscopy. Presumably they are one of the constituent parts of neurofibrils. Neurotubules, like microtubules in cells other than neurons, are 200-300 Å in diameter and have a dense wall about 60 Å thick and a lighter core. Many neurotubules have a thin central filament.

NGF   nerve growth factor.

nicotin´ic   pertaining to the action of a nicotine-like alkaloid. Nicotinic receptors are activated by ACh and low concentrations of nicotine and are blocked by high concentrations of nicotine and by atropine. These receptors occur exclusively at motor end plates in skeletal muscle and with muscarinic receptors in autonomic ganglia and certain CNS areas. *See also* muscarinic.

Nissl, Franz Alexander (1860-1919)   German neuropathologist and psychiatrist of Heidelberg, best known for his discovery of the cytoplasmic bodies, *Nissl granules* (chromatophilic substance), in nerve cell bodies (1894), and the stains which reveal them.

NMDA   N-methyl D-aspartate.

N-methyl D-aspartate (NMDA)   chemical used to detect molecules indicating the presence of receptors which are important in the biochemical reactions on which learning and memory depend, and especially rich in the hippocampus.

NMR   nuclear magnetic resonance, also known as magnetic resonance imaging (MRI). *See* tomography.

nociceptor /no-sĭ-sep´tor/ [*adj.* **nociceptive**] [L. *nocere* to injure; *capere* to take]   receptor sensitive to damaging or noxious stimuli. Firing of nociceptors almost always causes pain, but the firing of other receptors can also cause pain if they fire rapidly and often enough.

node, atrioventric´ular (AV node) [nodus atrioventricularis, NA]   structure composed of specialized cardiac muscle fibers, located in the interatrial septum beneath the endocardium of the right atrium just above the opening of the coronary sinus. It is supplied by parasympathetic fibers, mainly from the left vagus nerve, which slow the ventricles, and sympathetic fibers from the cervical and upper four or five thoracic chain ganglia, mainly on the left side, which increase the rate and force of the contraction of the ventricles. *Syn:* node of Aschoff, Tawara, or Aschoff-Tawara.

node (of) Ranvier [nodus neurofibrae, NA]   *See* Ranvier *and* Fig. R-1.

node, sinua´trial (sinoatrial) (sinus node) (SA node) [nodus sinuatrialis, NA]   structure composed of specialized cardiac muscle fibers, located in the upper part of the sulcus terminalis of the heart just anterior to the opening of the superior vena cava. It is the pacemaker of the heart and is supplied by parasympathetic fibers mainly from the right vagus nerve which slow the heart, and sympathetic fibers from the cervical and upper four or five thoracic chain ganglia mainly of the right side which increase the rate and force of the heart. *Syn:* node of Keith, Flack, or Keith and Flack; Koch's node.

no´dose [L. *nodosus*; from *nodus* knot]   pertaining to the nodose ganglion, the inferior ganglion of the vagus nerve.

nod´ule [nodulus, NA], CEREBELLUM, [L. *nodulus* little knot]   most caudal segment of the cerebellar vermis (Figs. C-2, V-6). *See also* vermis cerebelli.

no´dus neurofi´brae [NA]   node of Ranvier. *See* Ranvier *and* Fig. R-1.

Nomina Anatomica (NA)   terms approved by the International Anatomical Nomenclature Committee (Nomina Anatomica, '83). Throughout this text [NA] is used to indicate not only the approved anatomical terms (NA) but also the approved histologic (NH) and embryologic (NE) terms. *For an account of the historical background of the Nomina Anatomica, see* O'Rahilly ('89).

noradren´aline   norepinephrine.

noradrener´gic   releasing norepinephrine.

norepineph´rine (NE)   a catecholamine, an inhibitory neurotransmitter liberated at all sympathetic postganglionic nerve endings except those innervating sweat glands. It is present in the adrenal medulla but in much smaller amounts than epinephrine. It is the neurotransmitter formed in the cell bodies and released by the terminals of certain brain stem nuclei, including the locus coeruleus, whose axons project widely throughout the brain and into the spinal cord. *Syn:* noradrenaline; levarterenol. *See also* neurotransmitters.

notch, cerebellar, anterior, cerebellum   *See* incisure, cerebellar, anterior.

notch, cerebellar, posterior, cerebellum   *See* incisure, cerebellar, posterior.

notch, preoccip´ital (occipital), cerebrum   *See* incisure, preoccipital.

notch, tentor´ial   *See* incisure, tentorial.

noyau centre médian (of Luys), dorsal thalamus   *See* nucleus, centromedian.

nuclear magnetic resonance (NMR)   magnetic resonance imaging. *See* tomography.

Nuclear Yellow   trademark for a fluorescent tracer, used in marking the nuclei of nerve cell bodies. *See also* tracer, fluorescent.

nucleus /noo´kle-us/   **1.** vesicular organelle which contains the chromatin material and, in neurons, a prominent nucleolus.
2. group of nerve cell bodies within the CNS.

nucleus, abducens (abducent) /ab-du´sens/ [nucleus abducens (nucleus nervi abducentis), NA], pons   motor nucleus of VI, a somatic motor nucleus located in the dorsomedial part of the pontine tegmentum. Its fibers pass ventrally and caudally to emerge lateral to the pyramidal tract between the pons and medulla and continue as the abducens nerve to supply the lateral rectus muscle of the eye. *Syn:* external oculomotor nucleus. *See also* Fig. F-2, Table C-2.

nucleus, abducens, acces´sory, pons   *See* nucleus, facial, accessory.

nucleus, accessory [nucleus accessorii (nucleus nervi accessorii), NA], cord   special visceral motor nucleus located in the dorsolateral and lateral parts of the ventral horn of spinal cord segments (C1-C5 or C6). Its fibers cross the lateral funiculus to emerge midway between the dorsal and ventral roots, dorsal to the dentate ligament, and collect to form the spinal accessory nerve. Fibers from the most rostral part of the nucleus supply the sternocleidomastoid muscle. Those that arise more caudally supply the upper part of the trapezius muscle. *See also* nerve, accessory, bulbar *and* spinal; Table C-1.

nucleus, accessory, bul´bar, medulla   old term for nucleus ambiguus.

nucleus, accessory oculomo´tor, midbrain   *See* nucleus, oculomotor, accessory.

nucleus, accessory, spinal, cord   *See* nucleus, accessory.

nucleus accum´bens sep´ti (nucleus leaning against the septum), cerebrum   one of the nuclei of the precommissural septum, and a part of the ventral striatum. It is located ventromedial to the anterior horn of the lateral ventricle and is continuous laterally under the lateral ventricle with the head of the caudate nucleus.

nucleus (of) a´la ciner´ea, medulla   *See* nucleus, dorsal efferent.

nucleus alar´is, medulla   *See* nucleus, dorsal efferent.

nucleus ambiguus /am-big´u-us/ [NA], medulla   slender, intermittent column of special visceral motor cells present in all but the most caudal part of the medulla. It is located in the ventrolateral part of the medulla, about halfway between the spinal nucleus of V and the dorsomedial corner of the inferior olivary complex. Caudally it lies nearer the olivary nuclei and rostrally closer to the spinal nucleus. It supplies motor fibers to skeletal musculature derived from the third and fourth visceral arches, *viz.* the stylopharyngeus muscle (via the glossopharyngeal nerve), most of the muscles of the pharynx, larynx (in part), and upper esophagus (via the vagus nerve), and most of the muscles of the larynx (via the bulbar accessory nerve). *Syn:* ventral motor nucleus; ventral nucleus of the vagal nerve. *See also* Fig. F-2; Table C-1.

nucleus, ang´ular, pons   *See* nucleus, vestibular, superior.

nucleus (of the) an´sa lenticular´is [nucleus ansae lenticularis, NA], CEREBRUM nucleus consisting of scattered cells or small cell groups along the ansa lenticularis and inferior thalamic peduncle. The entopeduncular nucleus and the nucleus of the ansa peduncularis are sometimes considered subdivisions of this complex. These nuclei, together, constitute the nucleus basalis of lower forms.

nucleus (of the) ansa peduncular´is, CEREBRUM nerve cells located ventral to the globus pallidus, along the ansa lenticularis, and considered a subdivision of the nucleus of the ansa lenticularis.

nuclei, anterior [nuclei anteriores, NA], DORSAL THALAMUS the anterior nuclear group of the dorsal thalamus comprises the anteroventral nucleus (the largest of the group), the anteromedial, and the anterodorsal nuclei. They are located within the anterior tubercle of the thalamus, next to the interventricular foramen (Fig. V-5). Their main connections are afferent fibers (and some efferent fibers) in the mamillothalamic tract and efferent fibers to the cingulate gyrus through the anterior thalamic radiation. *See also* thalamus, dorsal.

nucleus, anterior, HYPOTHALAMUS *See* nucleus, hypothalamic, anterior.

nucleus, anterior ventral, DORSAL THALAMUS *See* nucleus, ventral anterior, of the dorsal thalamus.

nucleus, anterodorsal (AD) [nucleus anterodorsalis, NA], DORSAL THALAMUS small nucleus (almost vestigial in man) belonging to the anterior nuclear group of the dorsal thalamus. When present, it consists of darkly stained, closely packed cells dorsal to the anteroventral nucleus. *See also* nuclei, anterior, of the dorsal thalamus.

nucleus, anterolateral, CORD *See* nucleus, ventrolateral, *def.* 1.

nucleus, anteromedial **1.** CORD *See* nucleus, ventromedial, *def.* 1.

2. (AM) [nucleus anteromedialis, NA], DORSAL THALAMUS small nucleus of the anterior nuclear group of the dorsal thalamus, located ventral and medial to but not sharply separated from the anteroventral nucleus. It receives fibers from the mamillary body and sends fibers to the cingulate gyrus, mainly area 24 near the anterior part of the corpus callosum. *See also* nuclei, anterior, of the dorsal thalamus.

nucleus anteroprincipal´is, DORSAL THALAMUS the anteromedial and anteroventral nuclei of the dorsal thalamus, taken together, or sometimes just the anteroventral nucleus. *See also* nuclei, anterior, of the dorsal thalamus.

nucleus, anteroventral (AV) [nucleus anteroventralis, NA], DORSAL THALAMUS largest of the three anterior nuclei of the dorsal thalamus, it makes up the greater part of the anterior tubercle of the thalamus. It is partially enclosed, on its ventral and lateral sides, by fibers of the internal medullary lamina and covered on its ventricular surface by fibers of the anterior thalamic radiation. Its main afferent connections are by way of the mamillothalamic tract. Its efferent fibers terminate in the cingulate gyrus, mainly in area 23 over the corpus callosum. *See also* nuclei, anterior, of the dorsal thalamus.

nuclei, arcuate /ar´ku-āt/ any of several nuclei which are curved in shape or whose efferent fibers take a curved course. **1.** (arcuate nucleus of Flechsig), DORSAL THALAMUS ventral posteromedial nucleus of the dorsal thalamus. Sometimes this term is applied to just the medial part of this nucleus in which the ascending gustatory fibers end.

2. [nucleus arcuatus (infundibularis), NA], HYPOTHALAMUS small subependymal nucleus in the intermediate hypothalamic area (tuberal region), within the posterior periventricular nucleus. Fibers from this nucleus can be traced into the median eminence, where they terminate near sinusoids of the hypophysial portal system.

3. [nuclei arcuati, NA], MEDULLA nerve cells adjacent to the pyramid in the medulla, which send their fibers to the cerebellum via the ventral external arcuate fibers and the striae medullares of the fourth ventricle. These cells are sometimes designated the ventral arcuate nucleus to distinguish them from cells of the lateral arcuate nucleus near the lateral surface of the medulla. The rostral, larger part of this nucleus which becomes continuous with the pontine gray is also called the nucleus precursorius pontis. The nucleus conterminalis, dorsal to the pyramid, is sometimes considered a subdivision of this nucleus.

nucleus, arcuate, lateral, MEDULLA small group of nerve cells lateral to the spino-cerebellar tracts in the medulla. Its axons join the ventral external arcuate fibers.

nucleus, arcuate, ventral, MEDULLA *See* nucleus, arcuate, *def.* 3.

nuclei, auditory, PONS, MEDULLA *See* nuclei, cochlear, ventral *and* dorsal.

nuclei (of the) autonomic nervous system nuclei of the brain stem and spinal cord from which preganglionic nerve fibers arise, for termination in an autonomic ganglion. They include: the Edinger-Westphal (accessory oculomotor) nucleus (III nerve), superior salivatory (and lacrimal) nuclei (VII nerve), inferior salivatory nucleus (IX nerve), dorsal efferent nucleus (X nerve), intermediolateral (lateral horn) and intermediomedial nuclei (T1-L2/3), and sacral parasympathetic nuclei (S2-S4).

nucleus, ba´sal (of Meynert), CEREBRUM prominent group of large cells in the ventral part of the substantia innominata, near the ventral surface of the brain. Loss of cells in this region appears to be an important feature of Alzheimer's disease. *Syn:* basal nucleus of the substantia innominata; nucleus of Ganser. *For additional information, see* Tagliavini ('87).

nuclei basa´les [NA], CEREBRUM *See* ganglia, basal.

nucleus basal´i, CEREBRUM nucleus in lower forms which corresponds to a combination of the nucleus of the ansa lenticularis medially and the entopeduncular nucleus laterally of higher forms.

nuclei, bed, of the hippocam´pal and the anterior com´missures, CEREBRUM small precommissural septal nuclei, located among the fibers of the commissures named.

nucleus, caudate /kaw´dāt/ [nucleus caudatus, NA], CEREBRUM one of the basal ganglia, made up of a head which forms the lateral wall of the anterior horn of the lateral ventricle, a body overlying the lateral part of the dorsal thalamus, and a tail located above the inferior horn of the lateral ventricle (Fig. C-1). The caudate nucleus and the putamen, together, constitute the striatum or neostriatum. Lesions of the caudate nucleus are associated with chorea.

nucleus, central **1.** [nucleus centralis, NA], CORD cell group in the ventral horn of the cervical spinal cord (phrenic nucleus) and lumbosacral spinal cord (lumbosacral nucleus).

2. DORSAL THALAMUS *See* nucleus, centromedian.

3. (of the oculomotor nerve), MIDBRAIN median cell group of the oculomotor nucleus, which is thought to supply the medial rectus muscles and subserve convergence. *Syn:* nucleus impar; nucleus medianus anterior; nucleus of Perlia.

nucleus, central inferior [nucleus centralis inferior], PONS, MEDULLA median cell group, one of the raphe nuclei in the caudal part of the pontine tegmentum and at the pontomedullary junction. It may represent a rostral part of the nucleus raphe magnus. *Syn:* inferior central tegmental nucleus. *See also* nuclei (of the) raphe.

nucleus, central lateral [nucleus centralis lateralis, NA], DORSAL THALAMUS   one of the intralaminar nuclei of the dorsal thalamus. It is composed of cells of various shapes and sizes, and is located between the dorsomedial nucleus medially and the ventral posterolateral nucleus laterally, in a position rostral and dorsal to the centromedian nucleus and posterior to the nucleus paracentralis. *See also* nuclei, intralaminar, of the dorsal thalamus.

nucleus, central medial, DORSAL THALAMUS   **1.** [nucleus centralis medialis, NA] one of the intralaminar nuclei of the dorsal thalamus, located next to the medial part of the paracentral nucleus, rostral and dorsal to the centromedian nucleus.
2. term sometimes used for the central median nucleus of the median group. *See also* nuclei, intralaminar *and* median, of the dorsal thalamus.

nucleus, central median (medial), DORSAL THALAMUS   small nucleus of the median group of the dorsal thalamus, the largest in the interthalamic adhesion (when present) and adjacent thalamic area. Fibers from this nucleus have been traced to the amygdala. *See also* nuclei, median, of the dorsal thalamus.

nucleus, central superior, PONS   median cell group, one of the raphe nuclei, a relatively large cluster of serotonin-containing cells in the rostral part of the pontine tegmentum (Fig. N-5, medial raphe nucleus). It receives descending fibers from the forebrain. Its efferent fibers spread out to end widely in various parts of the forebrain and midbrain, especially the interpeduncular nucleus, the mamillary bodies, and the hippocampal formation. Other fibers distribute to the cerebellum, locus coeruleus, and pontine reticular gray. *Syn:* median nucleus of the raphe; Bechterew's nucleus; superior central tegmental nucleus. *See also* nuclei (of the) raphe.

nucleus central´is, DORSAL THALAMUS   *See* nucleus, centromedian, of the dorsal thalamus.

nucleus central´is central´is, DORSAL THALAMUS   *See* nucleus, centromedian, of the dorsal thalamus.

nucleus centralis lateralis superior, DORSAL THALAMUS   term sometimes applied to an intralaminar cell group dorsomedial to the central lateral nucleus in the dorsal thalamus of the monkey. It overlies the dorsomedial nucleus and corresponds to the nucleus circularis in man. *See also* nuclei, intralaminar, of the dorsal thalamus.

nucleus, centrome´dian (CM) [nucleus centromedianus, NA], DORSAL THALAMUS   largest of the intralaminar nuclei, it is enclosed by fibers of the internal medullary lamina in the posterior part of the thalamus (Fig. N-8). Although not all its connections are firmly established, it is thought to receive collaterals of various ascending sensory systems, such as the medial lemniscus and the paleospinothalamic tract, and to send efferent fibers to the caudate nucleus and putamen. It may also be part of the recruiting mechanism of the cerebral cortex. *Syn:* central nucleus; nucleus centralis; nucleus centralis centralis; nucleus centrum medianum. *See also* nuclei, intralaminar, of the dorsal thalamus.

nucleus cen´trum median´um, DORSAL THALAMUS   *See* nucleus, centromedian, of the dorsal thalamus.

nuclei, cerebel´lar [nuclei cerebelli, NA], CEREBELLUM   nuclear masses located within the cerebellum from which most of the efferent fibers of the cerebellum arise, *viz.* the dentate, emboliform, globose, and fastigial nuclei (Fig. N-2).

nuclei, cerebellar, deep, CEREBELLUM   collective term for all the cerebellar nuclei.

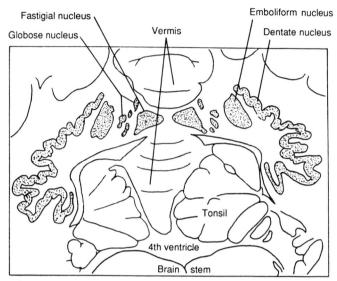

Fastigial nucleus   Emboliform nucleus

Globose nucleus   Vermis   Dentate nucleus

Tonsil

4th ventricle

Brain stem

Fig. N-2. A horizontal section through the cerebellum to show the relative positions of the cerebellar nuclei.

nucleus, cerebellar, lateral, CEREBELLUM   *See* nucleus, dentate.

nucleus, cer´vical, lateral, CORD   nucleus present in the cat but absent in man. It is located in the lateral funiculus of the spinal cord, lateral or ventrolateral to the dorsal horn, and may be a relay station to the cerebellum or to the thalamus.

nucleus, chief sensory, of V, PONS   *See* nucleus, pontine trigeminal.

nucleus circular´is, DORSAL THALAMUS   term sometimes applied to a small intralaminar nucleus in the dorsal thalamus. It is located dorsomedial to the central lateral nucleus, capping the dorsomedial, nucleus and corresponds to the nucleus centralis lateralis superior of the monkey. *See also* nuclei, intralaminar, of the dorsal thalamus.

nuclei, cochlear /kok´le-ar/ [nuclei cochleares, NA], PONS, MEDULLA   two nuclei, the dorsal and ventral cochlear nuclei, in the most rostral part of the medulla and adjoining pons, near the lateral recess of the fourth ventricle and next to the inferior cerebellar peduncle. *See* Table C-2.

nucleus, cochlear, anterior [nucleus cochlearis anterior, NA], PONS, MEDULLA   *See* nucleus, cochlear, ventral.

nucleus, cochlear, dorsal [nucleus cochlearis dorsalis (posterior), NA], MEDULLA   small-celled nucleus located dorsal or dorsolateral to the inferior cerebellar peduncle in the rostral part of the medulla. It receives cochlear nerve fibers. Its axons pass medially under the floor of the fourth ventricle, deep to the stria medullaris or through the inferior cerebellar peduncle. Some fibers cross the median plane and pass ventrolaterally to join the lateral lemniscus; others probably enter the homolateral lateral lemniscus. These fibers, with and without synapses in course, end mainly in the inferior colliculus, partly in the medial geniculate nucleus. *See* Table C-2.

nucleus, cochlear, posterior, MEDULLA   *See* nucleus, cochlear, dorsal.

nucleus, cochlear, ventral [nucleus cochlearis ventralis (anterior), NA], PONS, MEDULLA large-celled nucleus located ventrolateral to the inferior cerebellar peduncle in the rostral part of the medulla and the caudal pons. It receives cochlear nerve fibers. Its axons pass ventromedially into the trapezoid body and, with or without synapses along the way, enter the lateral lemnisci of both sides. They end mainly in the inferior colliculi, partly in the medial geniculate nuclei. *See* Table C-2.

nucleus, commis´sural (commissu´ral) [nucleus commissuralis, NA], CORD caudal extension of the nucleus parasolitarius which joins its counterpart of the other side across the median plane, dorsal to the central canal in the most rostral sections of the spinal cord. It is part of the dorsal gray commissure and Rexed's lamina X.

nucleus conterminal´is, MEDULLA inconstant group of nerve cells between the inferior olivary nucleus and the pyramid in the medulla, separated from but presumably a subdivision of the nearby arcuate nucleus.

nucleus (of) cor´pus restifor´me, MEDULLA *See* nucleus, cuneate, accessory.

nucleus cu´neate [nucleus cuneatus, NA], MEDULLA, [L. *cuneus* wedge] nucleus composed of medium and small cells in the lateral part of the posterior column in the closed medulla. It receives tactile and proprioceptive fibers from the upper half of the body by way of the fasciculus cuneatus. Axons from most of the cells in this nucleus cross the median plane in the sensory decussation, ascend in the medial lemniscus, and terminate in the ventral posterolateral nucleus of the dorsal thalamus. *Syn:* Burdach's nucleus.

nucleus, cuneate, acces´sory [nucleus cuneatus accessorius, NA], MEDULLA large-celled nucleus located dorsolateral and rostral to the cuneate nucleus. It receives fibers from the fasciculus cuneatus. Dorsal superficial arcuate fibers arising from this nucleus enter the inferior cerebellar peduncle and terminate in the cerebellar vermis. *Syn:* lateral or external cuneate nucleus; nucleus of corpus restiforme; nucleus of Monakow.

nucleus, cuneate, external, MEDULLA *See* nucleus, cuneate, accessory.

nucleus, cuneate, lateral, MEDULLA *See* nucleus, cuneate, accessory.

nucleus, den´tate [nucleus dentatus, NA], CEREBELLUM largest and most lateral of the deep cerebellar nuclei, located in the cerebellar white matter (Fig. N-2). Axons from these cells make up most of the superior cerebellar peduncle as dentorubral and dentothalamic tract fibers. Some fibers leave the peduncle and descend in the central tegmental tract to end in the inferior olivary nucleus (Fig. O-1). *Syn:* lateral cerebellar nucleus. *See also* Fig. F-2.

nucleus (of the) descending tract of V, PONS, MEDULLA *See* nucleus, spinal, of the trigeminal nerve (of V).

nucleus (of the) dia´gonal band (of Broca), CEREBRUM nerve cells associated with the diagonal band (stria diagonalis). It is one of the nuclei of the precommissural septum.

nucleus, dorsal (of Clarke), CORD *See* nucleus, thoracic. In this context *dorsal* means *thoracic* and is used with reference to the position of the nucleus primarily in the thoracic spinal cord.

nucleus, dorsal ef´ferent (motor) [nucleus vagalis dorsalis (nucleus dorsalis nervi vagi), NA], MEDULLA parasympathetic nucleus of the medulla, lateral or dorsolateral to the hypoglossal nucleus in the open medulla and dorsal to the hypoglossal nucleus in the closed medulla. It is composed of small cells supplying preganglionic fibers by way of the vagus (and bulbar accessory) nerves to terminal ganglia for relay to viscera of the thorax and abdomen. *Syn:* nucleus of ala centralis; nucleus alaris. *See also* reflexes, vagal *and* Fig. R-9; Table C-1.

nucleus, dorsal lateral [nucleus lateralis dorsalis, NA], DORSAL THALAMUS   *See* nucleus, lateral dorsal, of the dorsal thalamus.

nucleus, dorsal motor, MEDULLA   *See* nucleus, dorsal efferent.

nucleus, dorsal sensory, PONS, MEDULLA   *See* gray, dorsal visceral.

nucleus, dorsal tegmen´tal (of Marburg), MIDBRAIN, PONS   conspicuous, small-celled nucleus in the medioventral part of the periaqueductal gray of the caudal midbrain and extending caudally into the pontine isthmus. It is interconnected with the mamillary bodies and receives fibers from the habenula and the interpeduncular nucleus. It contributes fibers to the dorsal longitudinal fasciculus which distributes to the visceral motor nuclei of the brain stem. *Syn:* nucleus of Gudden.

nucleus, dorsal, (of the) trap´ezoid body, PONS   *See* nucleus, olivary, superior.

nucleus, dorsal va´gal, MEDULLA   *See* nucleus, dorsal efferent.

nucleus dorsal´is, CORD   *See* nucleus, thoracic.

nucleus dorsalis corpor´is trapezoi´dei [NA], PONS   dorsal nucleus of the trapezoid body. *See* nucleus, olivary, superior.

nucleus dorsalis ner´vi glossopharyn´gei [NA], MEDULLA   *See* nucleus, salivatory, inferior.

nucleus dorsalis nervi va´gi [NA], MEDULLA   *See* nucleus, dorsal efferent.

nucleus dorsalis superficial´is, DORSAL THALAMUS   *See* nucleus, lateral dorsal.

nucleus dorsocaudal´is, DORSAL THALAMUS   *See* nucleus, lateral posterior.

nucleus dorso-interme´dius externus, DORSAL THALAMUS   *See* nucleus, lateral posterior.

nucleus, dorsolateral [nucleus dorsolateralis, NA], CORD   column of nerve cells in the lateral division of the ventral horn of the cervical and lumbosacral enlargements, in a position indicated by its name (Fig. N-6). Its fibers supply the muscles of the forearm and leg. The cells located most laterally supply muscles of postaxial origin (predominantly extensors). Those located more medially supply muscles of preaxial origin (predominantly flexors). *Syn:* posterolateral nucleus.

nucleus, dorsolateral tegmen´tal, MIDBRAIN, PONS   *See* nucleus, tegmental, laterodorsal.

nucleus, dorsomedial   1. [nucleus dorsomedialis, NA], CORD   column of nerve cells in the medial division of the ventral horn in a position indicated by its name, mostly at thoracic and upper lumbar spinal cord levels (Fig. N-6). Fibers from these cells are thought to supplement those from the ventromedial nucleus in the innervation of trunk musculature. *Syn:* posteromedial nucleus.

2. (DM) [nucleus medialis dorsalis, NA], DORSAL THALAMUS   largest nucleus of the medial nuclear group, about 18 to 20 mm in length, located medial to the internal medullary lamina in the midregion of the dorsal thalamus (Fig. N-8). It consists of an anteromedial part of large and medium-sized cells (nucleus medialis fibrosus) and a posterolateral part of small cells (nucleus medialis fasciculorum). It is interconnected with other thalamic nuclei, and with the orbital and the prefrontal cortex of the frontal lobe. Other areas with connections to this nucleus are the striatum, the amygdala, and the preoptic and hypothalamic areas. Impulses relayed forward from the dorsomedial nucleus to the prefrontal cortex are non-specific and are believed to modify general "feelings" or "affective tone" and to constitute an important factor in behavior and personality. *Syn:* medial nucleus. *See also* thalamus, dorsal.

3. HYPOTHALAMUS   *See* nucleus, hypothalamic, dorsomedial.

nucleus, dorso-oralis, DORSAL THALAMUS   dorsal part of the ventral lateral nucleus of the dorsal thalamus.

nucleus, Edinger-Westphal [nucleus oculomotorius accessorius, NA], MIDBRAIN   the parasympathetic nucleus of the oculomotor nerve. *See also* Edinger.

nucleus, embol´iform [nucleus emboliformis, NA], CEREBELLUM, [Gr. *embolos* plug] nucleus located close to the hilus of the dentate nucleus (Fig. N-2). Its efferent fibers, and those from the globose nucleus, enter the superior cerebellar peduncle, cross the median plane in the caudal part of the midbrain, and end in the red nucleus. Some fibers, after giving off collaterals in the red nucleus, are thought to continue and end in the ventral lateral nucleus of the dorsal thalamus. The emboliform nucleus corresponds to the anterior part of the nucleus interpositus of the cat.

nucleus eminen´tiae ter´etis, MEDULLA   one of the parahypoglossal nuclei, located dorsomedial to the hypoglossal nucleus. *Syn:* nucleus funiculi teretis.

nucleus, entopedunc´ular [nucleus entopeduncularis, NA], CEREBRUM   relatively small nerve cell group medial to the inner segment of the globus pallidus, and to the fibers of the ansa lenticularis as it curves around the internal capsule. It is sometimes considered a subdivision of the nucleus of the ansa lenticularis and serves as a way station for fibers of this tract. The entire nerve cell complex is also sometimes called the entopeduncular group. The so-called entopeduncular nucleus of the cat represents both the entopeduncular nucleus of man and the inner segment of the globus pallidus.

nucleus, external oculomo´tor, PONS   *See* nucleus, abducens.

nucleus, facial [nucleus facialis (nucleus nervi facialis), NA], PONS   motor nucleus of VII; special visceral motor nucleus located in the ventrolateral part of the pontine tegmentum. Its fibers pass dorsomedially and ascend in the genu of the facial nerve, pass laterally over the rostral tip of the abducens nucleus, and descend ventrolaterally, passing between the facial nucleus and the spinal nucleus of V to emerge, with other fibers of the facial nerve, at the pontomedullary junction, just medial to the vestibulocochlear nerve at the cerebellopontine angle. Its fibers supply muscles derived from the second visceral arch, mainly the muscles of facial expression but also including the stapedial muscle, the stylohyoid muscle, and, by way of the accessory facial nucleus, the posterior belly of the digastric muscle. *See also* Table 2 *and* Figs. F-2, R-4, R-8.

nuclei (of the) facial nerve, MAINLY PONS   several nuclei which contribute fibers to or receive fibers from the facial nerve. They are: the facial, superior salivatory, and parasolitary nuclei, and the dorsal visceral gray. Facial nerve fibers also end in the spinal and, to some extent, the pontine nuclei of the trigeminal nerve. *See* Table C-2.

nucleus, facial, acces´sory, PONS   small cluster of cells in the pontine tegmentum between the main facial nucleus and the abducens nucleus, thought to supply the posterior belly of the digastric muscle. *Syn:* accessory abducens nucleus; dorsal facial nucleus.

nucleus, facial, dorsal, PONS   *See* nucleus, facial, accessory.

nucleus fasciculo´sus, DORSAL THALAMUS   small cell group in the region where the inferior thalamic peduncle crosses the internal medullary lamina.

nucleus (of) fascic´ulus solitar´ius, PONS, MEDULLA   *See* nucleus solitarius. *See also* gray, dorsal visceral *and* nucleus parasolitarius.

nucleus (of) fasciculus solitarius, dorsal, PONS, MEDULLA   *See* gray, dorsal visceral.

nucleus (of) fasciculus solitarius, ventral, MAINLY MEDULLA   *See* nucleus parasolitarius.

nucleus, fastigial /fas-tij ′ī-al/ [nucleus fastigii (fastigiatus), NA], CEREBELLUM   most
medial of the cerebellar nuclei, underlying the vermis on either side of the
fastigium of the fourth ventricle (Fig. N-2). Most efferent fibers cross the median
plane and enter the uncinate fasciculus. Others (uncrossed) enter the juxtarestiform body. They end mainly in the lateral, inferior, and superior vestibular nuclei,
brain stem reticular gray, and to some extent in the cervical spinal cord. *Syn:*
nucleus tecti; roof nucleus.

nucleus, fil ′iform, HYPOTHALAMUS   *See* nucleus, paraventricular.

nucleus funic ′uli lateral ′is, MEDULLA   *See* nucleus, reticular, lateral.

nucleus funiculi ter ′etis, MEDULLA   *See* nucleus eminentiae teretis.

nucleus, geniculate, lateral (dorsal part) /jen-ik ′u-lāt/ [nucleus geniculatus lateralis
(pars dorsalis), NA], DORSAL THALAMUS   laminated nucleus in the caudal part of the
diencephalon, rostral and lateral to the medial geniculate nucleus. It is one of the
metathalamic nuclei in the posterior nuclear group of the dorsal thalamus and
constitutes the thalamic center for the visual system. It is somewhat horseshoe-
shaped, with the hilum directed ventromedially. There are alternating layers of
cells and fibers with six layers of cells, numbered 1 to 6 from the hilum. The cells
of layers 1 and 2 are relatively large. Those of layers 3 to 6 are smaller. Optic
nerve fibers enter at the hilum. Uncrossed fibers end in layers 2, 3, and 5. Those
which cross in the optic chiasm end in layers 1, 4, and 6 (Fig. N-3). Fibers from
the macular part of the retina end in the posterolateral part of the nucleus, away
from the hilum. Those from the more peripheral parts of the retina end ventro-

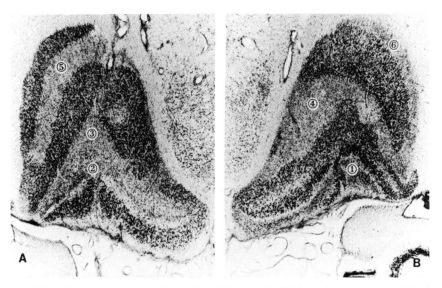

Fig. N-3. Photomicrographs of the right (A) and left (B) lateral geniculate nuclei of
a monkey that was blind in the right eye. Normally retinogeniculate fibers that cross
in the optic chiasm end in layers 1, 4, and 6, and those which do not cross end in layers
2, 3, and 5. In this specimen layers 2, 3, and 5 in the right nucleus (A) and 1, 4, and
6 in the left nucleus (B), related to the blind eye, are degenerated. Preparation
courtesy of the late Dr. George Clark, Medical University of South Carolina.

medially, nearest the hilum. Fibers from the superior retinal quadrants end in the outer half of the nucleus and those from the inferior quadrants end in the inner half of the nucleus; consequently the two halves of the two nuclei "see" the four quadrants of the visual field. Efferent fibers from the nucleus enter the optic radiation and terminate in the occipital cortex, primarily in area 17, and to a lesser extent in area 18. *See also* Fig. R-2; nuclei, posterior, of the dorsal thalamus.

nucleus, geniculate, lateral (ventral part) [nucleus geniculatus lateralis (pars ventralis), NA], DORSAL THALAMUS   this nucleus, a part of the metathalamus, is small or absent in man. It may or may not receive optic tract fibers. In forms where present, it has been said to receive fibers from the superior colliculi and to send fibers to the midbrain tegmentum. *See also* thalamus, dorsal.

nucleus, geniculate, medial (dorsal part) [nucleus geniculatus medialis (pars dorsalis), NA], DORSAL THALAMUS   small-celled, principal part of the medial geniculate nucleus, a part of the metathalamus, located in the posterior part of the dorsal thalamus, ventromedial to the lateral geniculate nucleus. It extends caudally to a position lateral to the rostral part of the midbrain. It is the thalamic center for the auditory system. Fibers from the inferior colliculus and the lateral lemniscus enter from the medial side via the brachium of the inferior colliculus and carry impulses from both cochleae. Efferent fibers, the auditory radiation, pass rostrally and laterally into the sublenticular part of the posterior limb of the internal capsule for termination in the transverse temporal gyri. Destruction of one nucleus does not eliminate hearing from either ear, but there may some loss of auditory acuity from the ear on the side opposite the lesion. *See also* nuclei, posterior, of the dorsal thalamus.

nucleus, geniculate, medial (ventral part) [nucleus geniculatus medialis (pars ventralis), NA], DORSAL THALAMUS   large-celled part of the medial geniculate nucleus, a part of the metathalamus, located ventrolateral to the principal nucleus. It is thought to be related to the reception of vestibular impulses. *See also* thalamus, dorsal.

nucleus, glo´bose [nucleus globosus, NA], CEREBELLUM   nucleus composed of several small groups of cells in the cerebellum, overlying the fourth ventricle and just lateral to the fastigial nucleus (Fig. N-2). Its efferent fibers join the superior cerebellar peduncle, decussate in the caudal part of the midbrain tegmentum, and end predominantly in the red nucleus, but some fibers, after giving off collaterals, are thought to continue and end in the ventral lateral nucleus of the dorsal thalamus. The globose nucleus corresponds to the posterior part of the nucleus interpositus in the cat.

nuclei (of the) glossopharyn´geal nerve, MAINLY MEDULLA   several nuclei which contribute fibers to or receive fibers from the glossopharyngeal nerve. They are: the nucleus ambiguus, the dorsal visceral gray, and the inferior salivatory and parasolitary nuclei. Glossopharyngeal nerve fibers also end in the spinal and, to some extent, the pontine nuclei of the trigeminal nerve. *See* Table C-1.

nucleus, grac´ile [nucleus gracilis, NA], MEDULLA   nucleus composed of medium and small cells in the medial part of the posterior column in the closed medulla. It receives tactile and proprioceptive fibers from the lower half of the body by way of the fasciculus gracilis. Axons from most of its cells cross the median plane in the sensory decussation, ascend in the medial lemniscus, and terminate in the ventral posterolateral nucleus of the dorsal thalamus. *Syn:* nucleus of Goll.

nucleus, gus´tatory   1. PONS, MEDULLA   *See* gray, dorsal visceral.

2. DORSAL THALAMUS   small-celled subdivision of the ventral posteromedial nucleus of the dorsal thalamus.

nuclei, haben´ular [nuclei habenulae, NA], EPITHALAMUS   medial and lateral nuclei located in the habenula, in the dorsal posterior part of the wall of the third ventricle. *See also* habenula; Fig. H-1.

nucleus, hypoglos´sal [nucleus hypoglossalis (nucleus nervi hypoglossi), NA], MEDULLA motor nucleus for the hypoglossal nerve, supplying tongue muscles (all but the palatoglossus). It is located on either side of the median plane in the hypoglossal trigone on the floor of the fourth ventricle, and ventrolateral to the central canal in the closed medulla. *See also* Fig. F-2; Table C-1.

nuclei, hypothalam´ic   *See* hypothalamus, and the individual hypothalamic nuclei (Fig. N-4).

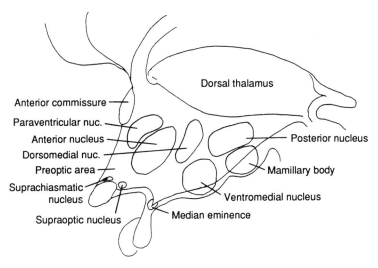

Fig. N-4.   Diagram to show the relative positions of the major hypothalamic nuclei in or near the wall of the third ventricle. *See also* Fig. V-5.

nucleus, hypothalamic, anterior [nucleus hypothalamicus anterior, NA], HYPOTHALAMUS An indistinct, small-celled nucleus in the anterior hypothalamic area, it blends imperceptibly with the medial preoptic area (Fig. N-4). It is important in the regulation of body temperature against heat. A lesion results in hyperthermia. *Syn:* parvicellular hypothalamic nucleus; fundamental gray substance of the hypothalamus.

nucleus, hypothalamic, dorsal [nucleus hypothalamicus dorsalis, NA], HYPOTHALAMUS *See* area, hypothalamic, dorsal.

nucleus, hypothalamic, dorsomedial [nucleus hypothalamicus dorsomedialis, NA], HYPOTHALAMUS   nucleus in the intermediate hypothalamic area, dorsal and somewhat rostral to the ventromedial hypothalamic nucleus (Fig. N-4) with which it functions in relation to emotional expression and food intake. It receives orbitohypothalamic and fimbria-fornix fibers from the orbital cortex and hippocampus respectively, and sends fibers to the cranial parasympathetic nuclei via the dorsal longitudinal fasciculus. Some fibers descend to the spinal cord. A destructive lesion leads to disagreeable behavior.

nuclei, hypothalamic, magnocel´lular, HYPOTHALAMUS   the supraoptic and paraventricular nuclei, located in the anterior hypothalamic area (Fig. N-4).

nucleus, hypothalamic, parvicel´lular, HYPOTHALAMUS   *See* nucleus, hypothalamic, anterior.

nucleus, hypothalamic, posterior [nucleus hypothalamicus posterior, NA], HYPOTHALAMUS   scattered cells of various sizes in the posterior hypothalamic area (Fig. N-4). In addition to cells in other hypothalamic areas these cells play a part in autonomic regulation and in the regulation of body temperature. A lesion results in an inability to maintain an adequate body temperature and the body temperature drops in a chilly environment. If the lesion extends into the lateral hypothalamic area, also interrupting the descending fibers from the anterior hypothalamic nucleus, a total lack of temperature regulation (poikilothermism) is possible.

nucleus, hypothalamic, ventromedial [nucleus hypothalamicus ventromedialis, NA], HYPOTHALAMUS   somewhat ovoid nuclear mass, the largest in the intermediate hypothalamic area (Fig. N-4). Its main afferent connections are from the septal area and the anterior perforated substance (medial forebrain bundle), orbital cortex (orbitohypothalamic fibers), temporal lobe (stria terminalis and perhaps fornix), and globus pallidus (pallidohypothalamic fibers). It discharges mainly through hypothalamotegmental fibers to the midbrain and appears to be related to food intake, regulation of the ANS, and emotional expression. Bilateral lesions of this nucleus result in voracious eating and obesity. Both destructive lesions and stimulation of this area in animals also have been shown to produce aggressive and sometimes savage behavior.

nucleus im´par, MIDBRAIN   *See* nucleus, oculomotor, central.

nucleus, inferior central tegmental, PONS, MEDULLA   *See* nucleus, central inferior.

nucleus (of the) inferior colliculus /kol-lik´u-lus/ [nucleus colliculi inferioris (caudalis), NA], MIDBRAIN   oval nucleus (in section) in the inferior colliculus. It is a way station in the auditory system, receiving lateral lemniscus fibers and interconnected with its counterpart of the other side through the commissure of the inferior colliculus. Its efferent fibers contribute mainly to the brachium of the inferior colliculus for termination in the medial geniculate nucleus. A bilateral lesion of these colliculi results in almost total deafness.

nucleus, inferior, of the trigeminal nerve [nucleus inferior nervi trigemini, NA], PONS, MEDULLA   *See* nucleus, spinal, of the trigeminal nerve (of V).

nucleus, infundib´ular [nucleus infundibularis, NA], HYPOTHALAMUS   *See* nucleus, arcuate, *def*. 2.

nucleus intercala´tus   **1.** HYPOTHALAMUS   small nucleus in the posterior hypothalamic area, interposed between the medial and lateral mamillary nuclei. *Syn:* intermediate nucleus; dorsal (of Ingram) or ventral (of Le Gros Clark) division of the lateral mamillary nucleus (of Rose).

2. [NA], MEDULLA   one of the parahypoglossal nuclei, composed mostly of small cells, interposed between the hypoglossal nucleus and the dorsal efferent nucleus. *Syn:* nucleus of Staderini.

nucleus, interfor´nical, HYPOTHALAMUS   *See* nucleus, perifornical.

nucleus, intermediate, HYPOTHALAMUS   *See* nucleus intercalatus, *def*. 1.

nucleus, intermediate ventral, DORSAL THALAMUS   *See* nucleus, ventral posterior inferior, of the dorsal thalamus.

nucleus, intermediolat´eral [columna intermediolateralis, NA], cord   column of small nerve cell bodies of preganglionic sympathetic nerve fibers, located in the lateral horn in the thoracic and upper three lumbar segments of the spinal cord (Fig. N-6).

nucleus, intermediome´dial, cord   column of small nerve cell bodies of preganglionic sympathetic nerve fibers, located between the central canal and the lateral horn in the thoracic and upper three lumbar segments of the spinal cord (Fig. N-6).

nucleus interme´dius, cerebellum   *See* nucleus interpositus.

nucleus, interpedun´cular [nucleus interpeduncularis, NA], midbrain   median nucleus in the ventral and caudal midbrain tegmentum, between the bases of the two cerebral peduncles. It receives fibers from the habenula, the medial mamillary nucleus, and the central superior nucleus of the raphe, and sends fibers to the dorsal tegmental nucleus (Fig. H-1). *Syn:* Gudden's ganglion.

nucleus interpos´itus, cerebellum   nucleus located between the dentate and fastigial nuclei of the cerebellum in forms below primates. Its anterior part corresponds to the emboliform nucleus, and its posterior part to the globose nucleus of primates. *Syn:* nucleus intermedius.

nucleus, interstitial (of the medial longitudinal fasciculus) /in-ter-stish´al/ [nucleus interstitialis, NA], midbrain   nucleus composed of fairly large cells interspersed among the fibers of the medial longitudinal fasciculus in the rostral part of the midbrain. Its main afferent connections are fibers of the lenticular fasciculus from the globus pallidus and ascending fibers of the medial longitudinal fasciculus from the vestibular nuclei. Its efferent fibers enter the medial longitudinal fas-ciculus for discharge to motor nuclei of the brain stem and spinal cord (Fig. F-2). *Syn:* interstitial nucleus of Cajal.

nucleus, interstitial (of the posterior commissure), midbrain   subdivision of the nucleus of the posterior commissure, consisting of cells intermingled with the fibers of the commissure.

nuclei, intralam´inar [nuclei intralaminares, NA], dorsal thalamus   nuclei located along or within the internal medullary lamina of the dorsal thalamus, including the centromedian nucleus (the largest of the group), the paracentral and parafascicular nuclei, and the central medial and central lateral nuclei. These nuclei are said to receive fibers of the ascending reticular system and may have diffuse cortical connections, presumably in relation to arousal of the cerebral cortex. *See also* thalamus, dorsal.

nucleus juxtasolitarius /juks-tah-sol-ĭ-tar´ĭ-us/, mainly medulla   *See* nucleus parasolitarius.

nucleus, lac´rimal [nucleus lacrimalis, NA], pons   scattered cells along the descending limb of the (internal) genu of the facial nerve in the caudal and lateral pontine tegmentum. It is a subdivision of the superior salivatory nucleus and supplies preganglionic parasympathetic fibers by way of the intermediate division of the facial nerve (nervus intermedius) to the pterygopalatine ganglion, for relay to the lacrimal gland (Fig. R-6; Table C-2).

nuclei, lateral, dorsal thalamus   the dorsal tier of ventrolateral nuclei of the dorsal thalamus, comprising the lateral dorsal and lateral posterior nuclei, the pulvinar, and the suprageniculate nucleus. *See also* nuclei, ventrolateral, *def.* 2.

nucleus, lateral   1. dorsal thalamus   *See* nucleus, lateral posterior. *See also* nuclei, ventrolateral, *def.* 2.

2. MEDULLA   *See* nucleus, reticular, lateral.

nucleus, lateral dorsal (LD) [nucleus lateralis dorsalis, NA], DORSAL THALAMUS   small nucleus on the superior surface of the dorsal thalamus overlapping and merging with the anterior nuclei anteriorly, and extending posteriorly to the lateral posterior nucleus. It has been thought to be related to the cortex of the inferior parietal lobule, adjacent to the lateral sulcus, but its fibers may project mainly to the cingulate gyrus. *Syn:* nucleus dorsalis superficialis. *See also* nuclei, ventrolateral, *def.* 2.

nucleus (of the) lateral funic´ulus, MEDULLA   *See* nucleus, reticular, lateral.

nuclei (of the) lateral lemnis´cus [nuclei lemnisci lateralis, NA], MAINLY PONS   small groups of nerve cells adjacent to the lateral lemniscus, which receive fibers from and contribute fibers to it.

nucleus, lateral posterior (LP) [nucleus lateralis posterior, NA], DORSAL THALAMUS   largest nucleus in the dorsal tier of the ventrolateral group of dorsal thalamic nuclei. It is located lateral to the internal medullary lamina and extends from about the middle of the dorsal thalamus back to the pulvinar (Fig. N-8). It is interconnected mainly with the parietal lobe cortex behind the postcentral gyrus. *Syn:* lateral nucleus; nucleus dorsocaudalis; nucleus dorsointermedius externus. *See also* nuclei, ventrolateral, *def.* 2.

nucleus, lateral ventral, DORSAL THALAMUS   *See* nucleus, ventral lateral, of the dorsal thalamus.

nucleus lateral´is, HYPOTHALAMUS   *See* nucleus, mamillary, lateral.

nucleus, laterodor´sal tegmental, MIDBRAIN, PONS   *See* nucleus, tegmental, laterodorsal.

nucleus lateropolar´is, DORSAL THALAMUS   lateral two-thirds of the ventral anterior nucleus of the dorsal thalamus.

nucleus, lateroven´tral tegmental, MIDBRAIN, PONS   *See* nucleus, tegmental, ventrolateral.

nucleus, len´tiform (lentic´ular) [nucleus lentiformis (lenticularis), NA], CEREBRUM, [L. *lens* lens or lentil; *forma* shaped; L. *lenticula* small lens or lentil]   putamen and globus pallidus of the basal ganglia.

nucleus lim´itans, DORSAL THALAMUS   small band of oval to spindle-shaped cells in the caudal part of the diencephalon, close to the midbrain, dorsomedial to the suprageniculate nucleus, and between the pulvinar and the medial geniculate nucleus. It is sometimes considered a separate entity and sometimes a part of the posterior thalamic group. *See also* thalamus, dorsal.

nucleus linear´is, MAINLY MIDBRAIN   small rostrally placed nucleus of the raphe (Fig. N-5). *See also* nuclei (of the) raphe.

nucleus (of) locus coeruleus /lo´kus ser-oo´le-us/, PONS   group of nerve cells which underlie the locus coeruleus, visible as a blue spot on the floor of the fourth ventricle, in the dorsolateral part of the tegmentum of the pontine isthmus (Fig. V-4). The cells are medium-sized with pigment granules (probably melanin) in their cytoplasm. *Syn:* nucleus pigmentosus pontis; substantia ferruginia. *See also* locus coeruleus.

nucleus, lumbosa´cral, CORD   subdivision of the central nucleus, in the lumbosacral enlargement (L2-S2), between the medial and lateral cell groups of the ventral horn. The peripheral distribution of its fibers is not known.

nucleus magnocellular´is basal´is, CORD   *See* nucleus, thoracic.

nuclei, mam´illary [nuclei corporis mamillaris, NA], HYPOTHALAMUS   two nuclei, a large medial mamillary nucleus and a small lateral mamillary nucleus, which make up most of the mamillary body in the posterior hypothalamic area. The nucleus intercalatus is a small group of cells interposed between the medial and lateral nuclei. The main afferent connections of the mamillary nuclei are the fibers of the fimbria-fornix system and the mamillary peduncle (including the secondary ascending gustatory tract). Their main efferent connections include the mamillothalamic tract to the anterior nuclei of the dorsal thalamus, the mamillo-tegmental tract to the dorsal tegmental nucleus, and the mamillopeduncular tract to the interpeduncular nucleus. *See also* area, hypothalamic, posterior.

nucleus, mamillary, internal, HYPOTHALAMUS   *See* nucleus, mamillary, medial.

nucleus, mamillary, lateral (of Rose), HYPOTHALAMUS   small group of fairly large cells located lateral to the medial mamillary nucleus in the mamillary body in the posterior hypothalamic area. Both the dorsal division (of Ingram) and the ventral division (of Le Gros Clark) of this nucleus have also been called the nucleus intercalatus. *See also* nuclei, mamillary.

nucleus, mamillary, medial (internal), HYPOTHALAMUS   large, somewhat spherical nucleus in the posterior hypothalamic area. It is composed of small cells and makes up most of the mamillary body (Fig. H-1). *See also* nuclei, mamillary.

nucleus, mam´illo-infundib´ular, HYPOTHALAMUS   cell group in the posterior part of the lateral hypothalamic area.

nucleus(i), medial, DORSAL THALAMUS   **1.** [nuclei mediales, NA] the medial nuclear group of the dorsal thalamus, *viz.* the dorsomedial nucleus, cells along the habenulopeduncular tract and the parafascicular nucleus.
2. *See* nucleus, dorsomedial, *def.* 2. *See also* thalamus, dorsal.

nucleus medial´is dorsal´is [NA], DORSAL THALAMUS   *See* nucleus, dorsomedial, *def.* 2.

nucleus medialis fasciculor´um, DORSAL THALAMUS   small-celled part of the dorso-medial nucleus of the dorsal thalamus.

nucleus medialis fibro´sus, DORSAL THALAMUS   large-celled part of the dorsomedial nucleus of the dorsal thalamus.

nuclei, median [nuclei mediani, NA], DORSAL THALAMUS   group of nuclei which span the median plane in the interthalamic adhesion of the dorsal thalamus, or which are close to the surface in the wall of the third ventricle (Fig. N-8). They are poorly differentiated in man but prominent in lower forms. The largest are the paratenial and paraventricular nuclei near the dorsal part of the ventricular wall. Smaller nuclei, in the interthalamic adhesion and/or adjacent ventricular wall, are: the rhomboid nucleus, nucleus reuniens, and central median nucleus. These nuclei are thought to be concerned with visceral functions and may also play a part in facilitation and suppression of motor activity. Efferent fibers to the hypothalamus, the amygdala, some parts of the cerebral cortex, and other areas have been reported. *See also* thalamus, dorsal.

nucleus, median, of the raphe, PONS   *See* nucleus, central superior.

nucleus median´us anterior, MIDBRAIN   *See* nucleus, central (of the oculomotor nerve).

nucleus, mesencephal´ic, of the trigeminal nerve (of V) [nucleus mesencephalicus trigeminalis (nucleus mesencephalicus nervi trigeminalis), NA], MIDBRAIN, PONS   large unipolar cells located mostly lateral to the periaqueductal gray of the midbrain and ventrolateral to the fourth ventricle in the pontine isthmus. The single processes of these cells constitute the mesencephalic tract of V. Peripheral processes (dendrites) from these cells carry proprioceptive impulses mostly from the muscles of mastication by way of the trigeminal nerve but also from the periodontal ligaments of the teeth (for pressure) and from the temporomandibular joint. Axons of these neurons terminate mainly in the motor nuclei of V. *See* Table C-2.

nucleus mesencephal´icus profund´us, MIDBRAIN   scattered cells and clusters of cells in the midbrain tegmentum, subdivided into parts according to their positions in relation to the red nucleus. *Syn:* deep tegmental gray. *See also* nucleus, red, caudal.

nuclei, metathalam´ic, DORSAL THALAMUS   the lateral and medial geniculate nuclei. These nuclei, located in the caudal part of the dorsal thalamus, are the thalamic centers for the visual and auditory systems respectively. *See also* thalamus, dorsal.

nuclei, midline, DORSAL THALAMUS   *See* nuclei, median, dorsal, of the dorsal thalamus.

nucleus min´imus, MIDBRAIN   extremely small cells along the fiber bundles in the red nucleus. Their significance is not known.

nucleus, motor, of III, MIDBRAIN   *See* nucleus, oculomotor.

nucleus, motor, of IV, MIDBRAIN   *See* nucleus, trochlear.

nucleus, motor, of V [nucleus motorius trigeminalis (nucleus motorius nervi trigemini), NA], PONS   special visceral motor nucleus in the dorsolateral part of the pontine tegmentum. Its fibers pass ventrolaterally to emerge at a midpontine level and mark the lateral boundary of the pons. They supply the muscles of mastication, derived from the first visceral arch. *See also* Fig. F-2, Table C-2.

nucleus, motor, of VI, PONS   *See* nucleus, abducens.

nucleus, motor, of VII, PONS   *See* nucleus, facial.

nucleus niger /ni´jer/, MAINLY MIDBRAIN   *See* substantia nigra.

nucleus, oculomo´tor [nucleus oculomotorius (nucleus nervi oculomotorii), NA], MIDBRAIN   motor nucleus of III, the somatic motor nucleus in the midbrain whose fibers enter the oculomotor nerve to supply the levator palpebrae muscle and all the extraocular eye muscles except the superior oblique and lateral rectus muscles. *Syn:* common oculomotor nucleus. *See also* Fig. F-2; Table C-3.

nucleus, oculomotor, accessory, MIDBRAIN   **1.** [nucleus oculomotorius accessorius, NA] general visceral motor nucleus of the oculomotor nerve (Figs. R-2, R-4). *Syn:* Edinger-Westphal nucleus. The rostral part of this nucleus is the nucleus of Bernheimer. *See also* Edinger; Table C-3.
2. any of three midbrain nuclei closely associated with the oculomotor complex, *viz.* the interstitial nucleus of the medial longitudinal fasciculus, the nucleus of Darkschewitsch, and the (dorsal) nucleus of the posterior commissure.

nucleus, oculomotor, central, MIDBRAIN   midline cell group in the oculomotor nucleus, thought to play a role in convergence of the eyes. *Syn:* nucleus of Perlia; nucleus impar.

nucleus, olfactory, anterior, CEREBRUM   small nucleus partly within and adjacent to the olfactory bulb in mammals in which the olfactory system is well developed. In man it is limited to scattered cells along the olfactory stalk.

nuclei, ol´ivary, PONS, MEDULLA   the inferior and accessory olivary nuclei of the medulla, and the superior olivary nucleus of the pons.

nuclei, olivary, accessory, MEDULLA   either of two nuclei, the dorsal and medial accessory olivary nuclei, which are part of the inferior olivary nuclear complex.

nucleus, olivary, dorsal accessory [nucleus olivaris accessorius dorsalis (posterior), NA], MEDULLA   nucleus located dorsal to the most medial part of the rostral part of the inferior olivary nucleus. Its fibers terminate mainly in the contralateral anterior lobe vermis (Fig. O-1). *Syn:* lateral accessory olivary nucleus.

nucleus, olivary, inferior [nucleus olivaris inferior (caudalis), NA], MEDULLA   nucleus in the ventrolateral part of the medulla. It is shaped like a crumpled bag with its hilum directed medially or dorsomedially. Its fibers terminate mainly as climbing fibers in the cortex of the contralateral cerebellar hemisphere (Fig. O-1). A lesion of this nucleus causes palatal myoclonus. *Syn:* principal olive; principal olivary nucleus. *See also* tract, olivocerebellar.

nucleus, olivary, lateral accessory, MEDULLA   *See* nucleus, olivary, dorsal accessory.

nucleus, olivary, medial accessory [nucleus olivaris accessorius medialis, NA], MEDULLA nucleus located caudal and medial to the inferior olivary nucleus. Its fibers terminate mainly in the contralateral flocculus, caudal vermis, and fastigial nucleus of the cerebellum (Fig. O-1). *Syn:* ventral accessory olivary nucleus.

nucleus, olivary, principal, MEDULLA   *See* nucleus, olivary, inferior.

nucleus, olivary, superior [nucleus olivaris superioris (rostralis), NA], PONS   a complex of several small nuclei in the caudal and ventral part of the pontine tegmentum. Its constituent nuclei are: the lateral and medial superior olivary nuclei (the two largest portions), and the preolivary, retro-olivary, and periolivary nuclei. Better developed in carnivores than in man, the superior olive is thought to play a part in sound localization and in sharpening frequency resolution. It receives collaterals of fibers from the ventral cochlear nucleus and contributes fibers to the trapezoid body and the lateral lemniscus for auditory conduction. Other fibers, the olivocochlear bundle, pass dorsomedially in the peduncle of the superior olive, toward the floor of the fourth ventricle, where most cross the median plane and emerge with the fibers of the vestibular nerve. Some fibers end in the facial nuclei for the stapedial reflex (Fig. R-8). *Syn:* dorsal nucleus of the trapezoid body.

nucleus, olivary, ventral accessory, MEDULLA   *See* nucleus, olivary, medial accessory.

nucleus ovoi´deus, HYPOTHALAMUS   *See* nucleus, suprachiasmatic.

nucleus papillifor´mis, PONS   rostral continuation of the central inferior nucleus located next to the median plane in the caudal pontine tegmentum. Its connections and function are unknown.

nucleus, parabdu´cens, PONS   small cells next to or intermingled with the cells of the abducens nucleus and concerned with horizontal conjugate eye movements. Its fibers cross the median plane and ascend in the medial longitudinal fasciculus to end in the oculomotor nucleus for relay to the medial rectus muscle of the contralateral eye (Fig. F-2). It appears to correspond to the paramedian pontine reticular formation.

nucleus, parabigem´inal, MIDBRAIN   small, oval nucleus in the lateral midbrain, ventrolateral to the inferior colliculus. It has bilateral connections with the superior colliculus and appears to function with it in processing visual information.

nuclei, parabra´chial, MIDBRAIN, PONS   noradrenergic cells adjacent to the superior cerebellar peduncle in the region of the pons-midbrain junction. Among their connections they appear to receive afferent fibers from the nucleus raphe dorsalis and the area postrema and to be interconnected with the hypothalamus.

nucleus, paracen´tral [nucleus paracentralis, NA], DORSAL THALAMUS   one of the intralaminar nuclei of the dorsal thalamus, located lateral to the rostral part of the dorsomedial nucleus, over its rostral pole. The caudal part of the nucleus appears to fuse with the central lateral nucleus. It consists of fairly large, deeply staining neurons arranged along the internal medullary lamina or arranged in clusters, especially in its rostral portion. *See also* nuclei, intralaminar of the dorsal thalamus.

nucleus, parafascic´ular [nucleus parafascicularis, NA], DORSAL THALAMUS   one of the intralaminar nuclei of the dorsal thalamus, located medial to the caudal part of the centromedian nucleus and ventral to the caudal part of the dorsomedial nucleus. It was evidently so named because the habenulo-interpeduncular tract passes through it, presumably without synapse. This nucleus, composed of somewhat elongated cells with coarse chromatophilic substance, is regarded as a part of the ascending reticular system related to arousal of the cerebral cortex. It receives spinothalamic fibers and sends fibers to the putamen. It may also have diffuse cortical connections. *See also* nuclei, intralaminar, of the dorsal thalamus,

nuclei (gray), parahypoglos´sal (perihypoglossal), MAINLY MEDULLA   group of nuclei adjacent to the hypoglossal nucleus, *viz.* the nucleus prepositus, the nucleus intercalatus (of Staderini), the dorsal paramedian nucleus, the nucleus of the eminentia teres, and the sublingual nucleus (of Roller). At least some of these nuclei are thought to be interconnected with the cerebellum.

nucleus, parame´dian, dorsal [nucleus paramedianus dorsalis (posterior), NA], MAINLY MEDULLA   one of the parahypoglossal nuclei, composed of closely packed, small to medium-sized cells in the medulla and caudal pons in a position medial or dorsomedial to the hypoglossal and prepositus nuclei, and the caudal part of the abducens nucleus. It is said to show retrograde degeneration with lesions of the cerebellum.

nucleus paramedian´us oral´is, MEDULLA   subdivision of the dorsal paramedian nucleus in the rostral part of the medulla where the nucleus is particularly well developed.

nucleus parasolitar´ius [NA], MAINLY MEDULLA   subdivision of the nucleus solitarius located just ventral and lateral to the fasciculus solitarius. It is a receptive area for general visceral afferent fibers from the fasciculus solitarius. *Syn:* nucleus juxtasolitarius; parasolitary gray; ventral nucleus of fasciculus solitarius; ventral sensory nucleus. *See also* Tables C-1, C-2; reflexes, vagal *and* Fig. R-9.

nuclei, parasympathet´ic, sacral [nuclei parasympathici sacrales, NA], CORD   two small cell groups in spinal cord segments S2-S4, located in the dorsomedial part of the ventral horn and at the lateral margin of the gray between the dorsal and ventral horns. They supply preganglionic parasympathetic fibers, after relay in the pelvic ganglion, to the organs of the pelvis and, after synapsing in the myenteric plexus, for the descending and sigmoid colon and the rectum.

nucleus, parate´nial, DORSAL THALAMUS   small nucleus in the median group of the dorsal thalamic nuclei. It is located next to the stria medullaris thalami near the dorsomedial margin of the dorsal thalamus. It receives fibers from the stria medullaris and is said to send fibers to the globus pallidus, nucleus accumbens, and subcallosal gyrus. *See also* nuclei, median.

nucleus, paraventric´ular [nucleus paraventricularis, NA]   **1.** DORSAL THALAMUS   small nucleus of the median cell group, close to the ventricular surface near the stria medullaris. Fibers from this nucleus have been traced to the amygdala. *See also* nuclei, median.

2. HYPOTHALAMUS   one of the magnocellular hypothalamic nuclei, an elongated plate of large, deeply staining cells located close to the third ventricle in the anterior hypothalamic area (Fig. N-4). It is the major source of oxytocin and, to a lesser extent, of antidiuretic hormone, neurohormones which are carried to the neurohypophysis along the paraventriculohypophysial tract. Other fibers are said to go directly to the spinal cord, ending in the dorsal and lateral horns. *Syn:* filiform nucleus.

nucleus, parolfac´tory, lateral, CEREBRUM   *See* nucleus, lateral septal. *See also* septum, precommissural.

nucleus, parolfactory, medial, CEREBRUM   *See* nucleus, medial septal. *See also* septum, precommissural.

nucleus, perifor´nical, HYPOTHALAMUS   nucleus composed of fairly large cells adjacent to the column of the fornix in the intermediate and posterior hypothalamic areas. It is thought to contribute fibers to the dorsal longitudinal fasciculus. Stimulation of these cells in cats is said to increase food intake and also to increase blood pressure and trigger defense reactions. *Syn:* interfornical nucleus.

nuclei, perihypoglos´sal, MEDULLA   *See* nuclei, parahypoglossal.

nucleus, periol´ivary, PONS   cells located dorsal and medial to the medial part of the superior olivary nucleus, and considered a subdivision of that complex.

nucleus, periventricular, posterior [nucleus periventricularis posterior, NA], HYPOTHALAMUS   nucleus composed of small and medium-sized cells, arranged in vertical rows separated by fine fiber strands, in the intermediate hypothalamic area (tuberal region) next to the ventricular wall, and adjacent to the ventromedial nucleus. It contains the arcuate nucleus of the hypothalamus. *Syn:* periventricular gray.

nucleus, phrenic /fren´ik/ [nucleus phrenicus (nucleus nervi phrenici), NA], CORD   cervical part of the central nucleus of the spinal cord. Its cells, centrally placed in the ventral horn mainly in segments C3-C6, send fibers into the phrenic nerve to supply the diaphragm.

nucleus pigmento´sus pontis, PONS   *See* nucleus of locus coeruleus, *also* locus coeruleus.

nuclei, pontine [nuclei pontis, NA], PONS   cells of the pontine gray intermingled with bundles of nerve fibers in the base of the pons. Their axons constitute the fibers of the pontocerebellar tract.

nucleus, pontine trigeminal (of V) [nucleus pontinus nervi trigemini, NA], PONS   nucleus located lateral to the motor nucleus of V at the level of the incoming fibers of the trigeminal nerve. It receives tactile fibers from the face and oral cavity by way of the trigeminal nerve. Axons from cells in this nucleus ascend bilaterally in the dorsal secondary ascending trigeminal tract and contralaterally in the ventral secondary ascending trigeminal tract, to terminate in the ventral posteromedial nucleus of the dorsal thalamus. *Syn:* chief, principal, or superior, sensory nucleus of V. *See also* Table C-2.

nuclei, posterior [nuclei posteriores, NA], DORSAL THALAMUS   group of nuclei located in the posterior and caudal part of the diencephalon and consisting primarily of the pulvinar and the dorsal parts of the lateral and medial geniculate nuclei. *See also* thalamus, dorsal.

nucleus (of the) posterior commissure, MIDBRAIN   group of cells located adjacent to the posterior commissure. It is sometimes divided into a dorsal nucleus on either side of the median plane at the dorsal edge of the periaqueductal gray, an interstitial nucleus intermingled with the fibers of the commissure, and a ventral nucleus, the nucleus of Darkschewitsch (Fig. F-2).

nucleus (of the) posterior commissure, dorsal, MIDBRAIN   subdivision of the nucleus of the posterior commissure, located on either side of the median plane at the dorsal edge of the periaqueductal gray.

nucleus (of the) posterior commissure, ventral, MIDBRAIN   nucleus of Darkschewitsch. *See* Darkschewitsch.

nucleus, posterior lateral, DORSAL THALAMUS   *See* nucleus, lateral posterior, of the dorsal thalamus.

nucleus, posterior mar´ginal, CORD   *See* nucleus, posteromarginal.

nucleus, posterior ventral, DORSAL THALAMUS   *See* nucleus, ventral posterior, of the dorsal thalamus.

nucleus, posterolateral, CORD   *See* nucleus, dorsolateral.

nucleus, posterolateral ventral, DORSAL THALAMUS   *See* nucleus, ventral posterolateral, of the dorsal thalamus.

nucleus, posteromarginal (posterior marginal), CORD   thin layer of large cells arranged tangentially over the dorsal and dorsolateral surface of the substantia gelatinosa, in the dorsal horn of the spinal cord (Fig. N-6). It corresponds to Rexed's lamina I. *Syn:* pericornual magnocellular column.

nucleus, posteromedial, CORD   *See* nucleus, dorsomedial, *def.* 1.

nucleus, posteromedial ventral, DORSAL THALAMUS   *See* nucleus, ventral posteromedial, of the dorsal thalamus,

nucleus, postposterolateral, CORD   *See* nucleus, retrodorsolateral.

nucleus postre´ma, MEDULLA   nerve cells in the area postrema, *q.v.*

nucleus praecursor´ius pontis, PONTOMEDULLARY JUNCTION   *See* nucleus precursorius pontis.

nucleus praepositus /pre-poz´T-tus/, PONS, MEDULLA   *See* nucleus prepositus.

nuclei, precerebel´lar, MAINLY MEDULLA   several brain stem nuclei which send fibers to the cerebellum, including the accessory cuneate, arcuate, and lateral reticular nuclei and those of the inferior olivary complex.

nucleus precursor´ius (praecursorius) pontis, PONTOMEDULLARY JUNCTION   the most rostral part of the arcuate nucleus of the medulla, located adjacent to the pyramidal tract fibers.

nucleus prefasciculo´sus, DORSAL THALAMUS   term sometimes applied to the area rostral to the place where the inferior thalamic peduncle crosses the internal medullary lamina.

nucleus, pregenic´ulate, DORSAL THALAMUS   small, crescent-shaped cell group dorsal to and overlying the anterior part of the lateral geniculate nucleus.

nucleus, premam´illary, dorsal, HYPOTHALAMUS   more or less discrete cell group rostral to the mamillary nuclei in many mammals but reduced to scattered cells in man.

nucleus, preol´ivary, PONS   cells in the area ventral to the superior olivary nucleus and considered a part of that complex.

nucleus, preop´tic, lateral, HYPOTHALAMUS   lateral part of the preoptic area, sometimes regarded as an interstitial nucleus of the medial forebrain bundle.

nucleus, preoptic, medial, HYPOTHALAMUS   small, diffusely arranged cells that constitute the major part of the preoptic area.

nucleus prepos´itus (praepositus), PONS, MEDULLA   one of the parahypoglossal nuclei located on the floor of the fourth ventricle in the lateral part of the medial eminence between the hypoglossal nucleus caudally and the abducens nucleus rostrally.

nucleus, pretec´tal, MIDBRAIN   nucleus in the rostral part of the midbrain, dorsolateral to the posterior commissure and extending into the superior collicular eminence, rostral to the laminated portion. It is a way station in the light reflex (Fig. R-7).

nucleus, principal trigeminal, ᴘᴏɴs   *See* nucleus, pontine trigeminal.

nucleus pro´prius, ᴄᴏʀᴅ   area of the dorsal horn of the spinal cord, ventral and ventromedial to the substantia gelatinosa (Fig. N-6). It corresponds to Rexed's laminae III and IV and is present at all spinal cord levels. It contains some fairly large and other small cells, including the cells of origin for a number of ascending tracts. *Syn:* dorsal funicular gray; nucleus of Waldeyer.

nuclei (of the) raphe /ra´fe/ [nuclei raphae, NA], ʙʀᴀɪɴ sᴛᴇᴍ   series of cell groups along the raphe of the brain stem. The major nuclei are: the nucleus raphe dorsalis and the central superior nucleus rostrally and the nucleus raphe magnus in the medulla. Smaller, or not so well understood, nuclei, are: the nuclei linearis, raphe pontis, raphe pallidus, and raphe obscurus, also the central inferior nucleus

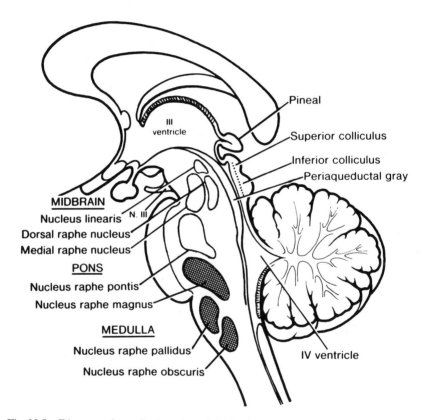

Fig. N-5. Diagram of a sagittal section of the brain stem to show the relative positions of the nuclei of the raphe. Those in the caudal part of the pons (nucleus raphe magnus) and in the medulla (cross-hatched) project to the spinal cord. The more rostral nuclei (clear) project to other parts of the brain (brain stem, cerebellum, and forebrain). From M.B. Carpenter and J. Sutin, *Human Neuroanatomy,* 8th ed., (c) 1983 (slightly adapted). Courtesy of the authors and Williams and Wilkins Co., Baltimore.

(Fig. N-5). The efferent fibers, largely serotonergic, distribute widely to the cerebrum and diencephalon, to the brain stem and cerebellum, and to the spinal cord. Ascending fibers and those ending in the brain stem arise mostly from the nucleus raphe dorsalis and the central superior nucleus. Fibers to the cerebellum arise from the central superior nucleus and nucleus raphe pontis. Those to the spinal cord are mainly from the nucleus raphe magnus. Among the functions ascribed to the raphe nuclear complex are regulation of sleep-waking rhythms, pain inhibition, and some aspects of behavior modulation. The raphe nuclei, their functions and connections, have been studied more extensively in the cat and the rat than in the human. *For additional information, see the individual nuclei named, also* Carpenter and Sutin ('83, pp. 406-409) *and* Steinbusch and Nieuwenhuys ('83, pp. 131-207).

nucleus raphe dorsal´is, MIDBRAIN, PONS   dorsal raphe nucleus; nucleus of closely packed, deeply staining cells in the ventral part of the periaqueductal gray and extending caudally from the level of the inferior colliculus into the pontine isthmus (Fig. N-5). Its two parts fuse across the median plane, giving the nucleus a butterfly shape in cross section. It is a major source of ascending, serotonergic fibers to the substantia nigra, lateral geniculate nucleus, neostriatum, olfactory bulb, piriform lobe cortex, and amygdala. Some fibers end in the norepinephrine-containing nuclei, locus coeruleus, and parabrachial nuclei. This nucleus and the central superior nucleus appear to be important in the regulation of sleep. Their destruction is said to produce total insomnia. *Syn:* supratrochlear nucleus. *See also* nuclei (of the) raphe.

nucleus raphe mag´nus, MEDULLA   major nucleus in the caudal part of the raphe (Fig. N-5). Its descending, serotonergic fibers project mainly to the spinal nucleus of the trigeminal nerve (pars caudalis) in the medulla and the dorsal horn of the spinal cord, and appear to inhibit the discharge of neurons related to the transmission of pain, and to be a part of the endogenous opiate system. *See also* nuclei (of the) raphe.

nucleus, raphe, median (medial), PONS   *See* nucleus, central superior and Fig. N-5.

nucleus raphe obscu´rus, MEDULLA   small nucleus of the raphe. Some fibers from this nucleus end in the locus coeruleus (Fig. N-5). *See also* nuclei (of the) raphe.

nucleus raphe pal´lidus, MEDULLA   small nucleus of the raphe. Fibers from this nucleus presumably supplement those from the nucleus raphe magnus and descend in the dorsolateral tract (of Lissauer) to end in the dorsal horn of the spinal cord (Fig. N-5). *See also* nuclei (of the) raphe.

nucleus raphe pon´tis, PONS   several small cell groups of the raphe, in the pontine tegmentum, dorsal and rostral to the central inferior nucleus and continuous with the central superior nucleus (Fig. N-5). It appears to be interconnected with the cerebellum. Fibers to the locus coeruleus also are said to arise, in part, from this nucleus. *See also* nuclei (of the) raphe.

nuclei, recruiting /re-kroo´ting/, DORSAL THALAMUS   *See* nuclei, thalamic, nonspecific.

nucleus, red [nucleus ruber, NA], MAINLY MIDBRAIN   large nucleus in the rostral part of the midbrain tegmentum and the caudal part of the ventral thalamus of the diencephalon. It receives fibers mainly from the cerebellum but also from the cerebral cortex, globus pallidus, ventral thalamus, and superior colliculus. From the red nucleus, according to some (but not all) observers, rubrothalamic fibers supplement the dentothalamic fibers to the ventrolateral thalamic nucleus. In man a small rubrospinal tract terminates in the cervical spinal cord. Other fibers synapse in nearby tegmental gray (caudal red nucleus) for relay to the spinal cord as part of a rubroreticulospinal system. A large number of fibers enter the central tegmental tract and end in the inferior olivary nucleus. *For additional information, see* Nathan and Smith ('82). Injury to the red nucleus results in hypotonicity and a postural tremor on the side opposite the lesion.

nucleus, red, caudal, MIDBRAIN   part of the deep tegmental gray of the midbrain, located at the level of the inferior colliculus. Fibers from this nucleus descend into the spinal cord, as part of the rubroreticulospinal tract. *Syn:* nucleus mesencephalicus profundus, pars lateralis caudalis.

nucleus, retic´ular [nucleus reticularis, NA], DORSAL THALAMUS   narrow layer of cells between the external medullary lamina of the dorsal thalamus and the internal capsule and continuous ventrally with the zona incerta (Fig. N-8). Although considered a part of the dorsal thalamus, it is said to be a derivative of the ventral thalamus. Its cells resemble those of adjoining thalamic nuclei. It is interconnected with other thalamic nuclei, particularly the intralaminar group. It may be a way station in the multisynaptic ascending reticular system and diffuse thalamocortical projection system. *See also* thalamus, dorsal.

nucleus, reticular, lateral, MEDULLA   nucleus located in the medulla oblongata, dorsolateral to the inferior olivary nucleus. Its caudal portion is a somewhat compact cluster of cells. In its rostral portion the cells are more diffusely arranged. Its afferent connections come from the cerebral cortex, red nucleus, fastigial nucleus, and spinal cord. Probably all its efferent fibers pass through the inferior cerebellar peduncle to end in the homolateral half of the cerebellum. *Syn:* nucleus of the lateral funiculus; lateral nucleus of the medulla.

nucleus, reticular, medial, MEDULLA   *See* gray, reticular, medial.

nucleus, reticular, spinal, CORD   cells interspersed among the fibers along the lateral margin of the dorsal horn in the cervical spinal cord.

nucleus retroambigual´is, MEDULLA   group of nerve cells intermediate in position between the accessory nucleus of the spinal cord and nucleus ambiguus of the medulla, sometimes considered the caudal end of the nucleus ambiguus.

nucleus, retrodorsolat´eral [nucleus retrodorsolateralis, NA], CORD   cell group in the lateral division of the ventral horn, dorsal or dorsolateral to the dorsolateral nucleus in the cervical and lumbosacral enlargements. Its fibers supply intrinsic muscles of the hand and foot. *Syn:* postposterolateral nucleus.

nucleus, retrofa´cial, PONS, MEDULLA   cluster of nerve cells interposed between the facial nucleus rostrally and the nucleus ambiguus caudally.

nucleus, retro-ol´ivary, PONS   cells located dorsal to the superior olivary nucleus, and considered a subdivision of that complex.

nucleus reuniens /re-u´nī-enz/ [NA], DORSAL THALAMUS   the most ventral of the median cell group, it extends along the ventricular surface of the dorsal thalamus from the anterior thalamic tubercle to the interthalamic adhesion. Fibers from this nucleus have been traced to the amygdala. *See also* nuclei, median, of the dorsal thalamus.

nucleus, rhomboid /rom´boid/ [nucleus rhomboidalis, NA], DORSAL THALAMUS   small cluster of cells in the median group of the dorsal thalamic nuclei. It lies partly in the interthalamic adhesion (when present) and adjacent thalamic area and indents the dorsomedial nucleus of the dorsal thalamus through most of its length. *See also* nuclei, median, of the dorsal thalamus.

nucleus, roof, CEREBELLUM   *See* nucleus, fastigial.

nucleus ruber [NA], MAINLY MIDBRAIN   *See* nucleus, red.

nuclei, sacral parasympathetic, CORD   *See* nuclei, parasympathetic, sacral.

nuclei, sal´ivatory, PONS, MEDULLA   two nuclei of the facial and glossopharyngeal nerves. They are concerned with the parasympathetic innervation of the glands of the head, *viz.* the salivary and lacrimal glands.

nucleus, salivatory, inferior [nucleus salivatorius inferior (caudalis), (nucleus dorsalis nervi glossopharyngei), NA], MEDULLA   parasympathetic nucleus of the medulla, rostral to the dorsal efferent nucleus. It is composed of small cells supplying preganglionic fibers by way of the glossopharyngeal nerve to the otic ganglion for relay to the parotid gland. It also provides preganglionic parasympathetic fibers to other ganglion cells for relay to the lingual (von Ebner's) glands at the back of the tongue. *See* Table C-1.

nucleus, salivatory, superior [nucleus salivatorius superior (cranialis), NA], PONS   parasympathetic nucleus located in the caudal part of the pontine tegmentum, medial to the fasciculus solitarius and rostral to the inferior salivatory nucleus. It is composed of small cells supplying preganglionic fibers by way of the intermediate division of the facial nerve (nervus intermedius) to the pterygopalatine ganglion for relay to the nasal and the palatine (and lacrimal) glands, also to the submandibular ganglion for relay to the sublingual gland, and to Langley's ganglion for the submandibular gland. *See* Table C-2; Fig. C-4; *and* nucleus, lacrimal.

nucleus, semilunar (of Friedemann), DORSAL THALAMUS   *See* nucleus, ventral postero-medial. Sometimes this term is applied to the entire nucleus and sometimes to just the medial part, in which the ascending gustatory fibers end.

nucleus, sensory, inferior, PONS, MEDULLA   *See* nucleus, spinal, of the trigeminal nerve.

nucleus, sensory, superior, PONS   *See* nucleus, pontine, of the trigeminal nerve.

nucleus, septal, dorsal, CEREBRUM   small nucleus in the dorsal part of the precommissural septum, dorsal to the medial and lateral septal nuclei.

nucleus, septal, lateral, CEREBRUM   one of the nuclei of the precommissural septum, continuous posteriorly with the scattered cells of the septum pellucidum. It receives mainly fornix fibers from the hippocampus and others from the amygdala. Efferent fibers enter the medial forebrain bundle to end in the lateral hypothalamic area. Other fibers join the stria medullaris and end in the habenula.

nucleus, septal, medial, CEREBRUM   one of the nuclei of the precommissural septum, continuous posteriorly with the nucleus of the diagonal band of Broca. Its afferent fibers arise mainly from the hippocampus and the amygdala, and its efferent fibers enter the stria medullaris. Other fibers join the medial forebrain bundle and the mamillary peduncle.

nucleus, septofim´brial, CEREBRUM   small nucleus ventral to the columns of the fornix where it overlies the anterior commissure.

nucleus, septohippocam´pal, CEREBRUM   a cellular strand on the underside of the corpus callosum, it is one of the hippocampal remnants left behind when the hippocampus is displaced posteriorly and inferiorly into the temporal lobe by the developing corpus callosum. Anteriorly it merges with the indusium griseum from above the corpus callosum and continues forward as the rudimentary anterior continuation of the hippocampus. *See also* rudiment, hippocampal.

nucleus, sexually dimor´phic, of the preoptic area, HYPOTHALAMUS   group of deeply stained cells identified in the preoptic area of the rat. It is concerned with the release of gonadotropins from the anterior lobe of the pituitary (Gorski *et al.*, '80).

nucleus solita´rius [NA], PONS, MEDULLA   gray matter associated with the fasciculus solitarius, in which visceral afferent fibers of the facial, glossopharyngeal, and vagus nerves end. It consists of two parts: the dorsal visceral gray (for taste) and the nucleus parasolitarius (for general visceral afferent fibers). *See* Tables C-1, C-2.

nuclei (of the) spinal cord   the nuclei and their approximate levels are as follows: Dorsal horn: posteromarginal, substantia gelatinosa, and nucleus proprius (all levels); secondary visceral substance and thoracic nucleus (T1-L3). Autonomic:

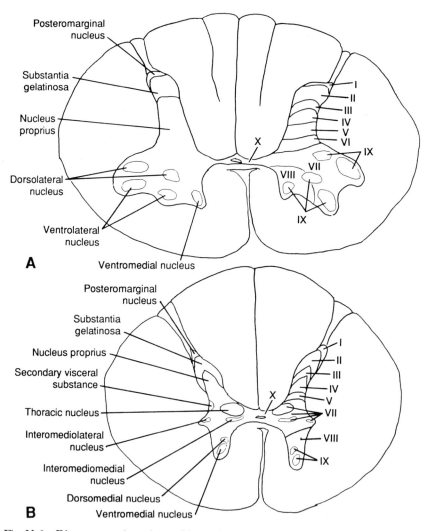

Fig. N-6.   Diagrams to show the positions of the spinal cord nuclei (reader's left side), and of the Rexed laminae (right side). A. cervical enlargement (C7). B. thoracic spinal cord (T7).

intermediomedial and intermediolateral (sympathetic, T1-L3); sacral parasympathetic (S2-S4).   Ventral horn (motor nuclei):   central (phrenic, C3/4-C5/6, and lumbosacral, L2-S2), ventromedial (all but C1, L5, S1), dorsomedial (C1, T1-L3), ventrolateral (C4-C8, L2-S1/2), dorsolateral (C4/5-T1, L2/3-S2/3), retrodorsolateral (C4/5-T1, S1-S3) (Fig. N-6).   *See also* individual nuclei *and* Rexed (for the Rexed layers of the spinal cord).

nucleus, spinal, of the trigeminal nerve (of V) [nucleus spinalis (inferior) nervi trigemini, NA], PONS, MEDULLA   nucleus in the dorsolateral part of the medulla and caudal portion of the pons and in the cervical spinal cord.   Rostrally it is continuous with the pontine nucleus of V.   Caudally it overlaps the substantia gelatinosa.   It is divided into three parts: the subnucleus rostralis, subnucleus interpolaris, and subnucleus caudalis.   It receives pain, temperature, and tactile fibers from the face by way of the spinal tract of V (Figs. O-2, T-2).   Axons from cells in this nucleus cross the median plane and ascend in the ventral secondary ascending tract of V to terminate in the ventral posteromedial nucleus of the dorsal thalamus.   *Syn:* nucleus of the spinal (descending) tract of V; spinal trigeminal nucleus; inferior sensory nucleus (of the trigeminal nerve).   *See also* Figs. R-3, R-4, R-6; reflexes, vagal *and* Fig. R-9; Tables C-1, C-2.

nucleus spinothalam´icus, CORD   cells of origin for the lateral and ventral spinothalamic tracts, mainly in the nucleus proprius of the dorsal horn of the spinal cord.

nucleus subcoeru´leus, PONS   scattered pigmented nerve cells near the nucleus of the locus coeruleus, apparently associated with it in function.

nucleus, subling´ual, MEDULLA   one of the parahypoglossal nuclei, a small cluster of fairly large cells located ventral to the hypoglossal nucleus.   *Syn:* nucleus of Roller.

nucleus, subme´dial (nucleus submedius), DORSAL THALAMUS   small, cigar-shaped group of medium-sized, deeply staining cells, located from the caudal tip of the anteroventral nucleus of the dorsal thalamus, to about the posterior limit of the interthalamic adhesion.   *See also* thalamus, dorsal.

nucleus, subputa´minal (of Ayala), CEREBRUM   lateral part of the sublenticular gray.

nucleus, subthalam´ic [nucleus subthalamicus, NA], VENTRAL THALAMUS   large biconvex nucleus in the ventral thalamus of the diencephalon (Fig. N-8).   It is an important way station in the extrapyramidal system and, with the basal ganglia, is concerned with the control of motor activity.   A destructive lesion of this nucleus results in a contralateral hemiballismus.   *Syn:* body or nucleus of Luys; corpus Luysii.   *See also* fasciculus, subthalamic.

nucleus, superior central tegmental, PONS   *See* nucleus, central superior.

nucleus, superior trigeminal, PONS   *See* nucleus, pontine trigeminal.

nucleus, suprachiasmat´ic, HYPOTHALAMUS   nucleus located adjacent to the third ventricle, and overlying the optic chiasm in the anterior hypothalamic area (Fig. N-4).   It receives direct axonal projections from the retina and relays impulses, by way of a series of neurons, to the pineal body (Fig. N-7).   It appears to function as a biological clock, concerned with the regulation and synchronization of circadian rhythms, and to play a role in the control of certain endocrine functions, particularly those that involve light.   *Syn:* nucleus ovoideus.   *See also* body, pineal.   *For additional information, see* Carpenter and Sutin ('81, pp. 497-500).

nucleus, suprageni´culate, DORSAL THALAMUS   small group of oval, deeply staining cells located in a wedge between the pulvinar and the pretectal area, medial to the medial geniculate nucleus.   It is sometimes considered a separate entity and sometimes one of the posterior nuclear group or lateral nuclei of the dorsal thalamus. *See also* thalamus, dorsal.

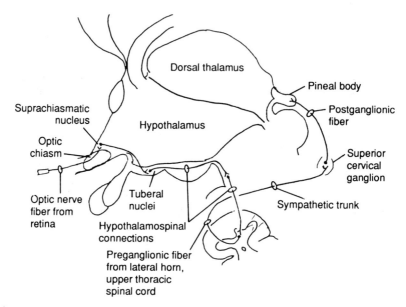

Fig. N-7. Diagram to illustrate the neuronal connections from the retina to the pineal body by way of the suprachiasmatic nucleus and the spinal cord, whereby environmental light adjusts the biological clock for circadian rhythms and modifies the secretory activity of the pineal body for the regulation of certain endocrine functions.

nucleus, supramam´illary, HYPOTHALAMUS   cells located dorsal to the mamillary nuclei in relation to the supramamillary decussation in the posterior hypothalamic area. Not well defined in man, it merges with the tegmental gray.

nucleus, supraop´tic [nucleus supraopticus, NA], HYPOTHALAMUS   one of the magnocellular hypothalamic nuclei, consisting of large, deeply staining cells located over the lateral border of the optic tract in the anterior hypothalamic area (Fig. N-4). The cells elaborate mainly the antidiuretic hormone (ADH). Other cells, to a lesser extent, produce oxytocin. These neurohormones are carried to the neurohypophysis along the supraopticohypophysial tract. *Syn:* basal optic ganglion; nucleus tangentialis.

nucleus, supraspi´nal, MEDULLA, CORD   rostral extension of the ventromedial nucleus of the spinal cord into the caudal part of the medulla.

nucleus, supratrigem´inal, PONS   dorsomedial extension of the pontine trigeminal nucleus. It functions in jaw reflexes and perhaps relays proprioceptive impulses to higher centers.

nucleus, supratroch´lear, MIDBRAIN   *See* nucleus raphe dorsalis.

nucleus tangentialis /tan-jen-she-al´is/   **1.** MEDULLA   scattered nerve cells along the lateral border of the lateral vestibular nucleus and the rostral end of the inferior vestibular nucleus.

2. HYPOTHALAMUS   *See* nucleus, supraoptic.

nucleus tec´ti, CEREBELLUM   *See* nucleus, fastigial.

nuclei, tegmen´tal [nuclei tegmenti, NA]   nuclei in the tegmentum of the brain stem, sometimes particularly the red nucleus.

nucleus, tegmental, dorsal (of Marburg), MIDBRAIN, PONS   conspicuous, small-celled nucleus in the medioventral part of the periaqueductal gray of the caudal midbrain and extending caudally into the pontine isthmus. It is interconnected with the mamillary bodies and receives fibers from the habenula and the interpeduncular nucleus. It contributes fibers to the dorsal longitudinal fasciculus, which distributes to the visceral motor nuclei of the brain stem (Fig. H-1). *Syn:* nucleus of Gudden.

nucleus, tegmental, laterodorsal (dorsolateral), MIDBRAIN, PONS   nucleus composed of nonpigmented cells in the laterodorsal tegmentum of the pontine isthmus and caudal midbrain and in the adjoining midbrain periaqueductal gray. It sometimes is considered a part of the nucleus of the locus coeruleus with which its cells are intermingled.

nucleus, tegmental, lateroventral, MIDBRAIN, PONS   *See* nucleus, tegmental, ventrolateral.

nucleus, tegmental, superior central, PONS   *See* nucleus, central superior.

nucleus, tegmental (reticular), ventrolateral, MIDBRAIN, PONS   nucleus located on the dorsal surface of the medial lemniscus in the tegmentum of the isthmus of the pons and caudal part of the midbrain. After a partial decussation at their level of origin, fibers arising from cells in this nucleus enter the ventral reticulospinal tract. *Syn:* lateroventral tegmental nucleus; reticular nucleus of Bechterew.

nuclei, thalam´ic, DORSAL THALAMUS   the dorsal thalamus consists of a number of nuclear groups, separated by fibrous laminae (Fig. N-8). An external medullary lamina separates the reticular nucleus from the ventrolateral group. An internal medullary lamina separates the medial from the ventrolateral groups. The latter is divided into a dorsal tier, the lateral nuclei, and a ventral tier, the ventral nuclei. Intralaminar nuclei are along or within the internal medullary lamina, which also encloses the centromedian nucleus posteriorly and partially surrounds the anterior nuclear group anteriorly. Nuclei of the median group are located in the interthalamic adhesion or next to the wall of the third ventricle. Other unclassified nuclei are: the submedial, suprageniculate, and limitans nuclei. *For the nuclear groups and their constituent nuclei, see* nuclei, anterior, intralaminar, lateral, medial, median, metathalamic, posterior, ventral, ventral posterior, *and* ventrolateral, *def.* 2. *See also* thalamus, dorsal.

nuclei, thalamic, diffuse, DORSAL THALAMUS   *See* nuclei, thalamic, nonspecific.

nuclei, thalamic, nonspecific, DORSAL THALAMUS   usually any of three groups of thalamic nuclei: the intralaminar, median, and reticular nuclei. They are sometimes also called the reticular, diffuse, or recruiting nuclei of the dorsal thalamus. *See also* thalamus, dorsal.

nucleus, thorac´ic [nucleus thoracicus, NA], CORD   large-celled nucleus in the dorsal horn of the spinal cord at levels about T1-L3 (Fig. N-6). It discharges through the dorsal spinocerebellar tract to the cerebellum. *Syn:* dorsal nucleus of Clarke; nucleus dorsalis.

nucleus, triangular, CEREBRUM   either of two small septal nuclei: 1. single median cell group located dorsal to the anterior commissure, between the two columns of the fornix.

2. small nucleus, bilaterally represented, constituting the ventral part of the septofimbrial nucleus.

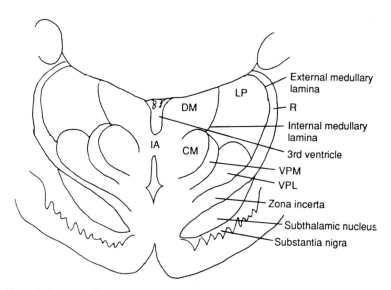

Fig. N-8.   Diagram of a coronal section of the diencephalon to show the position of some nuclear groups in the dorsal and ventral thalami.   In the dorsal thalamus are: CM-centromedian nucleus, DM-dorsomedial nucleus, IA-median nuclei in the interthalamic adhesion, LP-lateral posterior nucleus, R-reticular nucleus, VPL-ventral posterolateral nucleus, and VPM-ventral posteromedial nucleus.   In the ventral thalamus are: the zona incerta, the subthalamic nucleus, and the rostral part of the substantia nigra.

nuclei (of the) trigem´inal nerve   any of several nuclei which contribute to or receive fibers from the trigeminal nerve, *viz.* the motor, pontine, spinal, and mesencephalic nuclei of V. *See* Table C-2.

nucleus, trigeminal, spinal, PONS, MEDULLA   *See* nucleus, spinal, of the trigeminal nerve (of V).

nucleus, troch´lear [nucleus trochlearis, NA], MIDBRAIN   motor nucleus of IV; a somatic motor nucleus in the dorsal, caudal part of the midbrain tegmentum. Its fibers spiral dorsally and caudally around the periaqueductal gray, cross the median plane, and emerge from the dorsal surface of the brain stem at the junction of the pons and midbrain as the trochlear nerve, to supply the superior oblique muscle of the eye. *See also* Fig. F-2; Table C-3.

nuclei, tu´beral [nuclei tuberales, NA], HYPOTHALAMUS   two or three clusters of small cells in the lateral hypothalamic area, from a plane through the posterior end of the supraoptic nucleus to the rostral end of the mamillary body (Fig. N-7). They often produce small elevations on the ventral surface of the hypothalamus and are thought to belong to the neuroendocrine system. *Syn:* lateral tuberal nuclei.

nucleus, tuberomam´illary, HYPOTHALAMUS   cells located in the posterior part of the lateral hypothalamic area.

nuclei (of the) vagus nerve   any of several nuclei which contribute to or receive fibers from the vagus nerve, *viz.* the dorsal efferent nucleus, nucleus ambiguus, dorsal visceral gray, and nucleus parasolitarius. Vagus nerve fibers also end in the spinal nucleus and, to some extent, the pontine nucleus of the trigeminal nerve. *See also* Table C-1.

nucleus vagal´is dorsal´is [nucleus dorsalis nervi vagi, NA], MEDULLA   *See* nucleus, dorsal efferent.

nuclei, ventral, DORSAL THALAMUS   ventral tier of the ventrolateral nuclear group of the dorsal thalamus, comprising the ventral anterior, ventral lateral, and ventral posterior nuclei. *See also* nuclei, ventrolateral, *def.* 2.

nucleus, ventral anterior (VA) [nucleus ventralis anterior, NA], DORSAL THALAMUS   nucleus in the ventral tier of the ventrolateral nuclear group of the dorsal thalamus. It is located in the anterior part of the dorsal thalamus, lateral to the anterior nuclear group. Its main afferent fibers are from the medial segment of the globus pallidus and, to a lesser extent, from the contralateral cerebellar nuclei, both by way of the thalamic fasciculus. Its efferent fibers discharge primarily to the premotor area of the cerebral cortex (area 6), and to some extent to the motor area (area 4). It also serves as a waystation between the suppressor areas (4s and 6s) of the cortex and areas 4 and 6. It has other connections, especially with the intralaminar and median thalamic nuclei. It is concerned with the stabilization of cortically initiated movement and may also serve as a relay center for diffuse thalamocortical projection. *See also* nuclei, ventrolateral, *def.* 2.

nucleus, ventral intermediate, DORSAL THALAMUS   *See* nucleus, ventral posterior inferior, of the dorsal thalamus.

nucleus, ventral lateral (VL) [nucleus ventralis lateralis, NA], DORSAL THALAMUS   nucleus in the ventral tier of ventrolateral nuclear group. It is located in the dorsolateral part of the dorsal thalamus between the internal and external medullary laminae, posterior to the ventral anterior nucleus. More caudally it is lateral to the dorsomedial nucleus and dorsal to the ventral posterior nucleus. Posteriorly it is replaced by the lateral posterior nucleus. It receives thalamic fasciculus fibers mainly from the contralateral cerebellum (dentothalamic fibers) and to a lesser extent from the globus pallidus. Thalamocortical fibers from this nucleus go mainly to area 4 of the cerebral cortex, and, to some extent, to area 6. *See also* nuclei, ventrolateral, *def.* 2.

nucleus, ventral motor, MEDULLA   *See* nucleus ambiguus.

nuclei, ventral posterior (VP) [nuclei ventrales posteriores, NA], DORSAL THALAMUS   largest nuclear mass in the ventral tier of the ventrolateral nuclear group. It occupies the caudal half of the dorsal thalamus and is located lateral to the dorsomedial and centromedian nuclei, and ventral to the ventral lateral and lateral dorsal nuclei. Posteriorly it is replaced by the pulvinar. Its afferent fibers are the major sensory tracts for the body and the face and it constitutes the thalamic center for the related modalities. Its two main divisions are the ventral postero-medial nucleus (VPM) (for face) and the ventral posterolateral nucleus (VPL) (for body) (Fig. N-8). An adjoining small nucleus, the ventral posterior inferior nucleus (VPI), has vestibular connections. *Syn:* ventrobasal nucleus. *See also* nuclei, ventrolateral, *def.* 2; syndrome, thalamic.

nucleus, ventral, (of the) posterior commissure, MIDBRAIN   nucleus of Darkschewitsch.

See Darkschewitsch, *also* nucleus (of the) posterior commissure.

nucleus, ventral posterior inferior (VPI), DORSAL THALAMUS   small nucleus in the ventral tier of the ventrolateral nuclear group of the dorsal thalamus, one of the ventral posterior group. It is located ventral or ventrolateral to the ventral posterolateral and ventral posteromedial nuclei. Ascending vestibular fibers to this nucleus have been described, with efferent fibers to the parietal lobe. *Syn:* ventral intermediate nucleus.

nucleus, ventral posterolateral (VPL) [nucleus ventralis posterolateralis, NA], DORSAL THALAMUS   largest of the ventral posterior nuclei, located between the ventral posteromedial nucleus and the external medullary lamina in the dorsal thalamus (Fig. N-8). It relays impulses for pain, temperature, touch, and position from the body to the cerebral cortex. Fibers of the lateral and ventral spinothalamic tracts and the medial lemniscus terminate in this nucleus and efferent fibers (sensory radiations) end in the paracentral lobule and the upper part of the postcentral gyrus. *See also* nuclei, ventral posterior.

nucleus, ventral posteromedial (VPM) [nucleus ventralis posteromedialis, NA], DORSAL THALAMUS   crescent-shaped part of the ventral posterior nucleus, located between the ventral posterolateral nucleus laterally and the dorsomedial and centromedian nuclei medially in the dorsal thalamus (Figs. N-8, O-2). The larger lateral part (sometimes designated nucleus posteroventralis oralis) is concerned with the relay of sensation from the face and oral cavity. A smaller, medial part with small cells (VPMpc) is concerned with taste. *Syn:* arcuate nucleus (of Flechsig); semilunar nucleus (of Friedemann). *See also* nuclei, ventral posterior.

nucleus, ventral sensory, MAINLY MEDULLA   *See* nucleus parasolitarius.

nucleus, ventral, (of the) vagus nerve, MEDULLA   *See* nucleus ambiguus.

nucleus ventral´is anterior (VA) [NA], DORSAL THALAMUS   *See* nucleus, ventral anterior.

nucleus ventralis lateral´is (VL) [NA], DORSAL THALAMUS   *See* nucleus, ventral lateral, *def.* 2.

nucleus ventralis oral´is, DORSAL THALAMUS   the anterior part of this nucleus presumably corresponds to the ventral anterior nucleus of the dorsal thalamus, and the posterior part to the ventral lateral nucleus. *See also* nuclei, ventral.

nucleus ventralis posterolateral´is (VPL) [NA], DORSAL THALAMUS   *See* nucleus, ventral posterolateral.

nucleus ventralis posteromedial´is (VPM) [NA], DORSAL THALAMUS   *See* nucleus, ventral posteromedial.

nucleus ventralis posteromedialis oralis, DORSAL THALAMUS   lateral part of the ventral posteromedial nucleus. It receives fibers of the dorsal and ventral secondary ascending trigeminal tracts, carrying pain, temperature, and touch impulses from the face and oral cavity. Efferent fibers, part of the sensory radiations, end in the face area of the postcentral gyrus, just above the lateral sulcus.

nucleus, ventroba´sal, DORSAL THALAMUS   *See* nuclei, ventral posterior.

nucleus ventrocaudal´is, DORSAL THALAMUS   posterior part of the ventral posterior nucleus of the dorsal thalamus.

nucleus ventrocaudalis exter´nus, DORSAL THALAMUS   posterior part of the ventral posterolateral nucleus of the dorsal thalamus.

nucleus ventrocaudalis inter´nus, DORSAL THALAMUS   posterior part of the ventral posteromedial nucleus of the dorsal thalamus.

nucleus(i), ventrolateral   1. [nucleus ventrolateralis, NA], CORD   column of nerve cells in the ventral part of the lateral division of the ventral horn in the cervical and lumbosacral enlargements (Fig. N-6). Fibers from these cells are thought to innervate the muscles of the shoulder girdle and upper arm and those of the hip and thigh. The cells most laterally placed supply muscles of postaxial origin (primarily extensor muscles). Those located more medially supply muscles of preaxial origin (primarily flexor muscles). *Syn:* anterolateral nucleus.

2. [nuclei ventrolaterales, NA], DORSAL THALAMUS   group of nuclei that lie between the internal and external medullary laminae and extend almost the entire length of the dorsal thalamus. There is a dorsal tier, the lateral group, comprising the lateral posterior (Fig.N-8) and lateral dorsal nuclei, and a ventral tier, the ventral anterior, ventral lateral, and ventral posterior nuclei. Other terminologies for the subdivisions of this complex are also used. *See also* thalamus, dorsal.

nucleus, ventromedial   **1.** [nucleus ventromedialis, NA], CORD   column of nerve cells in the medial division of the ventral horn at most levels of the spinal cord (Fig. N-6). Fibers from these cell bodies are thought to supply neck, trunk, intercostal, and abdominal muscles. *Syn:* anteromedial nucleus.

2. HYPOTHALAMUS   *See* nucleus, hypothalamic, ventromedial.

nucleus ventro-oral´is externus, DORSAL THALAMUS   ventrolateral part of the ventral lateral nucleus of the dorsal thalamus.

nucleus ventro-oralis internus, DORSAL THALAMUS   ventromedial part of the ventral lateral nucleus.

nuclei, vestib´ular [nuclei vestibulares, NA], PONS, MEDULLA   nuclei underlying the vestibular area on the floor of the fourth ventricle, *viz.* the inferior, lateral, medial, and superior vestibular nuclei, in which fibers of the vestibular nerve fibers terminate. *See* Table C-2.

nucleus, vestibular, descending, MEDULLA   *See* nucleus, vestibular, inferior.

nucleus, vestibular, dorsal, PONS, MEDULLA   *See* nucleus, vestibular, medial.

nucleus, vestibular, inferior [nucleus vestibularis inferior (caudalis), NA], MEDULLA   special somatic afferent (proprioceptive) nucleus located in the dorsolateral part of the medulla, just medial to the inferior cerebellar peduncle. It receives mainly vestibular nerve fibers and fibers of the spinovestibular tract. Axons from most of its cells enter the medial vestibulospinal tract (medial longitudinal fasciculus) and descend to terminate on cells of the accessory nucleus and to some extent other ventral horn cells in the cervical spinal cord (Fig. F-2). *Syn:* descending vestibular nucleus; spinal vestibular nucleus.

nucleus, vestibular, lateral [nucleus vestibularis lateralis, NA], PONS, MEDULLA   nucleus located in the dorsal part of the tegmentum lateral to the medial vestibular nucleus in the region of the pontomedullary junction. Its main afferent connections are vestibular nerve fibers from the horizontal semicircular duct and fibers from the fastigial nuclei of the cerebellum. Its main efferent connections arise from the large cells of this nucleus and enter the ventrolateral vestibulospinal tract for distribution to ventral horn cells, mainly in the spinal cord enlargements. Other efferent fibers enter the medial longitudinal fasciculus and supplement those from the medial vestibular nucleus (Fig. F-2). *Syn:* Deiter's nucleus; nucleus vestibularis magnocellularis.

nucleus, vestibular, medial [nucleus vestibularis medialis, NA], PONS, MEDULLA   largest of the vestibular nuclei, located in the dorsal part of the tegmentum in the area of the pontomedullary junction. Its main afferent connections are vestibular nerve fibers from the horizontal semicircular duct. Its efferent fibers include connections to the contralateral abducens and parabducens nuclei and descending fibers to ventral horn cells in the cervical spinal cord by way of the medial longitudinal fasciculi (Fig. F-2), and vestibulocerebellar fibers to the flocculonodular lobe and to the fastigial nuclei of the cerebellum. *Syn:* nucleus of Schwalbe; principal, triangular, or dorsal vestibular nucleus.

nucleus, vestibular, principal, PONS, MEDULLA   *See* nucleus, vestibular, medial.

nucleus, vestibular, spinal, MEDULLA   *See* nucleus, vestibular, inferior.

nucleus, vestibular, superior [nucleus vestibularis superior (rostralis), NA], PONS nucleus located in the dorsolateral tegmentum of the pons at the level of the abducens nucleus. Its main connections include afferent fibers from the superior and posterior semicircular ducts and efferent fibers to the oculomotor and trochlear nuclei through the homolateral medial longitudinal fasciculus (Fig. F-2), and vestibulocerebellar connections to the flocculonodular lobe and both fastigial nuclei. *Syn:* nucleus of Bechterew; angular nucleus.

nucleus, vestibular, triangular, PONS, MEDULLA   *See* nucleus, vestibular, medial.

Nuel, Jean Pierre (1847-1920)   Belgian physiologist and otologist of Ghent and Liège. *Nuel's space* is located between the outer pillar and the outer hair cells of the spiral organ of the cochlea.

nystagmus /nis-tag´mus/ [Gr. *nystagmos* a nodding; from *nystazein* to be sleepy] oscillating movements of the eyes, usually involuntary, and which may be normal or abnormal.

nystagmus, cerebellar   nystagmus resulting from a cerebellar lesion, usually involving the pyramis or the fastigial nucleus on one side.

nystagmus, horizontal   nystagmus in which the eyes move in a horizontal plane.

nystagmus, jerk   nystagmus in which there is a slow movement of the eyes in one direction and a quick return.

nystagmus, miner's   nystagmus which is thought to be induced by poor illumination or poor vision.

nystagmus, optokinet´ic   nystagmus induced by viewing a succession of moving objects. Purkinje (1825) presumably was the first to describe this type of nystagmus. *Syn:* railroad nystagmus.

nystagmus, pal´atal   *See* myoclonus, palatal.

nystagmus, pen´dular   nystagmus in which the oscillatory movements of the eyes are approximately equal in rate for the two directions.

nystagmus, railroad   *See* nystagmus, optokinetic.

nystagmus, vertical   nystagmus in which the eyes move in a vertical plane.

nystagmus, vestibular   nystagmus resulting from stimulation or irritation of the vestibular part of the internal ear, the vestibular nuclei, or their related tracts. This type of nystagmus, first described by Erasmus Darwin (1794), grandfather of Charles Darwin, consists of a slow (vestibular) component (a vestibulo-ocular reflex), in which the eyes are turned in the direction opposite the movement of the head (away from the side of vestibular stimulation), followed by a quick recovery. It is dependent on connections involving the medial longitudinal fasciculus (Fig. F-2).

O

Obersteiner, Heinrich (1847-1922)   Austrian neuropathologist and founder of the Neurologisches Institut at the University of Vienna. His studies encompassed both the clinical aspects and the underlying pathology of many neurologic and psychiatric disorders. The *Obersteiner-Redlich space* or *area* is the segment of a nerve root in the subarachnoid space between the brain or spinal cord and the place of transition from glia to neurolemma.

o´bex [NA], MEDULLA, [L. barrier]   small transverse fold overlying the caudal tip of the fourth ventricle at its junction with the central canal of the closed medulla (Fig. V-4).

oblongata /ob-long-gah´ta/ [*adj.* **oblongatal**]   *See* medulla oblongata.

occipital /ok-sip´it-al/, CEREBRUM   pertaining to the occipital lobe or its cortex.

oculomotor /ok-u-lo-mo´tor/ [L. *oculus* eye]   pertaining to the oculomotor nerve and nucleus and their connections.

Ogawa, Teizo (b. 1901)   Japanese neuroanatomist. *Ogawa's bundle* consists of fibers, presumed to originate in the nucleus of Darkschewitsch and the interstitial nucleus of the medial longitudinal fasciculus, that descend in the central tegmental tract to terminate in the dorsal and the medial accessory olivary nuclei.

olfac´tory [L. *olfacere* to smell]   pertaining to the sense of smell. *For* olfactory bulb, glomerulus, nerve, *and* ventricle, *see the nouns.*

oligoden´dria   oligodendroglia.

oligodendro´glia [Gr. *oligos* scanty; *dendron* tree; *glia* glue]   neuroglial cells of ectodermal origin, with small oval nuclei and fine cytoplasmic processes, located near nerve cell bodies and along nerve fibers throughout the CNS. They are thought to correspond to the satellite cells and neurolemma of the PNS, and to be responsible for the formation of myelin in the CNS. *Syn:* oligoglia; oligodendria.

oligogli´a   oligodendroglia.

olive [oliva, NA], ᴍᴇᴅᴜʟʟᴀ   protuberance on the ventrolateral surface of the medulla overlying the inferior olivary nucleus (Fig. O-1). *See* nucleus, olivary, inferior.

olive, dorsal accessory, ᴍᴇᴅᴜʟʟᴀ   *See* nucleus, olivary, dorsal accessory.

olive, inferior, ᴍᴇᴅᴜʟʟᴀ   *See* nucleus, olivary, inferior.

olive, medial accessory, ᴍᴇᴅᴜʟʟᴀ   *See* nucleus, olivary, medial accessory.

olive, principal, ᴍᴇᴅᴜʟʟᴀ   *See* nucleus, olivary, inferior.

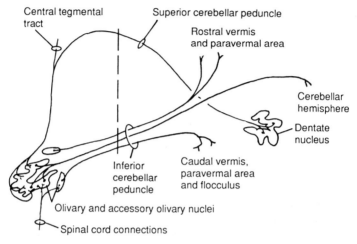

Fig. O-1.   Diagram to show the major connections of the inferior olivary and the dorsal and medial accessory olivary nuclei.

olive, superior, ᴘᴏɴs   *See* nucleus, olivary, superior.

onion-skin pattern   pattern by which trigeminal nerve fibers carrying pain from the face descend in the spinal tract of the trigeminal nerve and end in its spinal nucleus, so that those from the region around the lips end in the upper part of the closed medulla and those from the outer parts of the face end at successively more caudal levels as far as the fourth cervical spinal cord segment (Fig. O-2). *See also* nerve, trigeminal.

Onufrowicz, B. (Onuf)   The *nucleus of Onufrowicz* is the dorsal part of the superior vestibular nucleus. The *nucleus of Onuf* (1899) consists of motor neurons on the surface of the sacral ventral horn (S1-S3), which are said to supply muscles of the pelvic floor, including the urethral and anal sphincters.

Oort   The *nerve of Oort* is the olivocochlear bundle.

Opalski, Adam (1897-1963)   Polish physician. *Opalski cells* are oval-to-round cells (up to 35 μm in diameter) without processes. They have small, darkly staining, oval nuclei, usually centrally placed and occur primarily in the dorsal thalamus, globus pallidus, substantia nigra, and subthalamic nucleus but not in the striatum, in cases of hepatolenticular degeneration.

operculum /o-per´ku-lum/ [NA] [*pl.* opercula], ᴄᴇʀᴇʙʀᴜᴍ, [L. lid]   part of the cerebrum which overlies the insula and which forms the lips of the lateral sulcus.

operculum, frontal [operculum frontale, NA], ᴄᴇʀᴇʙʀᴜᴍ   part of the frontal lobe

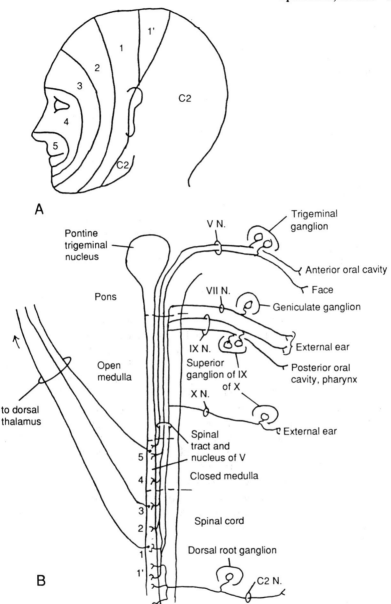

Fig. O-2.   Onion-skin pattern of the trigeminal nerve on the face (A), and the distribution of fibers for pain and temperature ending in the spinal nucleus of V in the closed medulla and upper cervical spinal cord (B). 1´ is the area of overlap of trigeminal and C2 fibers. There is also some overlap on the angle of the jaw (not shown in A). Fibers from the oral cavity and from the external ear are shown in B. Secondary fibers from the spinal nucleus of V ascend in the ventral secondary ascending trigeminal tract to end in the ventral posteromedial nucleus of the dorsal thalamus. *See also* Fig. N-1.

which overlies the insula and forms the anterior part of the upper lip of the lateral sulcus.

operculum, parietal [operculum parietale, NA], CEREBRUM   part of the parietal lobe which overlies the insula and forms the posterior part of the upper lip of the lateral sulcus.

operculum, temporal [operculum temporale, NA], CEREBRUM   part of the temporal lobe which overlies the insula and forms the lower lip of the lateral sulcus.

ophthalmoplegia, external /of-thal-mo-ple´jī-ah/ [*adj.* **ophthalmoplegic**] [Gr. *ophthalmos* eye; *plege* stroke]   paralysis of the extraocular eye muscles.

ophthalmoplegia, internal   paralysis of the ciliary muscle and constrictor muscle of the pupil of the eye.

ophthalmoplegia, internuclear   inability to turn the eye medially past the mid-position of the eye on horizontal conjugate gaze. It occurs with a lesion of the homolateral medial longitudinal fasciculus between the levels of the motor nuclei of VI and III, severing the fibers from the parabducens nucleus to the oculomotor nuclei (Fig. F-2). Convergence may be normal.

o´pioid   pertaining to certain substances produced by the nervous system, which have opium-like properties and inhibit pain transmission.

opis´thion [NA] [Gr. *opisthios* posterior]   mid-point of the posterior margin of the foramen magnum.

opisthot´onos (opisthotonus) [Gr. *opisthen* behind, backward; *tonos* tension]   an extensor posture in which the head and trunk are stiffly arched backward and all four limbs are rigidly extended, but without the pronation of the hands and plantar flexion of decerebrate rigidity. It is produced in man by an irritative lesion, usually meningitis or hemorrhage, of the ventral brain stem, involving the midbrain and upper pons (Penfield and Jasper, '54, pp. 379, 387).

Oppenheim, Hermann (1858-1919)   German neurologist of Berlin. *Oppenheim's disease* is amyotonia congenita, which he called dystonia musculorum deformans. *Oppenheim's sign,* dorsiflexion of the great toe in response to firm pressure downward along the anterior surface of the tibia, is indicative of injury to the corticospinal fibers. *See also* Babinski.

op´tic [Gr. *optikos*; from *ops* eye]   pertaining to the eye. *For* optic canal, chiasm, disk, foramen, papilla, nerve, radiation, tectum, thalamus, *and* tract, *see the nouns*.

optokinet´ic [from Gr. *opts-; kinesis* movement]   pertaining to eye movements in response to changes in position of an object in the visual field; also called *following* or *automatic* eye movements.

o´ra serrata /ser-ah´tah/ [NA], EYE, [L. *ora* margin; *serratus,* from *serra* a saw]   scalloped outer edge of the ciliary body, marking its junction with the retina.

organs, circumventricular   *See* organs, ventricular.

organ, paraventric´ular, HYPOTHALAMUS   the ventricular organ of the hypothalamus.

organ, pineal /pi-ne´-al, pin´e-al/, EPITHALAMUS   *See* body, pineal.

organ, spiral [organum spirale (cortiense), NA], EAR   end organ for hearing, located on the basilar membrane in the cochlear duct of the internal ear. *Syn:* organ of Corti; papilla or pars basilaris.

organ, subcommis´sural [organum subcommissurale, NA], MIDBRAIN   one of the ventricular organs. It is a plate of modified ependyma, consisting of tall, columnar, ciliated cells, neurosecretory in function, in the cerebral aqueduct just caudal to the posterior commissure. It appears to play a significant role in water intake.

organ, subfor´nical [organum subfornicale, NA], CEREBRUM   one of the ventricular organs. It is a small mass between the columns of the fornix at the level of the interventricular foramen. It consists of neuroglia and small nerve cells covered by ependyma and appears to be similar to the area postrema and the subcommissural organ. *Syn:* intercolumnar tubercle.

organ, ten´don   *See* spindle, neurotendinous.

organs, ventric´ular   small, specialized areas of tissue in the ventricular wall. They are: the subcommissural organ, subfornical organ (intercolumnar tubercle), area postrema, vascular organs of the hypothalamus (paraventricular organ) and of the lamina terminalis (supraoptic crest), and sometimes also including the hypophysis and pineal body (Peters *et al.*, '76, p. 275). In submammalian forms there are also the saccus vasculosus of certain fishes (Altner and Zimmermann, '72) and the paraphysis cerebri (J. Ariëns Kappers, '55). *Syn:* circumventricular organs. *For additional information, see* McKinley and Oldfield ('90).

organ, vomerona´sal   specialized epithelial cells lining a pocket in the nasal septum, from which the vomeronasal nerve arises. Although the vomeronasal organ and nerve are well developed in some subprimate mammals and submammals, and sometimes occur in the human embryo, they are not present in adult man. *Syn:* Jacobson's organ.

organum cortien´se [NA], EAR   organ of Corti. *See* organ, spiral.

orthodro´mic [Gr. *orthos* straight; *dromus* running]   conducting in the normal or conventional direction.

orthosympathet´ic   *See* sympathetic, *def.* 1.

os´sicles, EAR, [L. *ossiculum* little bone]   three small bones, *viz.* malleus, incus, and stapes, present in the tympanic cavity of the middle ear. They convey vibrations set up in the tympanic membrane to the oval window of the inner ear.

otalgia /o-tal´jĭ-ah/   earache.

o´tic   pertaining to the ear. *For* otic duct, fluid, ganglion, sac, *and* vesicle, *see the nouns.*

otoconia /o-to-ko´nĭ-ah/ [*sing.* otoconium], EAR   statoconia.

o´tocyst, EAR   *See* vesicle, otic.

o´tolite, EAR   *See* otolith, *def.* 1.

o´tolith, EAR   1. single calcareous body in the gelatinous membrane of the saccule of certain bony fishes. *Syn:* otolite; statolith.

2. sometimes used as a synonym for otoconium or statoconium. *See* statoconia.

oxyto´cin   neurohormone synthesized by the cells of the paraventricular (mainly) and supraoptic (to some extent) nuclei of the hypothalamus. Conjugated with a carrier protein, neurophysin, it is carried by axoplasmic flow along their axons and stored in their terminal swellings (Herring bodies) in the neurohypophysis, from which it is released into the vascular system. It stimulates contraction of the smooth muscle of the reproductive system and may play a number of roles in the endocrine regulation of reproduction. *Syn:* Pitocin. *See also* neurotransmitters *and* neuropeptides.

p

P, DORSAL THALAMUS   pulvinar.

Pacchioni, Antonio (1665-1726)   Italian anatomist of Rome and Tivoli. *Pacchionian bodies* (1705) are the enlarged arachnoid granulations in the superior sagittal sinus. *Pacchioni's foramen* is the incisure of the tentorium.

pachymeninx /pak-e-men´inks/ [NA] [Gr. *pachy* thick; *meninx* membrane]   *See* dura mater.

Pacini, Filippo (1812-1883)   Italian anatomist of Florence. A *Pacinian corpuscle* or *corpuscle of Vater-Pacini* (corpusculum lamellosum, NA) is a nerve ending having a multilayered connective tissue capsule. Such endings are located in subcutaneous connective tissue, mesentery, and other areas, and are thought to be sensitive to pressure. They were first described by Vater and later rediscovered (1830) and described (1844) by Pacini.

PAG, MIDBRAIN   periaqueductal gray, the area around the cerebral aqueduct.

pain, referred   pain originating in a visceral organ but felt in a somatic area innervated by the same segment of the CNS.

palaeo- [Gr. *palaios* old, ancient]   *See* paleo-.

paleocerebellum /pa-le-o-ser-ĕ-bel´um/ [NA], CEREBELLUM   old portion of the cerebellum, consisting mainly of parts of the vermis and adjacent parts of the cerebellar hemispheres, particularly those areas in which the spinocerebellar tract fibers end. Included are the vermis of the anterior lobe (possibly excluding some or all of the lingula), the pyramis, and some of the uvula of the posterior lobe vermis. *Syn:* spinocerebellum. *See also* archicerebellum; neocerebellum.

paleocor´tex (palaeocortex) [NA], CEREBRUM   piriform lobe cortex. *See also* paleopallium.

paleo-ol´ive, MEDULLA   older portion of the inferior olivary nucleus, including the dorsal and medial accessory olivary nuclei and the medial part of the inferior olivary nucleus.

paleopal´lium, CEREBRUM   piriform lobe cortex and its underlying white matter; uncus and adjacent part of the parahippocampal gyrus.

paleostria´tum, CEREBRUM   *See* globus pallidus.

paleothal´amus, DIENCEPHALON   older part of the dorsal thalamus, comprising the median thalamic nuclei (including the interthalamic adhesion), and the intralaminar nuclei. Although small in man, these nuclei constitute the largest part of the dorsal thalamus in lower forms.

palilal´ia   speech disorder characterized by involuntary repetition of words or phrases.

pallesthe´sia [Gr. *pallein* to shake; *aisthesis* sensation]   vibratory sensibility.

pal´lidum, (dorsal), CEREBRUM, [L. *pallidus* pale]   *See* globus pallidus.

pallidum, ventral, CEREBRUM   medial part of the sublenticular gray, ventral to the globus pallidus.

pal´lium, CEREBRUM, [L. cloak]   cerebral cortex and its underlying white matter; sometimes used loosely as a synonym for cerebral cortex.

palsy, bul´bar /pawl´ze/   weakness or paralysis of muscles supplied by a cranial nerve, after injury to the cell bodies or fibers of the lower motor neurons which supply them.

palsy, cer´ebral   any type of neurologic disorder resulting from damage to the nervous system in utero, at birth, or early in life.

palsy, oc´ular   paralysis or weakness of one or more of the extrinsic muscles of the eyeball.

palsy, pseudobulbar /soo-do-bul´bar/   an upper motor neuron paralysis or weakness of muscles supplied by a cranial nerve, after injury to the pyramidal tract fibers which supply the cranial nerve motor nucleus of the involved muscles.

Papez, James Wenceslaus (1883-1958)   eminent American neuroanatomist of Cornell University. He is most noted for his *Papez circuit* ('37), which consists of the connections by way of the fimbria-fornix from the hippocampus to the mamillary body, the mamillothalamic tract to the anterior nuclei of the dorsal thalamus, the anterior thalamic radiations to the cingulate gyrus, the cingulum back to the parahippocampal gyrus then to the hippocampus. Although Papez suggested that this circuit provided a mechanism for emotion, there is little evidence to this effect. However, his idea provided a powerful incentive for the development of the limbic system concept.

papil´la basila´ris, EAR   *See* organ, spiral.

papilla, op´tic, EYE   slight elevation in the optic disk of the retina, where the optic nerve fibers leave the eyeball.

paracu´sis [Gr. *para* next to or near, in this case denoting a departure from the normal; *akousis* hearing]   impaired hearing or auditory illusions. False paracusis (Willis's paracusis) is characterized by the ability to hear better in a noisy environment than in quiet surroundings.

parafloc´culus [NA], CEREBELLUM   small, inconstant segment within the posterolateral fissure of the cerebellar hemisphere (Fig. C-2). In some forms it is a fairly substantial part of the corpus cerebelli, but in man it is only occasionally present. *Syn:* accessory paraflocculus of comparative neuroanatomy.

paraflocculus, dorsal, CEREBELLUM   homologue in subprimate brains for the biventer of the primate cerebellum.

paraflocculus, ventral, CEREBELLUM   homologue in subprimate brains for the tonsil of the primate cerebellum.

paragang´lion [*pl.* **paraganglia**]   tissue such as that of the adrenal medulla (chrom-

affin paraganglia), or the tissue associated with certain blood vessels (nonchromaffin paraganglia).

paraganglion, aortic /a-or´tik/   *See* body, aortic.

paraganglion, carot´id   *See* body, carotid.

paraganglia, chro´maffin   chromaffin tissue in the adrenal medulla, and nests of
cells along the sympathetic trunk, in the celiac and pelvic plexuses and along the
abdominal aorta. This tissue has a common origin with the ganglion cells of the
sympathetic trunk and secretes epinephrine-like substances. *Syn:* chromaffin
bodies. The paraganglia along the aorta are also called Zuckerkandl's bodies.

paraganglion, cil´iary   paraganglion, probably nonchromaffin in type, located near
the ciliary ganglion in the orbit and described in the chimpanzee.

paraganglion, intrava´gal   *See* paraganglion, juxtavagal.

paraganglion, juxtavagal /juks-tah-va´gal/   nonchromaffin paraganglion associated
with the inferior ganglion of the vagus nerve. *Syn:* intravagal paraganglion.

paraganglia, nonchro´maffin   a number of small masses of tissue associated mainly
with the blood vessels and nerves (glossopharyngeal and vagus) derived from the
third and fourth visceral arches. They are histologically similar to one another and
consist of "epithelioid" cells in a highly vascular stroma. All are probably
chemoreceptors, able to detect changes in pH and CO_2 concentrations in blood,
and function in respiratory reflexes. They include: the carotid and aortic bodies,
glomus aorticum, glomus jugulare, paraganglion juxtavagale, and paraganglion
tympanicum. *For additional information, see* Lattes ('50).

paraganglion, tympan´ic   nonchromaffin paraganglion, located on the tympanic
branch of the glossopharyngeal nerve.

parageusia /par-ah-goo´zĭ-ah/ [Gr. *para* next to or near; *geusis* taste]   impaired
taste sensation, including hallucinations of taste.

parakoniocor´tex, CEREBRUM   cortex next to a sensory area, particularly Brodmann's
area 42 in the temporal lobe and probably area 52. *See* Fig. B-1.

paral´ysis, alternate   *See* hemiplegia, alternate.

paralysis, brachial cruciate (of Bell)   paralysis of both upper extremities, after a
lesion of the corticospinal tract fibers crossing in the rostral part of the pyramidal
decussation.

paralysis, crossed   *See* hemiplegia, crossed.

paralysis, flaccid /flak´sid/   paralysis in which the affected muscles receive too few
nervous impulses and are atonic, as following injury to a motor nerve.

paralysis, spas´tic   paralysis resulting from injury to the pyramidal and other
associated tracts, and accompanied by spasticity of the affected muscles,
particularly those of the extremities. *See* spasticity.

parame´dian pon´tine retic´ular forma´tion (PPRF), PONS   that part of the
reticular formation medial to the abducens nucleus, from which fibers arise, cross
the median plane, and ascend in the medial longitudinal fasciculus to the oculomotor nucleus for relay to the medial rectus muscle for horizontal conjugate
deviation of the eyes. It appears to be the same as the parabducens nucleus (Fig.
F-2).

paraneuron /par-ah-nu´ron/   any of a class of cells of neuroectodermal origin, with
certain characteristics common to both neurons and some endocrine cells. Some
cells are secretory and may release a neurotransmitter or hormonic substance.
Representative paraneurons include: paraganglia cells, pinealocytes, olfactory and
gustatory cells, amacrine cells of the retina, and the hair cells of the spiral organ.

paranode /par´ah-nŏd/ region of a myelinated nerve fiber next to a node of Ranvier, where the lamellae of the myelin sheath terminate.

parapha´sia language disorder in which there is substitution of an inappropriate syllable, or a real or nonsense word. When severe, the disorder constitutes jargon aphasia.

paraphysis cerebri /par-af´ĭ-sĭs ser´eb-ri/, CEREBRUM glandular structure present in some lower vertebrates, and occurring as a transient, rudimentary structure in the human embryo. It arises as an evagination from the roof of the third ventricle, just behind the interventricular foramen. Tumors which sometimes occur in this region have been said to arise from the paraphysis but are more likely of diencephalic origin (J. Ariëns Kappers, '55, p. 491).

paraplegia /par-ah-ple´jĭ-ah/ paralysis of both lower extremities or, rarely, paralysis of both upper extremities.

parasol´itary, MAINLY MEDULLA pertaining to the nucleus parasolitarius, the cellular area adjacent to the fasciculus solitarius.

parastri´ate, CEREBRUM pertaining to area 18 of the cerebral cortex, adjacent to area 17 (striate cortex) of the occipital lobe.

parasubic´ulum, CEREBRUM transitional cortex of the hippocampal formation between the presubiculum and the entorhinal area of the parahippocampal gyrus. *See also* subiculum.

parasympathet´ic pertaining to that part of the ANS whose preganglionic neurons arise in the brain and in the sacral part of the spinal cord. It is the craniosacral division of the ANS and is concerned with the maintenance of the body.

parasympathetic af´ferent pertaining to the general visceral afferent fibers which accompany the fibers of the parasympathetic division of the ANS.

parasympathetic, spinal postulated two-neuron chain for peripheral vasodilation. The first neuron has its cell body in the spinal cord, and its axon leaves the cord through the dorsal root to synapse in a dorsal root ganglion. The second neuron has its cell body in the dorsal root ganglion, and its axon ends in relation to subcutaneous blood vessels (Kuré *et al.*, '30).

parater´minal area (body or **gyrus)**, CEREBRUM *See* gyrus, paraterminal.

paraver´mal, CEREBELLUM pertaining to the area immediately adjacent to the vermis of the cerebellum, the most medial part of the cerebellar hemispheric cortex.

pare´sis (par´esis) [Gr. a letting go, slackening] **1.** mild or partial paralysis. **2.** one form of progressive dementia.

paresthe´sia abnormal spontaneous sensation, such as tingling.

pa´ries tympan´icus duc´tus cochlear´is [NA], EAR, [L. *paries* a wall] *See* membrane, spiral.

paries vestibular´is ductus cochlearis [NA], EAR *See* membrane, vestibular.

pari´etal, CEREBRUM pertaining to the parietal lobe or its cortex.

Parinaud, Henri (1844-1905) French ophthalmologist. *Parinaud's syndrome* (1883) consists of a paralysis of conjugate, vertical, optokinetic eye movements above the horizontal plane, as when a pineal tumor presses on the rostral part of the superior colliculi. Later, if the tumor enlarges and encroaches on adjoining areas, voluntary eye movements upward and even downward eye movements may be affected. *See also* tract, corticotectal, internal.

Parkinson, James (1755-1824) English physician of London, who first described (1817) the syndrome of paralysis agitans, *Parkinson's disease,* characterized by progressive rigidity, tremor, and other signs of basal ganglia dysfunction. A

Parkinson tremor, also called a "resting," "alternating," or "non-intention" tremor, usually occurs with a frequency of about 4 to 6 Hz and is characterized by rhythmic alternating contractions of the antagonistic muscles of a joint. It may involve the fingers (pill-rolling tremor); one or both arms and legs, the trunk, or the head.

parolfac´tory, CEREBRUM   pertaining to the parolfactory area of the frontal lobe.

pars basila´ris, EAR   *See* organ, spiral.

pars distal´is, HYPOPHYSIS   largest part of the adenohypophysis. Its glandular cells, in an extensive vascular mesh, produce a number of important hormones. *Syn:* anterior lobe of the pituitary gland. *See also* adenohypophysis.

pars interme´dia, HYPOPHYSIS   part of the adenohypophysis, derived from the posterior wall of Rathke's pouch, an evagination of the roof of the embryonic pharynx. In the adult it lies between the pars nervosa and the pars distalis, and is attached to both. In some species (but not in man) the cavity of Rathke's pouch is retained between pars dorsalis and pars intermedia. The pars intermedia is sometimes included in the posterior lobe of the pituitary gland and sometimes is called the middle lobe of the pituitary gland. *See also* adenohypophysis.

pars tuberal´is, HYPOPHYSIS   part of the adenohypophysis on the anterior surface of the infundibulum, which it partially encloses. It is continuous with the pars distalis and pars intermedia. *Syn:* pars infundibularis. *See also* adenohypophysis.

parvicel´lular [L. *parvus* small; *cellularis* cellular]   composed of small cells.

pathway, final common   lower motor neuron which receives impulses from multiple sources and is the sole mediator for impulses carried to voluntary striated muscles.

pathway, sensory   neuron chain by which a sensory modality is conducted from the periphery to the cerebral cortex. It is characteristically a 3-neuron chain, although there are exceptions. The primary neuron conducts impulses from the peripheral end organ to the CNS. The secondary neuron crosses the median plane and ends in the dorsal thalamus. The tertiary neuron ends in the cerebral cortex. *See* neuron, sensory, primary, secondary, *and* tertiary.

pattern, onion-skin   *See* onion-skin pattern.

Pavlov, Ivan Petrovitch (1849-1936)   great Russian physiologist noted for his work on digestion. In 1904 he received the Nobel Prize in medicine and physiology for his research establishing the importance of the autonomic nervous system and laying bare the details of the physiology of digestion. Later on his experiments on unconditioned and conditioned reflexes brought him additional renown.

ped´icle, cone, EYE   synaptic base of a retinal cone in the outer plexiform layer of the retina (layer 5), by which the cone synapses with the dendritic terminals of bipolar and horizontal cells of the retina.

pe´duncle [L. little foot]   usually a large band of nerve fibers in the brain, most frequently composed of multiple tracts. *Syn:* brachium.

peduncles, cerebel´lar [pedunculi cerebelli, NA], CEREBELLUM, BRAIN STEM   three fiber masses which connect the cerebellum and the brain stem bilaterally at the level of the pons, *viz.* the superior, middle, and inferior cerebellar peduncles (Figs. C-2, V-4). The superior and inferior peduncles contain fibers with connections above and below the level of the pons.

peduncle, cerebellar, inferior [pedunculus cerebellaris inferior (caudalis), NA]   bundle of nerve fibers interconnecting the cerebellum with the medulla and spinal cord, including connections with the vestibular complex, inferior olive, and reticular gray, and also containing fibers of the dorsal spinocerebellar, cuneatocerebellar, arcuatocerebellar, and cerebellomotorius tracts (Figs. C-2, O-1, V-4). Injury to one peduncle causes homolateral ataxia. *See also* body, restiform.

peduncle, cerebellar, middle [pedunculus cerebellaris medius (pontinus), NA] bundle of nerve fibers joining the pons and cerebellum and composed mostly of fibers of the pontocerebellar tract (Figs. C-2, V-4). *Syn:* brachium pontis.

peduncle, cerebellar, superior [pedunculus cerebellaris superior (rostralis), NA] bundle of nerve fibers interconnecting the cerebellum with the midbrain and diencephalon and composed mostly of fibers of the dentatorubral and dentato-thalamic tracts (Figs. C-2, O-1, V-4). Injury to one peduncle causes great hypotonicity and a postural tremor on the side of the lesion. *Syn:* brachium conjunctivum.

peduncle, cer´ebral [pedunculus cerebri, NA], MIDBRAIN   ventral part of each half of the midbrain, exclusive of the tectum. It consists of a dorsal part, the midbrain tegmentum, continuous with its counterpart on the other side across the median plane, and a ventral part, the basis pedunculi or crus cerebri, separated from its counterpart by the interpeduncular fossa (Fig. P-1). *See also* basis pedunculi.

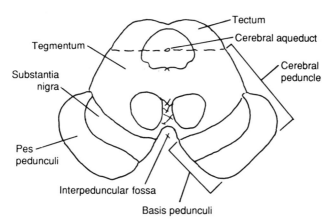

Fig. P-1.   Diagram to show the relationship of the parts in a cross section of the midbrain. The plane separating the tectum from the tegmentum of the cerebral peduncle is represented by the broken line through the cerebral aqueduct. The tegmentum spans the median plane, whereas the interpeduncular fossa separates the bases of the cerebral peduncles.

peduncle (of the) collic´ulus, inferior   *See* brachium, colliculus, of the inferior.

peduncle (of the) cor´pus callo´sum, CEREBRUM   *See* gyrus, subcallosal.

peduncle (of the) floc´culus [pedunculus flocculi, NA], CEREBELLUM   band of nerve fibers connecting the flocculus and the nodule of the cerebellum.

peduncle, mam´illary   bundle of fibers which connects the mamillary nuclei of the hypothalamus with nuclei of the midbrain and pons. It contains fibers which ascend from cells in the dorsal visceral (gustatory) gray and others which interconnect the dorsal and ventral tegmental nuclei and the mamillary body.

peduncle, olfac´tory, CEREBRUM   *See* band, diagonal (of Broca).

peduncle, ol´ivary, superior, PONS   fibers which arise from cells in the superior olive or the adjoining gray and pass dorsomedially toward the abducens nucleus. They belong to the olivocochlear bundle, which ends in the spiral organ.

peduncles, thalam´ic, FOREBRAIN   any of several fiber masses in the internal capsule and corona radiata, which interconnect the dorsal thalamus and the cerebral cortex, *viz.* the anterior, inferior, posterior, and superior thalamic peduncles. *See also* radiations, thalamic; radiations, sensory.

peduncle, thalamic, anterior, FOREBRAIN   *See* radiations, thalamic, anterior.

peduncle, thalamic, inferior (caudal), FOREBRAIN   **1.** [pedunculus thalami inferior (caudalis), NA] fibers in the anterior limb of the internal capsule and corona radiata connecting the dorsomedial thalamic nucleus with the orbital cortex and amygdala. *Syn:* ventral thalamic peduncle. *See also* ansa peduncularis.
2. *See* radiation, acoustic.

peduncle, thalamic, posterior, FOREBRAIN   *See* radiations, thalamic, posterior.

peduncle, thalamic, superior, FOREBRAIN   nerve fibers in the internal capsule and corona radiata, connecting the ventral nuclear complex of the dorsal thalamus with the cortex of the frontal and parietal lobes. They include the sensory radiations from the ventral posterior nuclei through the thalamolenticular part of the posterior limb to the postcentral gyrus, and thalamocortical fibers from the ventral anterior and ventral lateral nuclei through the genu of the internal capsule to the frontal lobe (Fig. C-1).

peduncle, thalamic, ventral, FOREBRAIN   *See* peduncle, thalamic, inferior, *def.* 1.

Penfield, Wilder Graves (1891-1976)   neurosurgeon born in Seattle Washington, later in Canada at McGill University. He made many contributions in the field of neurophysiology, especially including functions of the cerebral cortex.

pep´tides   *See* neuropeptides.

peptides, o´pioid   class of neurotransmitters encompassing the endorphins, which appear to function in response to stress. *See also* neurotransmitters.

periaqueduc´tal, MIDBRAIN, [Gr. *peri* around]   around the cerebral aqueduct.

perikar´yon [Gr. *peri*-; *karyon* nucleus]   cytoplasm of a nerve cell body, around the nucleus; sometimes incorrectly used as a synonym for nerve cell body.

per´ilymph [perilympha, NA], EAR   fluid contained in the spaces of the periotic labyrinth, surrounding the membranous labyrinth of the internal ear. *Syn:* liquor cotunnii; periotic fluid.

perineurium /per-ĭ-nu´rĭ-um/ [NA]   dense connective tissue which surrounds each fascicle of a nerve. The outer layer of the perineurial collagenous fibers is continuous with the dura mater. The deeper part is seen, with the electron microscope, to consist of concentric laminae, or sleeves, of flattened cells, endothelial in type with tight junctions, sometimes called *perineural epithelium*. This part, continuous with the pia-arachnoid, is probably of neural crest origin. Peripherally, as the nerve branches, the sleeves follow successive nerve fascicles, decreasing in number until the last one ends just before the axis cylinder passes into a nerve ending. *For additional information on the perineural epithelium, see* Shantha and Bourne ('68).

perio´tic fluid, EAR   *See* perilymph.

periph´eral nervous system (PNS)   the cranial and spinal nerves and all their branches, together with the autonomic and sensory ganglia.

peristri´ate, CEREBRUM   pertaining to the cortex anterior and adjacent to the parastriate area, in the posterior part of the parietal and temporal lobes; area 19.

Perlia, Richard (19th century)   German ophthalmologist. The *nucleus of Perlia* is the central nucleus of the oculomotor nerve, thought to play a role in convergence of the eyes.

persevera′tion   repetition of a word or other response, at first correctly, then in such a way that it is no longer relevant or appropriate.

pes hippocampi /pez hip-po-kam′pī/ [NA], CEREBRUM, [L. *pes* foot]   anterior part of the hippocampus, marked on its ventricular surface by shallow grooves which give it the appearance of an animal's paw.

pes pedun′culi, MIDBRAIN   fibrous part of the basis pedunculi of the midbrain, composed of pyramidal and corticopontine tracts (Fig. P-1). Sometimes basis pedunculi or crus cerebri is used as a synonym for this term. *See also* peduncle, cerebral.

PET   positron emission tomography. *See* tomography.

-petal   suffix denoting afferent conduction to the region indicated.

Petit, François Pourfour du (1664-1741)   French surgeon and anatomist of Paris. The *canal of Petit* (spatia zonularia, NA) consists of the spaces among the fibers of the suspensory ligament in the ciliary zonule of the eye.

petro′sal [L. like a rock]   pertaining to the inferior ganglion of the glossopharyngeal nerve, and to structures associated with the petrous part of the temporal bone.

Philippe, Claudien (1866-1903)   French pathologist. The *triangular field of Gombault and Philippe* is the sacral part of the septomarginal fasciculus.

photorecep′tor, EYE   light-sensitive (rod) or color-sensitive (cone) cell of the retina.

phrenic /fren′ik/ [Gr. *phren* diaphragm]   *For* phrenic nerve *and* nucleus, *see the nouns.*

pia-arachnoid /pī-ah-ah-rak′noid/   leptomeninges.

pia ma′ter [NA] [L. *pius* tender; *mater* mother]   innermost layer of the leptomeninges, which adheres to the brain and spinal cord and conforms to all the irregularities on their surfaces. *Syn:* intima pia. *See also* mater.

PICA   posterior inferior cerebellar artery.

Piccolomini, Archangelo (1526-1586)   Italian anatomist. The *fibers of Piccolomini* are the striae medullares on the floor of the fourth ventricle, fibers of the arcuatocerebellar tract.

Pick, Arnold (1851-1924)   Czech psychiatrist and neuropathologist, born of Austrian parents. *Pick's disease* (1892) consists of aphasia and presenile dementia, not unlike the clinical picture of Alzheimer's disease. There is cerebral atrophy of the frontal and temporal lobes. It is probably inherited as an autosomal dominant. *Pick's bundle* consists of corticobulbar fibers which accompany the corticospinal tract fibers through the pyramidal decussation then ascend to end in the nucleus ambiguus.

pillar (of the fornix) [crus fornicis, NA], CEREBRUM   posterior part of the fornix, between and continuous with the fimbria of the hippocampus in the temporal lobe and the body of the fornix in the margin of the septum pellucidum. Sometimes the columns of the fornix are called the *anterior pillars*, whereupon the bundles described here are designated the *posterior pillars*. *See also* Fig. P-2.

pineal /pin′e-al, pi-ne′al/ [L. *pinea* pine cone], EPITHALAMUS   *See* body, pineal.

pine′alocyte, EPITHALAMUS   parenchymatous cell of the pineal body. These cells have long processes and knoblike endings, and are arranged in cords or clusters in a bed of neuroglia.

Pinkus, F.   the *nerve of Pinkus* is the nervus terminalis.

pir´iform [L. pear-shaped]   *See* area, piriform.

Pitocin /pī-to´sin/   trademark for preparations of oxytocin.

pituitary gland (body)   *See* hypophysis.

placode, o´tic /plak´ōd/ [placoda otica, NA], ᴇᴀʀ   thickening of the surface ectoderm of the hindbrain, which appears early in the fourth week of embryonic
development and from which the membranous labyrinth develops.

pla´num temporal´e, ᴄᴇʀᴇʙʀᴜᴍ   triangular area on the superior surface of the
temporal lobe within the lateral sulcus. It is located between the transverse
temporal gyri (of Heschl) and the posterior margin of the Sylvian fossa.

plate, a´lar   that part of the mantle layer of the neural tube dorsal or dorsolateral
to the sulcus limitans. *Syn:* dorsal plate.

plate, ba´sal   that part of the mantle layer of the neural tube ventral or medial to
the sulcus limitans. *Syn:* ventral plate.

plate, brain   expanded rostral part of the neural plate from which the brain
develops.

plate, crib´riform   *See* lamina cribrosa.

plate, dorsal   *See* plate, alar.

plate, foot   terminal portion of a process of an astrocyte, which contributes to the
limiting membranes on the external and ventricular surfaces of the CNS and on
the surface of its blood vessels.

plate, floor   thin ventral wall of the neural tube.

plate, lateral   thickened side wall of the neural tube, the mantle layer of which
consists of an alar and a basal plate.

plate, motor end [terminatio neuromuscularis, NA]   specialized ending of a motor
neuron on a skeletal muscle fiber, whereby a nervous impulse can cause the
muscle fiber to contract. A slight elevation of the tissue occurs in the area of the
neuromuscular junction. The axolemma or presynaptic membrane of the axon is
separated from the sarcolemma or postsynaptic membrane of the muscle fiber by
a narrow synaptic cleft. When activated, presynaptic vesicles release acetylcholine
into the synaptic cleft, the sarcolemma of the muscle fiber becomes more
permeable to sodium ions, and a wave of depolarization continues along the
muscle fiber. The nervous impulse is promptly inactivated by cholinesterase. *See
also* vesicles, presynaptic.

plate, neu´ral   thickening of the ectoderm along the mid-dorsal surface of the
embryo, from which the neural tube is derived.

plate, quadrigem´inal, ᴍɪᴅʙʀᴀɪɴ   tectum.

plate, roof   thin, mid-dorsal membrane of the neural tube, from which the tela
choroidea of the third ventricle and the anterior and posterior medullary vela of
the fourth ventricle develop.

plate, ventral   *See* plate, basal.

plexus /plek´sus/ [L. something woven, a braid]   **1.** a network of nerve fibers or
nerve fiber bundles of the PNS.
2. a network of blood vessels.

plexus, aortic [plexus aorticus, NA]   plexus of autonomic nerve fibers along the
aorta.   Subdivisions of this plexus are named for the arteries which they
accompany.

plexus, brachial /bra´kī-al/ [plexus brachialis, NA]   nerve plexus derived from the
ventral primary rami of spinal nerves C5-T1, which gives rise to the nerves that
supply the upper extremity.

plexus, carot´id, external   plexus of postganglionic sympathetic fibers which arise from cells in the superior cervical ganglion and accompany the external carotid artery and its branches. Its fibers supply the structures served by the artery, particularly the salivary glands, ending on both mucous and serous acini, in major and minor glands. Stimulation causes vasoconstriction and the release, primarily, of stored macromolecules, producing a thick, low-volume saliva. *For additional information on the autonomic supply of salivary glands, see* nerve, facial.

plexus, carotid, internal   plexus of postganglionic sympathetic fibers which arise from cells in the superior cervical ganglion and accompany the internal carotid artery and its branches. Some fibers (the deep petrosal nerve) supply the nasopalatine glands. Other fibers enter the orbit and supply the lacrimal gland, the radial fibers of the iris for dilation of the pupil, and the smooth muscle of the upper eyelid, Müller's muscle, for maintaining an open eye (Fig. R-3).

plexus, celiac /se´lī-ak/   dense network of nerve fibers surrounding the celiac artery, and containing the celiac ganglia, one on each side. The greater and lesser splanchnic nerves join the plexus. In addition to the sympathetic fibers which end here or pass through the plexus, there are also parasympathetic fibers of the vagus nerve and visceral afferent fibers which pass through. *Syn:* solar plexus.

plexus, cer´vical [plexus cervicalis, NA]   plexus derived from the ventral primary rami of spinal nerves C1-C4. Its main branches include the phrenic nerve, motor branches to prevertebral and infrahyoid muscles of the neck, and cutaneous branches to part of the neck and head.

plexus, choroid /kor´oid/ [plexus choroideus, NA]   the secretory epithelium and associated blood vessels of the lateral, third, and fourth ventricles, which produce cerebrospinal fluid, or the blood vessels associated with the secretory epithelium of the ventricles.

plexus, choroid, of the fourth ventricle [plexus choroideus ventriculi quarti, NA], MEDULLA   The choroid plexus of the fourth ventricle is attached bilaterally along the margin of the posterior medullary velum. A part extends through the lateral aperture of the fourth ventricle for a short distance into the subarachnoid space.

plexus, choroid, of the lateral ventricle [plexus choroideus ventriculi lateralis, NA], CEREBRUM   The choroid plexus of the lateral ventricles is located in the body, collateral trigone, and inferior horn, and is attached along the fimbria-fornix on one side and the stria terminalis on the other, closing the choroid fissure.

plexus, choroid, of the third ventricle [plexus choroideus ventriculi tertii, NA], DIENCEPHALON   The choroid plexus of the third ventricle extends along the roof of the ventricle from the interventricular foramen to the pineal body and is attached to the stria medullaris thalami on each side.

plexus, hypogas´tric, inferior   pelvic plexus of autonomic and visceral afferent nerve fibers derived from the hypogastric nerves of the superior hypogastric plexus and from the pelvic nerves for distribution to organs of the pelvis.

plexus, hypogastric, superior   plexus of autonomic and visceral afferent nerve fibers anterior to the bifurcation of the aorta and the body of the L5 vertebra. It is derived from the aortic plexus and lower splanchnic nerves above, and continues caudally as the two hypogastric nerves. *Syn:* presacral nerve.

plexus, lumbosa´cral [plexus lumbosacralis, NA]   nerve plexus derived from the ventral primary rami of spinal nerves L2-S3, which gives rise to the nerves that supply the lower extremity.

plexus, myenter´ic   plexus of visceral afferent and efferent nerve fibers and cell bodies of parasympathetic postganglionic neurons between the circular and longitudinal layers of smooth muscle in the gastrointestinal tract. *Syn:* Auerbach's plexus.

plexus, retro-orb´ital   plexus of postganglionic parasympathetic fibers which arise from the pterygopalatine ganglion of the facial nerve for distribution to the lacrimal gland.

plexus, so´lar [L. *sol* sun]   *See* plexus, celiac. It was called *solar* plexus because its branches fan out "like the rays of the sun."

plexus, submuco´sal   plexus of visceral afferent and efferent nerve fibers and cell bodies of parasympathetic postganglionic neurons in the submucosal layer of the gastrointestinal tract. *Syn:* Meissner's plexus.

plexus, tympan´ic   plexus on the medial wall of the middle ear. It contains visceral afferent fibers of the glossopharyngeal nerve from the mucosal lining of the middle ear, mastoid air cells and auditory tube, preganglionic fibers of the glossopharyngeal nerve which enter the lesser petrosal nerve, and postganglionic sympathetic branches from the internal carotid plexus.

plexus, ver´tebral ve´nous [plexus venosus vertebralis, NA]   *See* veins, vertebral.

pneumoencephalog´raphy [Gr. *pneuma* air; *enkephalos* brain; *grapho* to write] procedure in which cerebrospinal fluid is replaced by air and followed by radiography to demonstrate the subarachnoid space and ventricles. Now computerized tomography is generally used for this purpose. *See also* tomography.

PNS   peripheral nervous system, the nerves and ganglia.

poikilothermism [Gr. *poikilos* varied; *therme* heat]   condition in which the body temperature varies with that of the environment.

polariza´tion   state of a nerve cell membrane in which the outer surface is positively charged and the inner surface is negatively charged, as in a resting potential.

pole, fron´tal [polus frontalis, NA], CEREBRUM   anterior tip of the frontal lobe of the cerebrum (Fig. C-3A,C).

pole, occip´ital [polus occipitalis, NA], CEREBRUM   posterior tip of the occipital lobe of the cerebrum (Fig. C-3A,C).

pole, temp´oral [polus temporalis, NA], CEREBRUM   anterior tip of the temporal lobe of the cerebrum (Fig. C-3A,C).

poliomyeli´tis   paralytic disease caused by a virus which destroys cells mainly in the ventral horn of the spinal cord (spinal polio) or motor nuclei of cranial nerves (bulbar polio).

pons /ponz/ [NA], METENCEPHALON, [L. bridge]   that part of the brain stem between the midbrain and the open medulla. It is derived from the metencephalon of the embryonic brain.   On the ventral surface of the pons are the conspicuous transverse fiber bundles, which connect this region with the cerebellar hemispheres on each side, and for which this region was named. The dorsal part of the pons provides the floor for the rostral part of the fourth ventricle (Fig. V-4).

pon´tine (pon´tile)   pertaining to the pons.

pontocerebel´lum, CEREBELLUM   part of the cerebellum which receives impulses derived mainly from the cerebral cortex and which are relayed to the cerebellum from the pons by way of the pontocerebellar fibers. *Syn:* neocerebellum.

po´rus acus´ticus exter´nus [NA], EAR   opening into the external auditory meatus on the outside of the skull.

porus acusticus inter´nus [NA], EAR   opening into the internal auditory meatus of the temporal bone in the posterior cranial fossa.

pos´itron emis´sion tomog´raphy (PET) *See* tomography.

postcen´tral, CEREBRUM, CEREBELLUM posterior to either the central sulcus of the cerebrum or the central lobule of the cerebellar vermis.

postcommis´sural (postcommissu´ral) posterior to the anterior commissure of the cerebrum.

postganglion´ic pertaining to a neuron or part of a neuron whose cell body is located in an autonomic ganglion and whose axon terminates in relation to smooth muscle, cardiac muscle, or a gland.

postrolan´dic, CEREBRUM posterior to the central sulcus of the cerebrum. *Syn:* postcentral.

poten´tial, ac´tion electrical manifestation of a nervous impulse. There is a sudden large influx of sodium ions with a rise in membrane potential to a positive state (depolarization), immediately followed by an efflux of potassium ions across the cell membrane and a return to its resting, negative state (repolarization).

potential, diffu´sion voltage difference reflecting the net diffusion of ions.

potential, equilib´rium voltage difference across a membrane, equal in force but opposite in direction to the concentration force affecting a given ion species.

potential, evoked nervous system's response to some sensory input. It may result from natural or from electrical or chemical stimulation of sensory or motor neurons and be recorded on an oscilloscope or EEG. Such recordings are used in the study of neurophysiological phenomena or, in clinical practice, to determine the health of the nervous system.

potential, exci´tatory postsynap´tic (EPSP) change in membrane potential, a small depolarization, which occurs in a postsynaptic neuron in response to an excitatory presynaptic volley. When the pre-excitatory change in the cell membrane reaches the threshold level, the neuron discharges.

potential, gen´erator *See* potential, receptor.

potential, inhib´itory postsynap´tic (IPSP) change in membrane potential, a hyperpolarization, which occurs in a postsynaptic neuron in response to an inhibitory presynaptic volley. During this time there is a change in the permeability of the cell membrane to potassium and chlorine ions and the excitability of the neuron is diminished.

potential, mem´brane voltage difference between the inside and outside of a cell, including the state and changes that occur in the concentration and transfer of sodium and potassium ions across nerve cell membranes as they relate to nerve conduction.

potential, recep´tor change in the membrane potential at the peripheral endings of afferent neurons. It serves to transduce the energy of an external stimulus into the electrical energy which the neuron uses for transmission of impulses. *Syn:* generator potential.

potential, res´ting physiologic state in which a nerve cell, not conducting an impulse, is positively charged outside and negatively charged inside its cell membrane. *Syn:* steady potential.

potential, steady *See* potential, resting.

PPRF, PONS paramedian pontine reticular formation.

precen´tral, CEREBRUM, CEREBELLUM anterior to either the central sulcus of the cerebrum or the central lobule of the cerebellar vermis.

precommis´sural (precommissu´ral) anterior to the anterior commissure of the cerebrum.

precul´men, CEREBELLUM   subdivision of the cerebellar vermis between the lingula and the culmen. *Syn:* central lobule.

precu´neus [NA], CEREBRUM   segment of the parietal lobe on the medial surface of the cerebrum, anterior to the parieto-occipital sulcus (Fig. C-3B). *Syn:* quadrate lobule.

prefron´tal, CEREBRUM   pertaining to the prefrontal area of the frontal lobe of the cerebrum, anterior to the premotor area.

preganglion´ic   pertaining to a neuron or part of a neuron whose cell body is located within the CNS and whose axon synapses in an autonomic ganglion.

premo´tor, CEREBRUM   pertaining to Brodmann's area 6, the cortical area anterior to the motor area, area 4.

preoccip´ital, CEREBRUM   pertaining to Brodmann's area 19, the cortical area anterior and adjacent to the parastriate area, mostly in the parietal and temporal lobes. *Syn:* peristriate.

preop´tic, HYPOTHALAMUS   pertaining to the region in or adjoining the part of the third ventricle immediately anterior to the optic chiasm. *See* area *and* recess, preoptic.

prepir´iform, CEREBRUM   pertaining to the area adjoining the lateral olfactory stria on the under surface of the frontal lobe.

prerolan´dic, CEREBRUM   anterior to the central sulcus of the cerebrum. *Syn:* precentral.

prerubrum, DIENCEPHALON, MIDBRAIN   *See* field, prerubral.

presbyopia /prez-bĭ-o´pĭ-ah/ [Gr. *presbys* old man; *ops* eye]   loss of elasticity of the lens of the eye with advancing age so that it is no longer possible for the lens to change its shape in accommodation for near vision.

pressorecep´tor [L. *pressus* past participle of *premere* to press; *recipere* to receive]   baroreceptor.

presubic´ulum, CEREBRUM   subdivision of the hippocampal formation between the subiculum and the entorhinal cortex, Brodmann's area 27. Sometimes the area of transition between the presubiculum and the entorhinal cortex is designated parasubiculum.

presynap´tic   pertaining to a neuron or part of a neuron that transmits impulses into a synapse.

pretec´tum, DIENCEPHALON, MIDBRAIN   *See* area, pretectal.

pretrigem´inal, PONS   pertaining to the region rostral to the motor and the pontine nuclei of V, particularly the pontine isthmus.

Probst, M. (late 19th-early 20th century)   *Probst's bundle* is a bundle of nerve fibers along the medial wall of the cerebrum in brains lacking a corpus callosum. It is probably composed of fornix fibers and association fibers. The *tract of Probst* is a fiber bundle continuous with the mesencephalic tract of V, at levels caudal to the motor and pontine nuclei of V. The *commissure of Probst* is the commissure of the lateral lemniscus in the pontine isthmus.

process /pros´ses, pro´ses/   filamentous extension of a nerve cell body, which may be either an axon or a dendrite.

process, ciliary /sil´ĭ-ar-ĭ/ [processus ciliari s, NA], EYE   one of about 70-75 little, leaf-like projections, about 2.0 mm × 0.5 mm, on the surface of the ciliary body. They consist of a core of delicate connective tissue and capillaries, covered with a double layer of epithelium, a deeper, pigmented layer, and a superficial, nonpigmented layer which secretes aqueous humor.

process, infundibular, HYPOPHYSIS   pars nervosa of the neurohypophysis.

process, protoplasmic /pro-to-plaz´mik/   thick, short, rough process of a multipolar nerve cell body; a dendrite, similar in structure to the cytoplasm of the cell body.

prom´inence, spiral [prominentia spiralis, NA], EAR   ridge on the spiral ligament in the cochlear duct, between the stria vascularis and the cells of Claudius of the spiral organ.

propriocep´tion [*adj.* **proprioceptive**] [L. *proprius* one's own; *capere* to take]   that class of impulses that arise from afferent nerve endings located in skeletal muscles (Figs. L-1, R-5, S-2), tendons, or joints, or in the vestibular portion of the internal ear.

propriocep´tor   one of the peripheral nerve endings for proprioception.

propriospi´nal   limited to or contained within the spinal cord.

prosencephalon /pro-zen-sef´al-on/ [NA] [Gr. *pros* before; *enkephalos* brain]   forebrain; most rostral subdivision of the embryonic brain, from which the telencephalon and diencephalon are derived.

prosopagno´sia [Gr. *prosop* face; *agnosia* ignorance]   inability to recognize faces, after bilateral lesions on the inferior surface of the occipital lobe.

prosubic´ulum [L. *pro* before; *subiculum* support], CEREBRUM   4-layered cortex in the floor of the hippocampal fissure, between the cornu ammonis and the subiculum (Fig. C-7). It constitutes an area of transition between the two.

prothal´amus, HYPOTHALAMUS   rostral one-third of the preopticohypothalamic area, containing the preoptic and anterior hypothalamic areas and separated from the remainder of the hypothalamus by the fornix. *See also* area, preoptic.

protoneu´ron   first neuron in a reflex arc.

protopath´ic   pertaining to the appreciation of gross pain, tactile, and temperature sensations.

psalterium /sal-ter´ĭ-um/, CEREBRUM, [Gr. *psalterion* harp]   fibers of the hippocampal commissure, under the corpus callosum and between the crura (pillars) of the fornix, so named for its presumed resemblance to an ancient lyre (Fig. P-2). *Syn:* lyra of David.

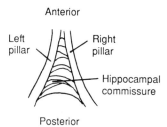

Fig. P-2.   Psalterium. The hippocampal commissure and the pillars (crura) of the fornix, as viewed from above, after removal of the corpus callosum, suggesting the appearance of an ancient lyre.

pseudounipolar neuron /soo-do-u-nĭ-po´lar/   *See* neuron, unipolar.

pterion /ter´ĭ-on/ [NA] [Gr. *pteron* wing]   point at which the greater wing of the sphenoid bone meets the frontal, the parietal, and the squamous part of the temporal bones. In the infant it is the site of the small anterolateral fontanelle. It overlies the middle meningeal artery or its anterior branch, and is an important neurosurgical landmark. It is also useful as a guide in the lateral approach to the sella turcica and parasellar structures.

pterygopalatine /ter-ĭ-go-pal´at-ĕn/ [Gr. *pteryx, pterygos* wing; L. *palatum* palate] related to, or in the region of, the pterygoid process of the sphenoid bone and the palatine bone. *See* ganglion, pterygopalatine.

ptosis /to´sis/   drooping of the upper eyelid. This condition may occur because of paralysis of the levator palpebrae muscle, as in an oculomotor nerve paralysis, or as a result of impairment of the sympathetic nerve supply to the smooth muscle of the upper eyelid (Müller's muscle), as in Horner's syndrome.

pul´vinar (pulvi´nar) [NA], DORSAL THALAMUS, [L. *pulvinus* pillow]   posterior part of the dorsal thalamus, which projects into the subarachnoid space, above and lateral to the rostral part of the superior colliculus. It is sometimes considered one of the posterior group of dorsal thalamic nuclei and sometimes one of the lateral group. It has also been subdivided into a number of subnuclei. The cells are predominantly medium-sized and lightly staining, but some of other sizes also occur. The anterior part of the pulvinar is believed to be interconnected with the parietal lobe cortex, and the more posterior part with the temporal and occipital lobe cortices. *See also* nuclei, posterior.

pu´pil [pupilla, NA], EYE   circular aperture in the center of the iris, which by changes in its diameter regulates the amount of light admitted to the eye.

Purkinje, Johannes (Purkyně, Jan Evangelista) (1787-1869)   Czech anatomist and physiologist, active in Breslau and Prague. A *Purkinje cell* (neuronum piriforme, NA) (1837) is a large cell of the *Purkinje cell layer* (stratum neuronorum piriformium, NA) between the molecular and granular layers of the cerebellar cortex (Figs. C-8, C-9). The dendrites of these cells ramify in a single plane in the molecular layer. They are activated by climbing fibers and parallel fibers but inhibited by the basket cells and the stellate cells of the molecular layer. The axons of these cells terminate as inhibitory fibers, mostly on the cells of the deep cerebellar nuclei. He also described the *Purkinje fibers* of the heart (1839).

puta´men [NA], CEREBRUM, [L. shell]   lateral part of the lentiform nucleus (Fig. C-1), composed mostly of small and medium-sized cells. One of the basal ganglia, it is continuous anteriorly, around the anterior limb of the internal capsule, with the head of the caudate nucleus. Lesions of the putamen produce athetoid movements on the opposite side of the body. *See also* striatum; corpus striatum.

pyr´amid   **1.** [pyramis, NA], MEDULLA   protuberance on the ventral surface of the medulla, overlying the pyramidal tract.
2. petrous part of the temporal bone.
3. [pyramis vermis, NA], CEREBELLUM   a subdivision of the posterior lobe of the cerebellar vermis.
4. CEREBRUM   pyramidal cell of the cerebral cortex.

pyramid, double, CEREBRUM   elongated cell of the cornu ammonis having a rich dendritic process at each end. Its axon arises from the cell body or from a dendrite and enters the alveus and fimbria. *Syn:* Ammon's pyramids.

pyramid, posterior   old term for fasciculus gracilis.

pyr´amis vermis [NA], CEREBELLUM   lobule of the posterior lobe of the cerebellar vermis, between the uvula and the tuber (Figs. C-2, V-6). *See also* vermis cerebelli.

pyr´iform (piriform)   *See* area, piriform.

q

quadrantanop´sia (quadrantano´pia) blindness in one quarter of the visual field.

quadriplegia /kwod-rĭ-ple´jĭ-ah/ [L. *quattuor* four; Gr. *plege* stroke] paralysis of all four limbs. *Syn:* tetraplegia.

Queckenstedt, Hans Heinrich Georg (1876-1918) German physician. *Queckenstedt's test* (1916) is used to determine the patency of the spinal subarachnoid space. When pressure is applied to the jugular veins, venous pressure is increased. When there is no blockage in the subarachnoid space, there is a simultaneous rise in CSF pressure, but if there is a block in the subarachnoid space, cerebrospinal fluid pressure is unchanged.

quermem´bran delicate membrane which covers the axis cylinder at each node of Ranvier, in the gap between internodal segments.

Quincke, Heinrich Irenaeus (1842-1922) German physician, noted for his introduction of spinal puncture as a diagnostic tool and as a therapeutic measure.

r

radia′tion, acou′stic (auditory) [radiatio acustica, NA], FOREBRAIN thalamocortical fibers of the auditory system. They arise from cells in the medial geniculate nucleus, pass through the sublenticular part of the posterior limb of the internal capsule (Fig. C-1), and terminate in the transverse temporal gyri, areas 41 and 42, on the upper surface of the temporal lobe within the lateral sulcus. *Syn:* geniculotemporal tract; inferior thalamic peduncle.

radiation, fron′tal, FOREBRAIN *See* forceps, minor.

radiation, occip′ital, FOREBRAIN *See* forceps, major.

radiation, olfac′tory (of Zuckerkandl), FOREBRAIN *See* band, diagonal (of Broca).

radiation, op′tic [radiatio optica, NA], FOREBRAIN thalamocortical fibers of the visual system. They arise from cells in the lateral geniculate nucleus and pass through the posterior limb of the internal capsule to the calcarine cortex, area 17, in the occipital lobe (Fig. C-1). *Syn:* geniculocalcarine tract. *See also* loop, temporal, of the optic radiation.

radiation, sen′sory, FOREBRAIN nerve fibers which arise from cells in the ventral posterior nuclei of the dorsal thalamus and pass through the thalamolenticular part of the posterior limb of the internal capsule (Fig. C-1) and the corona radiata, to end in areas 3, 1, and 2 of the postcentral gyrus. They are a part of the superior thalamic peduncle.

radiation, tegmen′tal, MIDBRAIN fibers which extend rostrally on the lateral surface of the red nucleus.

radiations, thalam′ic, FOREBRAIN thalamocortical and corticothalamic fibers in the internal capsule and corona radiata. *See also* peduncles, thalamic.

radiations, thalamic, anterior [radiationes thalamicae anteriores, NA], FOREBRAIN nerve fibers which pass through the anterior limb of the internal capsule (Fig. C-1), interconnecting the anterior and dorsomedial nuclei of the dorsal thalamus with the cingulate and prefrontal cortices. *Syn:* anterior thalamic peduncle.

radiations, thalamic, posterior [radiationes thalamicae posteriores, NA], FOREBRAIN nerve fibers in the postlenticular part of the posterior limb of the internal capsule (Fig. C-1) and in the corona radiata, which interconnect the cortex of the parietal and occipital lobes with the lateral thalamic nuclei, pulvinar, and superior colliculus. *Syn:* posterior thalamic peduncle.

Ramón y Cajal, Santiago   *See* Cajal, Santiago Ramón y.

ra´mus anastomot´icus [L. *ramus* branch]   *See* ramus communicans.

ramus, anterior ascending, CEREBRUM   branch of the lateral sulcus which separates the triangular from the opercular part of the inferior frontal gyrus.

ramus, anterior horizontal, CEREBRUM   branch of the lateral sulcus which separates the orbital from the triangular part of the inferior frontal gyrus.

ramus commu´nicans [NA]   **1.** small branch interconnecting the ventral primary ramus of a spinal nerve with the sympathetic trunk of the same side. **2.** This term is also used for any branch that connects one nerve with another. *Syn:* ramus anastomoticus.

ramus, gray   ramus communicans composed of postganglionic fibers whose cell bodies are located in the ganglia of the sympathetic trunk and which terminate in visceral structures underlying or associated with the skin. Those to the sweat glands, cutaneous blood vessels, and perhaps sebaceous glands are unmyelinated (C fibers). Those to the piloerector muscles are thinly myelinated (B fibers).

ramus, pri´mary   one of the two initial branches, dorsal and ventral, into which each spinal nerve divides as it leaves its intervertebral foramen. This branching of the sacral spinal nerves, however, occurs within the sacrum, and the dorsal and ventral sacral rami emerge through the dorsal and pelvic sacral foramina, respectively.

ramus, primary, dorsal   dorsal division of a spinal nerve, innervating the genuine muscles of the back and the overlying cutaneous area.

ramus, primary, ventral   ventral division of a spinal nerve innervating the musculature of the extremities and of the trunk (other than the genuine muscles of the back) and the associated cutaneous areas.

ramus, white   ramus communicans composed of thinly myelinated preganglionic fibers (B fibers), which arise from cells in the thoracolumbar spinal cord and which terminate in ganglia of the sympathetic trunk or prevertebral sympathetic ganglia.

Ranson, Stephen Walter (1880-1942)   eminent American neuroanatomist of Northwestern University, whose text, *The Anatomy of the Nervous System,* in its many editions was for many years the bible for innumerable medical and graduate students of neuroanatomy.

Ranvier, Louis Antoine (1835-1922)   French histologist. A *node of Ranvier* (1878) (nodus neurofibrae, NA) is an interruption of the myelin sheath of a myelinated nerve fiber between two internodal segments. At the nodes of peripheral nerve fibers the neurolemma dips in to cover the axis cylinder. Nodes also occur in the central nervous system but are less conspicuous features (Fig. R-1). *See also* segment, internodal.

raphe /ra´fe/ [NA], BRAIN STEM, [Gr. *rhaphe* seam]   intersection of fibers along the median plane of the brain stem. *See also* nuclei (of the) raphe *and* Fig. N-5.

RAS   reticular activating system.

Rathke, Martin Heinrich (1793-1860)   German anatomist of Danzig and Königsberg. *Rathke's pouch* is the craniobuccal or neurobuccal pouch, a dorsal, median epithelial pocket in the stomodeal ectoderm, from which the adenohypophysis develops. It forms a closed, double-layered sac which loses its connection with the stomodeum. The thin posterior wall of the sac fuses with the pars nervosa and becomes the pars intermedia. The anterior wall thickens to form the pars distalis. An extension upward onto the infundibular stalk becomes the pars tuberalis. Although the lumen of the sac is retained in some forms, it nearly or completely disappears in man.

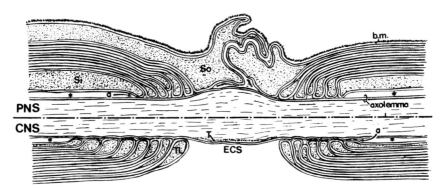

Fig. R-1.   Node of Ranvier, showing the nodal region in the PNS (above) and the CNS (below). In the PNS, but not in the CNS, interdigitating processes of an outer collar (So) of cytoplasm cover the axolemma of the nerve fiber, and the sheath is covered externally by a basement membrane (bm). In the CNS there is no such barrier and in some regions there is considerable extracellular space (ECS) where synapses may occur. From R.P. Bunge, Glial cells and the central myelin sheath, 1968, *Physiological Reviews,* vol 48: 197. Courtesy of the author and The American Physiological Society, Bethesda.

Raynaud, Maurice (1834-1881)   French physician noted for his description (1862) of a disorder, *Raynaud's disease*, characterized by ischemia and cold sensitivity of the extremities.

receptor   *See* ending, nerve.

recess, fastigial /fas-tij ´T-al/, HINDBRAIN   fastigium of the fourth ventricle.

recess, infrapin ´eal (infrapine ´al), DIENCEPHALON   that part of the ambient cistern between the pineal body and the superior colliculi (Fig. C-6).

recess, infundib ´ular [recessus infundibuli (infundibularis), NA], DIENCEPHALON   extension of the third ventricle ventrally into the infundibular stalk between the optic chiasm and the mamillary bodies (Fig. V-5).

recess, lateral [recessus lateralis, NA], HINDBRAIN   lateral conical part of the fourth ventricle, leading to the lateral aperture (Fig. V-3).

recess, op ´tic [recessus opticus, NA], DIENCEPHALON   that part of the third ventricle superior and anterior to the optic chiasm (Fig. V-5). *Syn:* preoptic recess; supraoptic recess.

recess, pin ´eal (pine ´al) [recessus pinealis, NA], DIENCEPHALON   posterior part of the third ventricle, just anterior to the pineal body and between the habenular commissure above and the posterior commissure below.

recess, preop´tic, DIENCEPHALON   *See* recess, optic.

recess, supraop´tic, DIENCEPHALON   *See* recess, optic.

recess, suprapin´eal (suprapine´al) [recessus suprapinealis, NA], DIENCEPHALON   that part of the third ventricle in a pocket of the tela choroidea extending posteriorly above the pineal body (Fig. V-5).

recess, triang´ular, DIENCEPHALON   anterior part of the third ventricle, between the two columns of the fornix and above the anterior commissure, as seen in a coronal section of the brain.

recessus tec´ti, HINDBRAIN   fastigium of the fourth ventricle (Fig. V-3).

Recklinghausen, Friedrich Daniel von (1833-1910)   German pathologist at the University of Strassburg, noted especially for his study of neurofibromatosis, *von Recklinghausen's disease* (1822).

recruitment /re-kroot´ment/   process of increasing the number of active motor units.

re´flex   automatic stereotyped response to a stimulus, dependent upon intact connections of the relevant afferent and efferent neurons.

reflexes, abdom´inal   superficial reflexes, contraction of the underlying abdominal muscles upon stroking the skin of the abdomen, dependent on afferent and efferent connections of spinal cord segments T7-T9 for the upper area, T9-T11 for the middle area, and T11-T12 for the lower area.

reflex, accommodation   changes that occur in the adaptation of the eye for near vision (Fig. R-2). *See* accommodation.

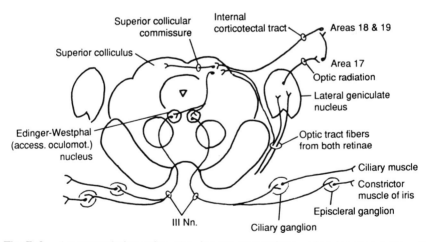

Fig. R-2. Accommodation reflex, showing the connections underlying contraction of the ciliary muscle to permit increased convexity of the lens and constriction of the pupils, in accommodation of the eye for near vision.

reflex, Achilles tendon /ah-kil´ēz/   plantar flexion of the foot by contraction of the muscles of the calf of the leg, on percussion of the Achilles tendon just above the calcaneus. It is a stretch reflex, dependent on afferent and efferent connections of the spinal cord segments L5-S2, but mainly S1. *Syn:* ankle jerk; triceps surae reflex; gastrocnemius-soleus reflex.

reflex, acoustic   *See* reflex, stapedial.

reflex, a´nal   contraction of the external rectal sphincter muscle upon touching the perianal area, dependent on afferent and efferent connections of spinal cord segments S2-S4.

reflex, axon /ak´son/   vasodilation restricted to an area of cutaneous stimulation, such as the local reddening of the skin after a scratch, or following pressure on the bridge of the nose by glasses. It is thought to be mediated through the distal portions of peripheral nerve fibers because the response still occurs after the nerve fibers to the region have been severed but not after the fibers have had time to degenerate.

reflex, Babinski   *See* Babinski.

reflex, bi´ceps   flexion at the elbow by contraction of the biceps muscle, on percussion of the biceps tendon, dependent on afferent and efferent connections of spinal cord segments C5 (mainly) and C6 (to some extent).

reflex, blink   closure of the eyes in response to a bright light or sudden visual stimulus. It is dependent on afferent connections from the retina through the optic nerve with relay to the visual cortex, then to the pons for efferent connections through the facial nerve.

reflex, brachioradial´is   flexion at the elbow and supination of the hand by contraction of the brachioradialis muscle on percussion of the brachioradialis tendon at the distal end of the radius. It is dependent on afferent and efferent connections of spinal cord segments C5 (partly) and C6 (mainly). *Syn:* radial periosteal reflex; radial jerk.

reflex, bulbocaverno´sus   contraction of the bulbocavernosus muscle upon pinching the penis, dependent on afferent and efferent connections of spinal cord segments S3 and S4.

reflex bundle   *See* fasciculus proprius.

reflex, carot´id body   respiratory reflex with afferent fibers from the carotid body, carried by the glossopharyngeal nerve. Activation increases inspiration.

reflex, carotid si´nus   reflex concerned with the maintenance of normal blood pressure. It is dependent on afferent fibers of the glossopharyngeal nerve, with receptors in the wall of the carotid sinus. *See also* tract, reticulospinal, medial.

reflex, ciliospinal /sil-ĭ-o-spi´nal/   dilation of the pupils in response to pain, primarily from the face or oral cavity but also from the neck or shoulder region by way of the trigeminal nerve and upper cervical spinal nerves. Secondary connections go to the superior colliculus. Descending fibers of the lateral tectotegmentospinal tract end in the upper thoracic spinal cord, and pre- and postganglionic sympathetic fibers activate the dilator muscle of the iris. Dilation of the pupil, in response to fear, results from activation of the external corticotectal tract from the temporal lobe (Fig. R-3).

reflex, clasp knife   an abnormal response in which rapid passive movement of a limb results first in little or no resistance, followed by an abrupt "catch," then a sudden release and cessation of resistance. The sudden muscular contraction is thought to be a stretch reflex response and the release to result from activation of an inhibitory reflex. Such a response in a hemiplegic patient is considered indicative of spasticity. *See also* reflex, stretch *and* inhibitory; Fig. R-5.

reflex, consen´sual   reflex in which the response occurs on the side contralateral to the stimulation.

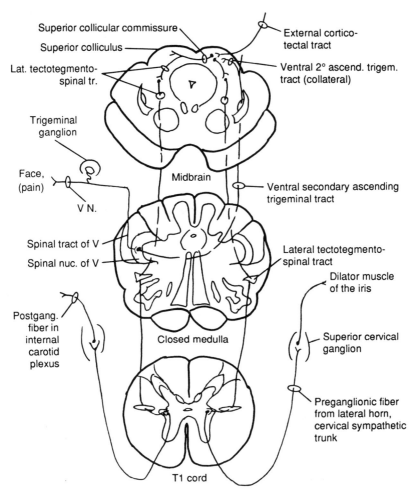

Fig. R-3. Ciliospinal reflex, showing the connections underlying reflex dilation of the pupils in response to pain in the face (or oral cavity) (V nerve), neck or shoulder region (cervical nerves, not shown), or to fear (external corticotectal tract).

reflex, cor´neal   closure of the eyes in response to touching the cornea. It is dependent on afferent connections through the ophthalmic division of the trigeminal nerve to the spinal nucleus of V in both the open and closed medulla, and efferent connections through the facial nerve in the pons (Fig. R-4).

reflex, cremaster´ic   a superficial reflex in which there is elevation of the scrotum on stroking the skin on the inner side of the thigh, dependent on afferent and efferent connections of spinal cord segments L1 and L2 and the ilioinguinal and genitofemoral nerves. This reflex is lost after lesions of the corticospinal tract.

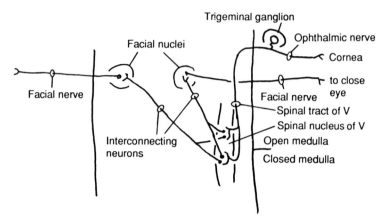

Fig. R-4. Corneal reflex, showing the connections for closing the eyes in response to corneal stimulation.

reflex, crossed exten´sion   extension of the contralateral lower extremity to support the body, when the homolateral lower limb is flexed in response to a superficial stimulus, as when a dog scratches a flea on his shoulder. This reflex, multisynaptic and intersegmental, does not usually occur in man. *See also* reflex, scratch.

reflex, deep   motor response to stimulation of sensory endings in muscles, tendons and joints. *See also* reflexes, stretch *and* inhibitory (Fig. R-5).

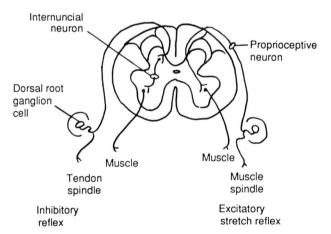

Fig. R-5. Deep reflexes. The stretch reflex, shown on the right, is an excitatory reflex, consisting of a 2-neuron chain, its afferent fiber arising in a neuromuscular spindle. *See also* Fig. S-2. The inhibitory reflex, on the left, is a 3-neuron reflex, and arises from a neurotendinous spindle.

reflex, del´toid   abduction of the upper arm by contraction of the deltoid muscle, on percussion of the insertion of the deltoid muscle, dependent on afferent and efferent connections of spinal cord segments C5 and C6.

reflex, direct   reflex in which the response occurs on the side stimulated.

reflex, exci´tatory stretch   *See* reflex, stretch.

reflex, flex´ion   contraction of flexor muscles in response to a stimulus such as pain, a withdrawal response away from the stimulus. Such reflexes also play a part in stepping.

reflex, gag   contraction of the pharyngeal musculature in response to stimulation of the soft palate or pharyngeal mucosa. It is dependent on afferent connections through the glossopharyngeal nerve and efferent connections through the vagus nerve. *Syn:* pharyngeal, palatal, or uveal reflex.

reflex, gastrocnemius /gas-trok-ne´mĭ-us/   *See* reflex, Achilles tendon.

reflex, glu´teal, superfic´ial   contraction of the gluteal muscles upon stroking the overlying skin, dependent on afferent and efferent connections of spinal cord segments L5-S2.

reflex, hand flexor   *See* reflex, wrist flexion.

reflex, Hering-Breuer   *See* Hering; *also* reflexes, respiratory.

reflex, inhib´itory   reflex inhibition of the contraction of a muscle resulting from stimulation (stretching) of the endings in the tendon of the same muscle. Neurotendinous endings have a relatively high threshold and respond only when the stretch is extreme. Unlike excitatory stretch reflexes, which are monosynaptic, inhibitory reflexes are disynaptic, having an interneuron interposed between the afferent and efferent neurons (Fig. R-5). *See also* reflex, clasp knife. *Syn:* inverse myotatic reflex.

reflex, inverse myotat´ic   *See* reflex, inhibitory.

reflex, jaw-closing   stretch reflex in which closing of the jaw occurs in response to stretching the chewing muscles (except the external pterygoid), as in tapping the chin. Both afferent and efferent fibers are in the trigeminal nerve. The afferent neurons have their cell bodies in the mesencephalic nucleus of V and the efferent fibers arise from cells in the motor nucleus of V. The response is minimal in healthy individuals but conspicuous after lesions of the corticospinal tract. *Syn:* masseter or mandibular reflex; jaw jerk.

reflex, jaw-opening   reflex opening of the jaw in response to pressure on the teeth. Both afferent and efferent fibers are in the trigeminal nerve. The afferent neurons have their cell bodies in the mesencephalic nucleus of V and the efferent fibers arise from cells in the motor nucleus of V.

reflex, lac´rimal   reflex lacrimation in response to corneal irritation. It is dependent on afferent fibers of the trigeminal nerve from the cornea and efferent fibers from the lacrimal nucleus, a subdivision of the superior salivatory nucleus of VII (Fig. R-6).

reflex, light   constriction of the pupil in response to light striking the retina. It is dependent on afferent connections from the retina, through the optic nerve and tract to the pretectal nucleus with relay to the Edinger-Westphal (accessory oculomotor) nuclei, and efferent connections through the oculomotor nerves to the ciliary ganglia for relay to the circular muscle of the iris of both eyes. Normally there is both a direct and consensual reflex response (Fig. R-7).

reflex, mandib´ular   *See* reflex, jaw-closing.

reflex, mass   flexion of the lower limbs, evacuation of the bladder and bowels, and sweating of the skin below the level of the lesion, after severe injury of the spinalcord. *Syn:* Riddoch's reflex.

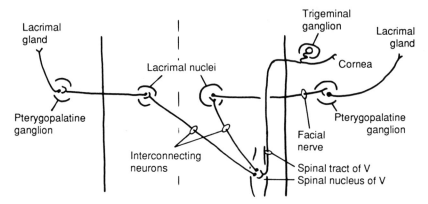

Fig. R-6. Lacrimal reflex, showing the neuronal connections for lacrimation in response to corneal irritation.

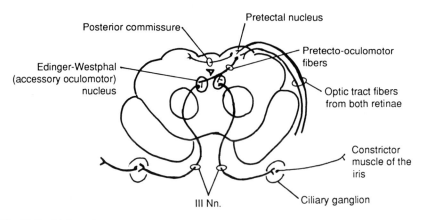

Fig. R-7. Light reflex, showing the neuronal connections for constriction of the pupils in response to light.

reflex, masse´ter *See* reflex, jaw-closing.

reflex, monosynap´tic reflex in which the afferent neurons synapse directly on the efferent neurons, without any intercalated neurons. Stretch reflexes are of this type (Fig. R-5).

reflex, multisynap´tic reflex involving at least a 3-neuron chain, with one or more intercalated neurons between the afferent and efferent neurons. Reflexes which inhibit muscle contraction are of this type.

reflex, myotat´ic *See* reflex, stretch.

reflex, oculocar´diac   slowing of the heart, lowering of the blood pressure, and modification of the respiratory rhythm in response to compression of the eyeballs. It is dependent on afferent (pain) fibers in the trigeminal nerve and efferent fibers in the vagus nerve. *See also* reflexes, vagal, *and* Fig. R-9.

reflex, pal´atal   *See* reflex, gag.

reflex, patel´lar   stretch reflex involving extension at the knee on percussion of the patellar tendon. It is dependent on afferent and efferent connections of spinal cord segments L2-L4, mainly L4. *Syn:* knee jerk; quadriceps reflex.

reflex, pharyn´geal   *See* reflex, gag.

reflexes, post´ural   reflex adjustments whereby the body and head are maintained in an upright position. Such motor responses are dependent on afferent impulses from the utricle, from neuromuscular spindles, and/or from the retina.

reflex, plan´tar   flexion of the toes upon stroking the sole of the foot, dependent on afferent and efferent connections of spinal cord segments L5-S2.

reflex, quad´riceps   *See* reflex, patellar.

reflex, ra´dial perios´teal   *See* reflex, brachioradialis.

reflexes, respiratory   reflexes which control or modify respiration. Afferent fibers from the carotid body, carried by the glossopharyngeal nerve, activate inspiration and increase respiration. Those from the lungs, carried by the vagus nerve, block inspiration, thus preventing harmful overdistension of the lungs (Hering-Breuer reflex). *See also* Hering.

reflex, scratch   a homolateral flexor reflex, in response to a superficial cutaneous stimulus, as in a dog's response when he uses his hind leg to scratch a irritated spot on his body. *See also* reflex, crossed extension.

reflex, segmen´tal   reflex in which a stimulus, applied in the region of the sensory distribution of a spinal nerve, produces a response in muscles innervated by the same spinal cord segment.

reflex, stape´dial   reflex contraction of the stapedial muscle of the middle ear by way of facial nerve fibers, in response to auditory impulses transmitted by the cochlear nerve, after synapse in the cochlear nuclei, superior olive, and facial nucleus. It serves to dampen the effects of loud sounds. Damage to the efferent fibers of this reflex results in hyperacusis (Fig. R-8). *Syn:* acoustic reflex.

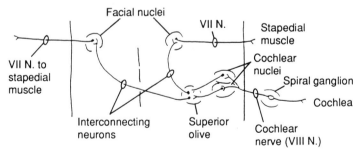

Fig. R-8.   Stapedial reflex, showing the neuronal connections for dampening the effects of loud sounds on the auditory apparatus.

reflex, stretch   a monosynaptic reflex in which stretching of a muscle activates its neuromuscular spindles and their afferent fibers, which, in turn, synapse directly on the motor neurons supplying the same muscle, causing it to contract. Such reflexes are important in the maintenance of normal muscle tone, especially in relation to posture (Fig. R-5). *Syn:* myotatic or tendon reflex. *See also* loop, gamma; reflex, clasp knife.

reflex, superficial /soo-per-fish´al/   motor response to stimulation of sensory endings in the skin. Abdominal, gluteal, and cremasteric reflexes are of this type. Such reflexes are lost after lesions of the corticospinal tract fibers.

reflex, supraor´bital   closure of the eye in response to percussion of the outer part of the supraorbital ridge. *Syn:* McCarthy reflex. Greater pressure on the ridge can also trigger a vagal response. *See also* reflexes, vagal.

reflex, ten´don   reflex contraction of a muscle, elicited by a sharp tap on its tendon; the receptor on the afferent limb of the reflex is, however, in the muscle itself and not in the tendon proper (Fig. R-5). *Syn:* stretch reflex; myotatic reflex.

reflex, tri´ceps   extension at the elbow by contraction of the triceps muscle on percussion of the triceps tendon where it crosses the olecranon fossa. It is dependent on afferent and efferent connections of spinal cord segments C6-C8, mainly C7.

reflex, triceps su´rae   *See* reflex, Achilles tendon.

reflex, u´veal   *See* reflex, gag.

reflexes, va´gal   reflex cardiac slowing or arrest in response to afferent impulses from any of a number of sources. It is a high-threshold reflex that may be prevented with a parasympathetic blocking agent such as atropine. It can be triggered by stimulation of the throat and pharynx, as in tonsillectomy (IX nerve), the introduction of an endotracheal tube (X nerve), heart or lung emboli (X nerve), stimulation of the external auditory meatus (V, VII, IX, &/or X nerves), or manipulation of the extraocular muscles (V nerve). Pressure on the supra-orbital ridge (V nerve) can be used to reduce tachycardia (Fig. R-9).

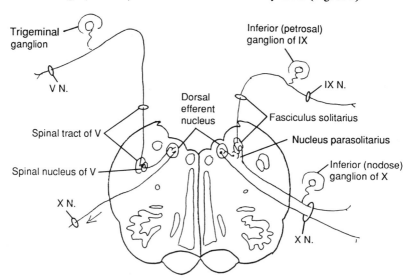

Fig. R-9. Vagal reflexes, showing the connections whereby stimulation of tissues in various regions can cause vagal slowing of the heart or cardiac arrest. *See the text.*

reflexes, vestib´ulo-oc´ular   reflex eye movements in response to changes in position of the head. Such responses are mediated by the vestibular nerve and nuclei, the medial longitudinal fasciculi, and the nuclei and nerves that supply the eye muscles (Fig. F-2). *See also* nystagmus, vestibular.

reflex, visceral   one mediated by visceral afferent and visceral efferent fibers so that a visceral organ responds to a stimulus from some internal structure.

reflex, wrist extension   contraction of the extensor muscles of the wrist upon tapping their tendons while the forearm is pronated and the muscles acting upon the wrist are relaxed. It is dependent on afferent and efferent connections of spinal cord segments C6-C8.

reflex, wrist flexion   contraction of the flexor muscles of the hand and fingers upon tapping the flexor tendons just above the wrist, with the hand supinated and the fingers relaxed. It is dependent on afferent connections of spinal cord segments C6-T1. *Syn:* hand flexor reflex.

Reichert, Carl Bogislaus (1811-1884)   German anatomist. The *substantia innominata (of Reichert)* was illustrated, but not named, in his atlas of the brain, published in 1859-1861.

Reil, Johann Christian (1759-1813)   German physician and anatomist. He first noted the insula, *island of Reil,* in 1796 and described it in 1809. He also named the corona radiata. Named for him were: *Reil's ansa,* the ansa peduncularis; the *ribbon of Reil,* the medial lemniscus; and the *triangle of Reil,* the lemniscal trigone.

Reissner, Ernst (1824-1878)   German anatomist of Dorpat, then Breslau. *Reissner's membrane* (1851) is the vestibular membrane of the cochlea.

releasing factors   *See* factors, releasing.

REM   rapid eye movements that characteristically occur during "deep" or "dream" sleep. During REM sleep the EEG consists mostly of low-voltage fast activity, similar to that during the waking state; consequently, REM sleep is also called *paradoxical sleep.*

Remak, Robert (1815-1865)   German neurologist who wrote the first account of the myelin sheath (1836) and identified unmyelinated nerve fibers, C-fibers, *fibers of Remak* (1838). The *ganglion of Remak* consists of clusters of parasympathetic ganglion cells on the heart wall. *Remak's reflex* is plantar flexion of the first three toes and sometimes the foot, and extension of the knee in response to stroking the upper anterior surface of the thigh.

Renshaw, Birdsey (1911-1948)   American neurophysiologist. *Renshaw cells* are small internuncial neurons in the ventral horn of the spinal cord. They presumably receive their afferent stimulation from axonal collaterals of neighboring motor neurons and in turn inhibit the same or other ventral horn motor neurons, thus constituting a negative feedback mechanism.

repolariza´tion   the concluding event in the nerve impulse in which the cell membrane returns to its resting, negative state.

RER   rough endoplasmic reticulum.

reser´pine   one of a group of drugs which reduce catecholamine activity. It is an alkaloid with sedative and tranquilizing properties, first used to lower blood pressure.

res´tiform [L. *restis* rope; *forma* form]   resembling a rope; pertaining to the restiform body.

rete mirabile /re´te mĭ-rab´il-e/ [NA] [L. *rete* a net; *mirabile* wonderful]   an arterial plexus interconnecting the intracranial (brain) vessels and the extracranial vessels, particularly the branches of the external carotid artery. It is characteristic of certain animals, e.g., cat, but not of monkey or man (Batson, '44).

retic´ular [L. *reticulum* small net, dim. of *rete*]   pertaining to certain areas of the brain stem and upper cervical spinal cord that have a net-like appearance in fiber-stained cross sections, and the tracts derived from these areas. *See* formation, reticular; tracts, reticulospinal.

ret´ina, EYE   inner layer of the eyeball, between the choroid on its outer surface and the vitreous body which it encloses. It develops from the optic cup and contains the sensory part of the eye. Its outermost layer (layer 1) develops from the outer layer of the optic cup. The nervous portion (layers 2 to 10) develops from the inner layer of the optic cup. The layers of the retina, beginning with the outermost, next to the choroid, are as follows:

layer 1, pigment layer [stratum pigmentosum, NA]   single layer of pigmented, cuboidal cells.

layer 2, layer of rods and cones [stratum neuroepitheliale, NA]   layer comprising the rod-shaped and cone-shaped dendritic processes of the photoreceptors. *Syn:* bacillary layer.

layer 3, outer limiting membrane [stratum limitans externum]   layer composed of processes of the Müller's cells, through which the rods and cones are connected to their cell bodies. *Syn:* external limiting membrane.

layer 4, outer nuclear layer [stratum nucleare externum, NA]   layer containing the cell bodies of the rods and cones. *Syn:* external nuclear layer; outer granular layer.

layer 5, outer plexiform layer [stratum plexiforme externum, NA]   synaptic layer containing the axons of the rods and cones, the dendrites of the bipolar cells, and the processes of the horizontal cells. *Syn:* outer molecular or reticular layer.

layer 6, inner nuclear layer [stratum nucleare internum, NA]   layer containing the cell bodies of the bipolar cells, the second link in the chain of retinal connections; also the nuclei of the Müller cells, which are supporting cells and neuroglial in type, and the cell bodies of the horizontal and amacrine cells, which are retinal association neurons. *Syn:* inner granular layer; outer ganglionic layer.

layer 7, inner plexiform layer [stratum plexiforme internum, NA]   synaptic layer containing the axons of the bipolar cells, the dendrites of the ganglion cells, and the processes of the amacrine cells. *Syn:* inner molecular or reticular layer.

layer 8, ganglion cell layer [stratum ganglionare, NA]   layer containing the large cell bodies of the neurons (the third link in the chain of retinal connections) whose axons compose the optic nerve. The parasol cells of the retina are also in this layer. *See also* cells, midget.

layer 9, optic nerve fiber layer [stratum neurofibrarum, NA]   layer composed of the axons of the ganglion cells which turn and run under the inner surface of the retina to the optic disk, where they leave the eyeball as the optic nerve. Retinal arteries and veins are also in this layer. *Syn:* stratum opticum.

layer 10, inner limiting membrane [stratum limitans internum, NA]   delicate membrane composed of processes of Müller's cells, on the inner surface of the retina.

retina, ciliary /sil´ī-ar-ī/, EYE   double layer of epithelium, derived from the optic cup, covering the ciliary body and its processes. *See also* epithelium, ciliary.

retina, iridial /ir-id ´ī-al/, EYE   double layer of epithelium on the posterior surface of the iris, derived from the optic cup. The cells of both layers are pigmented.

retina, light-insen´sitive, EYE   ciliary epithelium (ciliary retina) and the posterior epithelium of the iris (iridial retina), both derived from the optic cup.

retinal detachment   *See* detachment, retinal.

retinene /ret ´in-ēn/, EYE   a photopigment present in rhodopsin. *Syn:* visual yellow.

retrosubic ´ular, CEREBRUM   cortex posterior to the subiculum of the hippocampal formation.

Retzius, Anders Adolf (1796-1860)   Swedish anatomist and pathologist. *Retzius' gyrus* is the intralimbic gyrus.

Retzius, Gustaf Magnus (1842-1919)   Swedish anatomist and pathologist, son of Anders A. Retzius. He was noted for his studies of cerebral morphology, as well as for his contributions to the knowledge of sensory organs, nerve terminations, and the supporting tissues of the brain. The *foramina of Key and Retzius* are the lateral apertures of the fourth ventricle. The *sheath of Key and Retzius* is the endoneurium.

Rexed, Bror   contemporary Swedish neuroanatomist. Rexed layers of the spinal cord gray matter (Fig. N-6) are 10 laminae which he described for the cat (Rexed, '64) but which are characteristic of other species as well. They are arranged, roughly from dorsal to ventral, as follows:

lamina I   layer of marginal cells of various sizes applied to the surface of the substantia gelatinosa. *Syn:* posteromarginal nucleus; Waldeyer's layer.

lamina II   layer of small, closely packed cells, which caps the dorsal horn. *Syn:* substantia gelatinosa.

lamina III   layer of cells somewhat larger and less densely arranged than those in lamina II. It lies ventral to and within the concavity of lamina II and corresponds to the dorsal portion of the nucleus proprius.

lamina IV   layer of cells of various sizes, loosely arranged in the dorsal horn, ventral to lamina III. This layer contains many myelinated fibers. It corresponds to the ventral portion of the nucleus proprius. Laminae I-IV constitute the head of the dorsal horn.

lamina V   relatively thick layer in the neck of the dorsal horn. The medial two-thirds is paler than the lateral third and contains more cells of smaller size. The lateral portion, cut through by fiber bundles, is the reticular area of the spinal cord.

lamina VI   fairly broad layer at the base of the dorsal horn, prominent only in the enlargements. Its smaller medial portion contains smaller, more closely packed cells than the lateral part. The medial and lateral divisions of this layer correspond approximately to Cajal's internal and external basal nuclei.

lamina VII   layer that occupies most of the intermediate zone between the dorsal and ventral horns and, at appropriate levels, includes the thoracic nucleus, the intermediolateral nucleus (lateral horn), and the intermediomedial nucleus. In the enlargements it extends ventrally into the lateral part of the ventral horn, where it surrounds the lateral cell groups of lamina IX.

lamina VIII   layer that extends across the base and mid-portion of the thoracic ventral horn, but in the enlargements is confined to the medial half. It surrounds the medial cell groups of lamina IX.

lamina IX   somatic motor cell groups of the ventral horn, the axons from which enter the ventral roots and the spinal accessory nerve roots.

lamina X small area of gray matter around the central canal, consisting mainly of the dorsal and ventral gray commissures. The most rostral portion of the dorsal gray commissure contains the commissural nucleus.

rheobase /re´o-bās/ [Gr. *rheos* current] minimum current intensity necessary to excite a nervous impulse when allowed to flow for an indefinitely long period.

rhinal /ri´nal/, CEREBRUM, [Gr. *rhis* nose] pertaining to the rhinal sulcus, which separates a part of the rhinencephalon from the neocortex.

rhinencephalon /ri-nen-sef´al-on/ [NA], CEREBRUM, [Gr. *rhis*-; *enkephalos* brain] certain parts of the cerebrum, mainly on its basal surface, including the olfactory bulb and stalk, anterior olfactory nucleus, anterior perforated substance, olfactory gyri, parolfactory area, diagonal band of Broca and its nucleus, hippocampus, parahippocampal gyrus, and uncus. It corresponds to the limbic lobe, but usually excluding the cingulate gyrus and the isthmus of the cingulate gyrus. At one time the rhinencephalon was regarded as subserving the olfactory system but later it was shown that most of the area is unrelated to the sense of smell. *Syn:* rhinic lobe.

rhizotomy /ri-zot´o-mī/ [Gr. *rhiza* root; *tome* section] section of a peripheral nerve root, usually a sensory root for the relief of pain.

rhodopsin /ro-dop´sin/, EYE, [Gr *rhodon* rose, therefore red; *opsis* vision] purple-red pigment present in rods and important in maintaining the sensitivity of the rod system in twilight or dim light. It consists of retinine (an aldehyde form of vitamin A) and opsin, a protein. It is broken down by light and restored in the dark. *Syn:* visual purple.

rhombencephalon /rom-ben-sef´al-on/ [NA], HINDBRAIN, [Gr. *rhombos* rhomb or lozenge; *enkephalos* brain] most caudal subdivision of the developing brain, which later divides into the metencephalon and myelencephalon.

rhombic /rom´bik/, HINDBRAIN pertaining to the rhombencephalon. *See also* lip, rhombic.

rhomboid fos´sa, HINDBRAIN floor of the fourth ventricle.

Ribes, François, Sr. (1765-1845) French physician, noted especially for his studies of the anatomy and physiology of the eye and the ear. *Ribes' ganglion* is a tiny sympathetic ganglion sometimes occurring on the anterior communicating artery.

Ribes, François, Jr. (1800-1867) French physician. He determined that the membrane of the round window of the ear consists of three layers, an epithelium on each surface of an intervening layer of tissue.

Riddoch, George (1888-1947) British neurologist. *Riddoch's reflex* is the mass reflex.

rigidity, decerebrate /rī-jid´it-ī, de-ser´eb-rāt/ posture first described by Sherrington (1898) in cats after section of the brain stem just beneath the edge of the tentorium cerebelli. The antigravity or extensor muscles are stiffly contracted so that a cat assumes the position of a standing animal. In man the arms are held close to the body, internally rotated and extended at the elbow. The hands are hyperpronated. The legs are extended at the hips, knees, and ankles, and the toes are plantar flexed. This posture occurs after section of the brain stem between the red nucleus and the vestibular nuclei, presumably with release of the vestibulospinal tracts.

rigidity, decor´ticate posture in which the arms are flexed and adducted and the legs are extended. It occurs after a lesion of the frontal lobe cortex or the posterior limb of the internal capsule, but in which the red nuclei and its descending connections (rubrospinal and rubroreticulospinal tracts) and the (lateral) vestibulospinal tracts are spared.

rigidity, extrapyram´idal   increased resistance to passive movement, usually with cogwheel jerks but without the increased deep reflexes or the clasp-knife phenomenon characteristic of spasticity.

Robertson, Argyll   *See* Argyll Robertson, Douglas.

Robin, Charles Philippe (1821-1885)   French physician and histologist of Paris. He described in greater detail the spaces around brain blood vessels, *Virchow-Robin spaces,* which had previously been noted by Virchow.

rod, EYE   light-sensitive photoreceptor of the retina, specialized for vision in dim light. *See also* cone; *and see* microglia for rod cell.

rod´let   elongated straight or crescent-shaped intranuclear organoid of nerve cells, visible in fixed and in living material.

Rolando, Luigi (1773-1831)   Italian anatomist of Turin. He described the central sulcus of the cerebrum in his lectures at the University of Turin and in 1839, François Leuret named it the *fissure of Rolando* in his honor. Other structures associated with the central sulcus are: *Rolando's area,* the pre- and postcentral gyri, anterior and posterior to the central sulcus; the *Rolandic vein,* which lies along the central sulcus on the lateral surface of the cerebrum and empties into the superior longitudinal sinus, but which also usually communicates with one of the middle cerebral veins; the *Rolandic angle,* the acute angle formed by the central sulcus and the superior border of the frontal lobe; and the *upper Rolandic point,* a term sometimes applied to the tip of the central sulcus on the medial surface of the cerebrum. Also named for him are the *substantia gelatinosa (of Rolando)* in the dorsal horn of the spinal cord, the *tubercle of Rolando* for the trigeminal tubercle, and *Rolando's lobe* for the operculum.

Roller, Christian Friedrich Wilhelm (1844-1884)   German neurologist. The *nucleus of Roller* is the sublingual nucleus, one of the parahypoglossal nuclei. It consists of large cells located ventral to the hypoglossal nucleus. The *root of Roller* consists of the descending fibers of the vestibular root.

Romberg, Moritz Heinrich (1795-1873)   German neurologist. *Romberg's sign* (1840) consists of increased difficulty in maintaining one's balance while standing after closing the eyes, because of a loss of position sensibility. His contribution to neurology rests not only on his famous sign, now a routine part of a neurological examination; he is regarded as the founder of modern neurology. He had established a neurology clinic at the University of Berlin by 1837 and wrote the first major textbook of neurology, published 1840-1846.

root, anterior   *See* root, ventral.

root, dorsal (posterior)   aggregation of dorsal rootlets on each side of a spinal cord segment. The rootlets attach along the dorsolateral sulcus of the spinal cord. Peripherally, each dorsal root combines with a ventral root to form a spinal nerve as it enters an intervertebral foramen. Most dorsal root fibers are afferent and have their cell bodies in the related spinal ganglion, but efferent fibers have been described in the dorsal roots of lower forms and may also occur in man as a part of the postulated spinal parasympathetic system. *See also* Bell for the Bell-Magendie law.

root, mesencephal´ic, of V, MAINLY MIDBRAIN   *See* tract, mesencephalic trigeminal.

root, nerve   intramedullary part of a cranial nerve.

root, posterior   *See* root, dorsal.

root, ventral (anterior)   aggregation of ventral rootlets which emerge from the ventrolateral surface on each side of the spinal cord. Peripherally each ventral root combines with a dorsal root of the same cord segment to form a spinal nerve as it enters an intervertebral foramen. Most ventral root fibers are efferent and arise from cell bodies in the ventral and lateral horns, but now it is known that there are also some afferent (pain) fibers among them. *See also* Bell for the Bell-Magendie law.

rootlet   one fascicle of a dorsal or ventral root of a spinal nerve, or root of a cranial nerve.

Rose, Jerzy (b. 1909)   Polish neuroanatomist. The lateral mamillary nucleus is sometimes called the *lateral mamillary nucleus of Rose.*

Rosenthal, Friedrich Christian (1780-1829)   German anatomist. *Rosenthal's vein* is the basal vein, a tributary of the great cerebral vein.

rosette, cerebel´lar, CEREBELLUM   termination of a mossy fiber in contact with the clawlike dendritic terminals of granule cells in a cerebellar glomerulus in the granular layer of the cerebellar cortex. *See* Fig. C-9.

Rossolimo, Grigorij Ivanovich (1860-1928)   Russian neurologist. *Rossolimo's sign* or *reflex* is a stretch reflex which consists of plantar flexion of the toes in response to tapping the plantar surface of the toes and is indicative of injury to corticospinal fibers.

ros´trum corpor´is callo´si [NA], CEREBRUM   *See* corpus callosum, rostrum.

rough endoplas´mic retic´ulum (RER)   organelle present in many kinds of cells, and shown by electron microscopy to have ribosomes on its outer surface. In nerve cells such structures consist of large, flattened sacs which form lamellae and correspond to the chromatophilic substance (Nissl bodies) visible by light microscopy.

Roussy, Gustave (1874-1948)   Swiss physician, later of Paris. In addition to publication with Dejerine on the thalamic syndrome, he made other substantial contributions to the neurological literature.

ru´diments, hippocam´pal, CEREBRUM   cell groups left behind when the developing corpus callosum displaces the hippocampal formation posteriorly and down into the temporal lobe. They are: the indusium griseum, septohippocampal nucleus, anterior continuation of the hippocampus (represented in man by relatively few scattered cells), and fasciolar gyrus.

Ruffini, Angelo (1864-1929)   Italian anatomist. *Ruffini endings* or *corpuscles* (1898) are elongated, cylindrical nerve endings having a thin connective tissue capsule and containing nerve fibers. Those endings in the subcutaneous connective tissue are thought to be receptors for warmth. *Ruffini's subsidiary sheath* is the endoneurium.

Russell, James Samuel Risien (1863-1939)   British neurologist. *Russell's fasciculus* is the uncinate fasciculus of the cerebellum.

Ruysch, Frederick (1638-1731)   Dutch anatomist of The Hague, later Professor of Anatomy at Amsterdam. He used a wax injection technique to demonstrate small blood vessels in many parts of the body, including the eye. The *membrane* or *lamina of Ruysch* is the choriocapillary layer of the choroid of the eye.

S

S   sacral.

sac, endolymphat´ic [saccus endolymphaticus, NA], EAR   terminal part of the endolymphatic duct, located within the dura mater on the posterior surface of the petrous part of the temporal bone. *Syn:* otic sac.

sac, o´tic, EAR   *See* sac, endolymphatic.

saccades /sak-ădz´/ [*adj.* sacca´dic] [Fr. jerk; sudden check of a horse, from *saquer* to pull]   fast, essentially voluntary, eye movements by which the center of gaze is shifted from one point in the visual field to another.

saccule /sak´ūl/ [sacculus, NA], EAR, [L. *sacculus* little sack]   somewhat spherical subdivision of the membranous labyrinth, located anterior to the utricle in the vestibule of the bony labyrinth. It is connected with the utricle by the utriculosaccular duct and with the cochlear duct by the ductus reuniens. The saccular macula is in a nearly vertical position. It may respond to linear acceleration of the head and may also be sensitive to slow vibratory stimuli.

Sachs, Bernard (1858-1944)   American neurologist, of German parents. His description of the cerebral changes in amaurotic familial idiocy and that of Tay on the associated ocular manifestations led to the identification of *Tay-Sachs disease.*

sacral (S)   pertaining to one or more of the five sacral spinal cord segments or nerves, or to the sacrum.

sagulum, MIDBRAIN   group of elongated triangular cells, distributed irregularly along the external surface of the lateral lemniscus at levels between the trochlear nucleus and trochlear decussation.

St. Vitus' dance   early term used by Sydenham for the chorea which now bears his name. Originally the term pertained to outbreaks of wild, emotional dancing in frenzied religious spectacles in the middle ages.

sal´tatory [L. *saltatio* from *saltare* to leap]   pertaining to or characterized by dancing or leaping movements. *See* conduction, saltatory.

sand, brain, EPITHALAMUS   calcareous bodies in the pineal body. *See* acervulus cerebri.

Sapolini, Giuseppe (1812-1893)   The *nerve of Sapolini* is the nervus intermedius.

sat´ellite, nucle´olar [corpusculum chromatini sexualis, NA]   small dense mass first described in nerve cells, and characteristic of cells in females. It is located within the nucleus, next to the nucleolus or at the inner surface of the nuclear membrane. It is a mass of sex chromatin which contains the second, condensed X-chromosome and other material (Barr and Bertram, '49). *Syn:* Barr body.

Sattler, Hubert (1844-1928)   Austrian ophthalmologist. *Sattler's layer* is the inner part of the vascular layer of the choroid of the eye, containing the smaller blood vessels of the lamina.

sca´la me´dia, EAR   *See* duct, cochlear.

scala tym´pani [NA], EAR   perilymphatic space of the bony labyrinth of the cochlea, separated from the cochlear duct by the spiral membrane.

scala vestib´uli [NA], EAR   perilymphatic space of the bony labyrinth of the cochlea, separated from the cochlear duct by the vestibular membrane.

Scarpa, Antonio (1747-1832)   Italian anatomist of Pavia, a pupil of Morgagni's. He was a skillful surgeon and ophthalmologist, and a brilliant illustrator. He is best known for his work on the internal ear and his name is associated with a number of structures in this region. *Scarpa's ganglion* (1779) is the vestibular ganglion; *Scarpa's membrane* is the secondary tympanic membrane which occludes the round window of the ear; *Scarpa's fluid* is endolymph; and *Scarpa's nerve* is the nasopalatine nerve.

Schaffer, Károly (1864-1939)   pioneer Hungarian neuropathologist. *Schaffer collaterals* are recurrent branches which arise from the axons of pyramidal cells in the cornu ammonis. Given off in the stratum oriens, the branches turn back and enter the strata lacunosum and moleculare, where they synapse on the apical dendrites of adjacent pyramidal cells (Fig. C-7).

Schilder, Paul Ferdinand (1886-1940)   neurologist and psychiatrist, originally of Vienna, later practicing in the United States. He is noted for his description of diffuse cerebral sclerosis, *Schilder's disease,* a disease of children or young adults in which there is demyelination mainly of the cerebral white matter, with progressive dementia, spasticity, and blindness.

schizophrenia [Gr. *schizein* to split or cleave; *phren* mind]   severe, complex mental disorder sometimes of acute onset and sometimes having a slow, life-long course. It may include a personality change, when of sudden origin; delusions, often paranoid in nature; and/or hallucinations. There is also almost always some disturbance in the thinking processes. There is a hereditary factor involving chromosome 5 and perhaps other chromosomes. Other contributing factors include psychological stresses, especially early in life. *Syn:* formerly dementia praecox.

Schlemm, Friedrich (1795-1858)   German anatomist. The *canal of Schlemm* (1830) is the venous sinus of the sclera, although it had previously been noted by Fontana (1778). This channel encircles the cornea at the corneoscleral junction and is a link in the drainage of aqueous humor from the anterior chamber of the eye to the conjunctival veins.

Schmidt, Henry D. (1823-1888)   American anatomist and pathologist. The *clefts* or *incisures of Schmidt-Lanterman* are funnel-shaped formations within the myelin sheath of peripheral nerve fibers. *See* incisures, myelin.

Schultze, Maximillian Johann Sigismund (1825-1874)   German anatomist, noted for his description of the nerve endings in the retina. The *tract of Schultze* is the fasciculus interfascicularis.

Schütz, Hugo (19th century)   German anatomist. The *fasciculus of Schütz* (1891) is the dorsal longitudinal fasciculus.

Schwalbe, Gustav Albert (1844-1916)   German anatomist. The *nucleus of Schwalbe* is the medial vestibular nucleus. *Schwalbe's fissure* is the choroid fissure of the cerebrum.

Schwann, Theodor (1810-1882)   German anatomist and physiologist, a professor at Liège in Belgium. The *sheath of Schwann* (1839) is the neurolemma of peripheral nerve fibers.

scler´a [NA], EYE, [Gr. *skleros* hard]   dense, white, fibrous, connective tissue which, with the cornea, constitutes the external tunic of the eyeball. Its fibers are continuous anteriorly with those of the substantia propria of the cornea.

sclero´sis, amyotro´phic lateral (ALS)   progressive motor disease first described by Charcot and characterized by a combination of upper motor neuron and lower motor neuron signs. *Syn:* Lou Gehrig's disease.

sclerosis, disseminated   *See* sclerosis, multiple.

sclerosis, multiple   demyelinating disease in which sclerotic plaques develop in multiple locations throughout the CNS. It tends to strike young adults, particularly in the northern, colder climates. The disease is usually intermittently progressive with remissions. *Syn:* disseminated sclerosis.

sclerosis, tu´berous   disease inherited as an autosomal dominant with variable penetrance. There are cerebral lesions, skin lesions, and tumors in other organs. There is characteristically also epilepsy and mental retardation. *Syn:* epiloia; Bourneville's disease.

sec´tion, cross (transverse)   section at right angles to the longitudinal axis. In man a cross section of the spinal cord or brain stem is a section in the horizontal plane. A cross section of the cerebral hemispheres and diencephalon is in the vertical or frontal plane, at right angles to that of the brain stem and spinal cord.

section, frontal   section of the brain in the frontal or coronal plane, that is, one that crosses the median plane in a vertical direction, at right angles to the sagittal plane.

section, horizontal   section in a plane parallel to the horizon, and which separates superior and inferior portions. Thus a horizontal section of the forebrain is at right angles to a forebrain cross section but is the same as a cross section of the brain stem and spinal cord.

section, transverse   *See* section, cross.

seg´ment, init´ial ax´on   that portion of an axon devoid of myelin, between the axon hillock and the axis cylinder. Synapses on this part characteristically inhibit conduction along the axon.

segment, interno´dal   part of a myelinated nerve fiber between two nodes of Ranvier.

segment, spinal cord   block of spinal cord to which the root fibers of a given pair of spinal nerves attach.

segment, sympathet´ic   that part of the sympathetic trunk from which a specific gray ramus arises, whether or not the place is marked by a ganglion.

sel´la turcica /tur´sĭ-kah/ [NA] [L. *sella* saddle; *turcica* Turkish]   median saddle-shaped depression in the sphenoid bone, which contains the hypophysis.

sep´tum, dorsal median [septum medianum dorsale, NA], MEDULLA, CORD, [L. *saeptum* fence]   connective tissue septum extending ventrally between the two dorsal funiculi, from the mid-dorsal surface of the spinal cord and closed medulla ventrally to the gray matter.

septum pellucidum /pel-loo´sĭ-dum/ [NA], CEREBRUM, [pellucidum from L. *per* through; *lucere* to shine]   thin sheet of nervous tissue suspended between the corpus callosum and the body of the fornix and forming the medial wall of the anterior horn of the lateral ventricle. It may be fused into a single median structure or be divided into two sheets separated by a space, the cavum septi pellucidi. It is a part of the medial olfactory area and receives fibers from the medial olfactory stria. It is interconnected with the hippocampus and discharges to the epithalamus, and, by way of the fornix, to the precommissural septal and preoptic areas, and to the hypothalamus, especially its ventromedial nucleus. Stimulation of the septum pellucidum is said to produce contraction of the bladder. *Syn:* postcommissural septum; septum lucidum. *See also* area, septal; septum, precommissural.

septum, postcommis´sural (postcommissu´ral), CEREBRUM   *See* septum pellucidum.

septum pos´ticum, CORD   *See* septum, subarachnoid.

septum, precommis´sural (precommisu´ral) [septum precommissurale, NA], CEREBRUM   a major part of the septal area, consisting of a group of nuclei located between the anterior horn of the lateral ventricle and the medial surface of the frontal lobe. Its medial surface constitutes the parolfactory area (of Broca). It consists of: the medial and lateral septal nuclei, the nucleus of the diagonal band (of Broca), the dorsal septal nucleus, the nucleus accumbens, the bed nuclei of the hippocampal and anterior commissures, and certain other small cell groups. It is an important way station in the limbic system and is interconnected with the preoptic and hypothalamic nuclei on the one hand and the amygdala and hippocampus on the other. Following lesions in this area changes in behavior have been observed and also edema of the legs. *Syn:* septal verum. *For additional information, see* Andy and Stephan ('68).

septum, subarach´noid, CORD   thin meningeal partition from the arachnoid to the pia mater, along the mid-dorsal surface of the cervical and thoracic spinal cord, which divides the subarachnoid space longitudinally in this region. *Syn:* septum posticum.

septum ve´rum, CEREBRUM   *See* septum, precommissural.

seroto´nin   5-hydroxytryptamine (5-HT), an indolamine occurring in many cells of the body. It has many physiologic properties. Peripherally it inhibits gastric secretion but has an excitatory effect on smooth muscle and motoneurons. In the CNS it is synthesized from tryptophan and is a precursor of melatonin. It occurs mainly in cells of the raphe nuclei of the brain stem, from which it is transported to the forebrain, the cerebellum, other brain stem nuclei including the locus coeruleus, and the spinal cord. It appears to act mainly in sleep regulation, and as an inhibitory neurotransmitter in the substantia nigra and striatum and to suppress pain transmission in the spinal cord. *Syn:* enteramine; thrombocytin; thrombotonin. *See also* neurotransmitters.

sex chro´matin   *See* satellite, nucleolar.

sheath, axial /ak´sĭ-al/   inner layer of the double-layered connective tissue capsule of neuromuscular and neurotendinous spindles.

sheath, my´elin   *See* myelin.

sheath, neurolem´ma   *See* neurolemma.

sheath, nu´cleated   *See* neurolemma.

sheath, prim´itive   *See* neurolemma.

shepherd's crook, MIDBRAIN   *See* crook, shepherd's.

Sherrington, Sir Charles Scott (1857-1952)   great English neurophysiologist. In addition to his many contributions in this field, particularly in the analysis of motor activity, he was an outstanding teacher, whose many pupils became eminent clinicians and scientists in their own right. In 1932 he and Lord E.D. Adrian were awarded the Nobel Prize for medicine and physiology for their discoveries regarding neuron function.

SIF   small intensely fluorescent cells.

sign, segmen´tal   clinical manifestation indicative of a lesion at a particular level of the CNS.

sign, tract   clinical manifestation indicative of injury to a CNS tract.

single pho´ton emis´sion compu´terized tomog´raphy (SPECT)   *See* tomography.

si´nus, carot´id [sinus caroticus, NA]   dilation of the internal carotid artery, just above the bifurcation of the common carotid artery. Its wall contains receptors of glossopharyngeal nerve fibers which monitor blood pressure. *See* reflex, carotid sinus.

sinus, cav´ernous [sinus cavernosus, NA]   paired dural sinus located on the lateral surface of the body of the sphenoid bone. It consists of many venous channels. The internal carotid artery passes through it (Fig. A-1), accompanied by the internal carotid plexus and the abducens nerve. In its lateral wall are the oculomotor and trochlear nerves, and the ophthalmic and maxillary branches of the trigeminal nerve. The sinus receives blood primarily from the ophthalmic vein, sphenoparietal sinus, superficial middle cerebral vein, and several emissary veins.

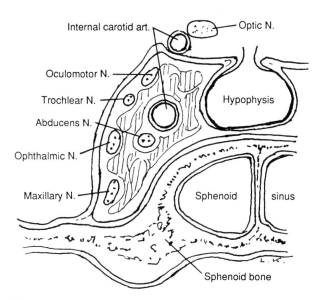

Fig. S-1.   Coronal section through the cavernous sinus, showing its relations and associated nerves and blood vessels. Drawing courtesy of Dr. L.G. Kempe.

It is connected with its contralateral counterpart by way of the intercavernous sinuses, and is drained by the superior and inferior petrosal sinuses. Because of its connections with the veins of the face, infections may be carried from the face, particularly the nose and the upper lip, by the facial vein into the cranial cavity and then to the brain. (Fig. S-1.)

sinus, cir´cular   anterior and posterior intercavernous dural sinuses and the two cavernous sinuses which they connect.

sinus (of the) du´ra ma´ter [sinus durae matris, NA]   any of the valveless venous channels located under or along the attachments of the dural folds or in the free edges of the folds. The main ones are: the cavernous, superior and inferior sagittal, transverse and sigmoid sinuses, straight, and superior and inferior petrosal sinuses.

sinus, intercav´ernous [sinus intercavernosus, NA]   either of two (anterior and posterior) dural sinuses interconnecting the cavernous sinuses of the two sides.

sinus, jug´ular   *See* bulb, jugular.

sinus, lateral   *See* sinus, transverse.

sinus, longitudinal, inferior   *See* sinus, sagittal, inferior.

sinus, longitudinal, superior   *See* sinus, sagittal, superior.

sinus, occip´ital [sinus occipitalis, NA]   small, median dural sinus in the attachment of the falx cerebelli from the margin of the foramen magnum to the confluence of the sinuses, and connecting with the veins of the internal vertebral plexus.

sinus, petro´sal, inferior [sinus petrosus inferior, NA]   paired dural sinus which connects the cavernous sinus with the internal jugular vein, along the junction of the petrous part of the temporal bone and the basal part of the occipital bone to the jugular foramen.

sinus, petrosal, superior [sinus petrosus superior, NA]   dural sinus along the anterior attachment of the tentorium cerebelli on the crest of the petrous part of the temporal bone. It connects the cavernous sinus medially and the junction of the transverse and sigmoid sinuses laterally.

sinus rec´tus [NA]   *See* sinus, straight.

sinus, sagittal, inferior /să´jĭ-tal/ [sinus sagittalis inferior, NA]   median dural sinus within the free edge of the falx cerebri, extending backward to the junction of the falx and the tentorium cerebelli, to empty into the straight sinus. *Syn:* inferior longitudinal sinus.

sinus, sagittal, superior [sinus sagittalis superior, NA]   median dural sinus extending along the attachment of the falx cerebri from the foramen cecum anteriorly, to the confluence of the sinuses, anterior to the internal occipital protuberance (Fig. C-6). It receives blood mainly from the superior cerebral veins, and usually empties into the right transverse sinus. *Syn:* superior longitudinal sinus.

sinus, sig´moid [sinus sigmoideus, NA]   paired dural sinus which, as a continuation of the transverse sinus, forms an S-curve in a groove leading down to the jugular foramen.

sinus, sphenoparietal /sfe-no-pah-ri´ĕ-tal/ [sinus sphenoparietalis, NA]   paired dural sinus located along the posterior edge of the lesser wing of the sphenoid bone. It empties into the cavernous sinus. *Syn:* Breschet's sinus.

sinus, straight [sinus rectus, NA]   median dural sinus along the attachment of the falx cerebri to the tentorium cerebelli (Fig. C-6). It is formed by the union of the inferior sagittal sinus and the great cerebral vein and empties usually into the left transverse sinus at the confluence of the sinuses.

sinus, tentor´ial   relatively constant channel in a venous plexus in the tentorium cerebelli. It empties into the junction of the straight sinus and the transverse sinus. *Syn:* sinus of Gibbs.

sinus, transverse [sinus transversus, NA]   paired dural sinus along the bony attachment of the tentorium cerebelli from the inferior occipital protuberance to the posterolateral tip of the petrous part of the temporal bone. The right sinus usually drains the superior sagittal sinus and the left the straight sinus. Each sinus also receives blood from the superficial veins of the occipital lobe and from the superior petrosal sinus. It empties into the sigmoid sinus. *Syn:* lateral sinus.

sinus, ve´nous, of the scler´a [sinus venosus sclerae, NA], EYE   channel which encircles the cornea at the corneoscleral junction. It drains aqueous humor from the spaces (of Fontana) in the trabecular meshwork at the iridocorneal angle and communicates with the venous system by way of the aqueous veins. *Syn:* canal of Schlemm.

si´phon (syphon), carot´id   segment of the internal carotid artery which curves forward and upward in the cavernous sinus, then passes through the meninges into the subarachnoid space and turns backward below the optic nerve before dividing into the anterior and middle cerebral arteries (Fig. A-1).

sleep paral´ysis   disorder characterized by inability to move or cry out, taking place on going to sleep or awakening.

sleeve, du´ral   connective tissue investment of each spinal nerve within the intervertebral space. It is continuous with the dura mater centrally and with the perineurium peripherally.

Smith, Grafton Elliott   *See* Elliott Smith, Grafton.

Snider, Ray S. (b. 1911)   American anatomist, noted for his contributions to cerebellar physiology.

Soemmering, Samuel Thomas (1755-1830)   German anatomist, born in Poland. He was a student of Wrisberg's early in his career. Both the substantia gelatinosa and the substantia nigra have been called *Soemmering's substance. Soemmering's nerve* is the pudendal nerve, and *Soemmering's yellow spot* or *fovea* is the macula lutea of the retina.

so´lar plexus   *See* plexus, celiac.

so´ma [*pl.* somata] [Gr. body]   *See* body, cell.

somat´ic af´ferent (SA)   *See* component, nerve.

somatic ef´ferent (SE)   *See* component, nerve.

somatostat´in   neuropeptide distributed widely, including sensory cells, the retina, and the cerebral cortex. In the hypothalamus it provides some control over the hormones secreted by the anterior lobe of the hypophysis and by the pancreas. It likely plays a role in pain perception and may also have other important functions as yet unknown. *See also* neurotransmitters.

somatotop´ic   organized according to a pattern of body representation.

somesthe´sis [*adj.* **somesthetic**]   the general somatic senses, *viz.* somatic pain, temperature, tactile, vibratory, and position sensibility.

Sommer, Wilhelm (1852-1900)   German physician of Allenberg, in Bavaria. In an 1880 study on epilepsy he described degenerative changes in the cornu ammonis, in the area beneath the ventricular surface and opposite the hippocampal fissure. In this area, now known as *Sommer's sector,* pyramidal cells appear to be especially sensitive to oxygen deficiency.

space, epidural /ep-ĭ-du´ral/ [cavitas (cavum) epiduralis, NA]   space between the spinal dura mater and the vertebral column, containing many thin-walled blood vessels and, particularly in its caudal portion, adipose tissue.

spaces (of the) iridocorne´al angle [spatia anguli iridocornealis, NA], EYE   small spaces in the trabecular meshwork of the pectinate ligament at the corneoscleral junction. Aqueous humor from the anterior chamber of the eye enters these spaces and is transported to the venous sinus of the sclera (canal of Schlemm) from which it enters the conjunctival veins. *Syn:* spaces of Fontana.

space, per´forated, anterior, CEREBRUM   *See* substance, perforated, anterior.

space, perforated, posterior, MIDBRAIN   *See* substance, perforated, posterior.

space, perio´tic, EAR   *See* labyrinth, periotic.

space, subarach´noid [cavitas (cavum) subarachnoidea, NA]   space between the arachnoid and the pia mater, containing cerebrospinal fluid, and through which pass the nerve roots and the blood vessels for the CNS.

space, subdu´ral [spatium subdurale, NA]   potential space between the dura mater and the arachnoid.

spaces, zonular [spatia zonularia, NA], EYE   spaces among the fibers of the suspensory ligament in the ciliary zonule of the eye. *Syn:* canal of Petit.

spasmus nu´tans /spaz´mus/   disorder of infants characterized by nystagmus, head movements, and torticollis.

spasticity /spas-tis ́ĭ-tĭ/   abnormal condition in which there is an increase in stretch reflex activity. Its clinical manifestations are hypertonia, especially in the antigravity muscles, hyperreflexia, clonus, and increased resistance to passive movement with the clasp-knife phenomenon.

special somat´ic af´ferent (SSA)   *See* component, nerve.

special somatic ef´ferent (SSE)   *See* component, nerve.

special vis´ceral afferent (SVA)   *See* component, nerve.

special visceral efferent (SVE)   *See* component, nerve.

SPECT   single photon emission computerized tomography. *See* tomography.

Sperry, Roger Wolcott (b. 1913)   American neurobiologist noted for his work on the "split brain." In 1981 he received the Nobel Prize for medicine and physiology for his research showing the different and specialized functions of the two cerebral hemispheres.

spher´ule, rod, EYE   synaptic base of a retinal rod, by which the rod synapses with the dendritic terminals of bipolar and horizontal cells of the retina.

spi´der cell   old term for astrocyte.

Spielmeyer, Walther (1879-1935)   German neuropathologist, who investigated the pathogenesis of certain psychiatric disorders, and the role of impaired blood flow as the cause of some neurologic lesions.

spi´na bifida /bif´id-ah, bi´fid-ah/   disorder characterized by a developmental defect in which there is failure of the vertebral column to close, with or without an associated defect of the spinal meninges and spinal cord.

spina bifida cystica /sis´tik-ah/   spina bifida in which there is herniation of the meninges (meningocele), spinal cord (myelocele), or both (meningomyelocele) through a vertebral defect.

spina bifida occul´ta   spina bifida which is limited to defective closure of the vertebrae, although the spinal cord is sometimes imperfectly developed. The skin overlying the defect is often marked by a tuft of hair.

spi´nal   pertaining to the spine and associated structures. *For* spinal column, cord, *and* nerve, *see the nouns.*

spinal parasympathet´ic *See* parasympathetic, spinal.

spindle, neuromus´cular (muscle) [fusus neuromuscularis, NA]   nerve ending in skeletal muscle. It consists of small, modified skeletal muscle fibers (intrafusal fibers), afferent nerve fibers with primary (anulospiral) and secondary (flower spray) receptors, gamma efferent nerve fibers with motor end plates, and capillaries, all contained within a two-layered connective tissue capsule. It is activated when the intrafusal fibers are stretched, and functions in stretch reflexes in the regulation of muscle tone and in proprioceptive sensibility (Figs. R-5, S-2). *See also* loop, gamma, Fig. L-1.

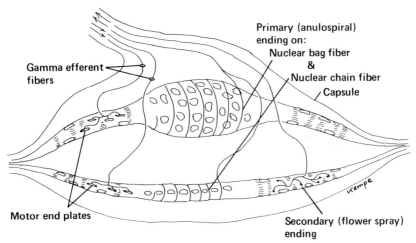

Fig. S-2.   Diagram of a neuromuscular spindle to show the two types of intrafusal fibers, the nuclear bag and nuclear chain fibers, and their motor and afferent nerve supply. Gamma efferent fibers end in small motor end plates on both types of fibers. The primary (anulospiral) endings on both types of fibers and the secondary (flower spray) endings on the nuclear chain fibers are stretch receptors. Drawing courtesy of Dr. L.G. Kempe. *See also* Fig. R-5.

spindle, neuroten´dinous (tendon) [fusus neurotendineus, NA]   nerve ending in tendons, having a double-walled connective tissue capsule and containing small tendon fibers. Impulses from neurotendinous spindles are carried to internuncial cells which in turn inhibit alpha motor neurons, causing relaxation of the muscle innervated (Fig. R-5). *Syn:* Golgi ending; Golgi tendon organ. *See also* reflex, inhibitory.

spines (gemmules or thorns), dendrit´ic [spinula (gemmula) dendritica, NA]   short, spiny processes, each of which receives one nerve ending. They are present on the dendritic branches of many neurons within the CNS, including Purkinje cells of the cerebellar cortex and pyramidal cells of the cerebral cortex.

spinocerebel´lum, CEREBELLUM   part of the cerebellum which receives impulses predominantly from the spinal cord, mainly by way of the spinocerebellar and cuneatocerebellar tracts. It consists of vermis portions of the anterior lobe (central lobule, culmen, and declive) and posterior lobe (pyramis and uvula). *Syn:* paleocerebellum.

spi´ral, EAR   pertaining to the structures and spaces of the cochlea which spiral around the modiolus. *For* spiral ganglion, lamina, ligament, limbus, organ, *and* sulci, *see the nouns.*

splanchnic /splank´nik/ [Gr. *splanchna* viscera]   *See* nerves, splanchnic.

sple´nium [NA], CEREBRUM, [Gr. *splenion* bandage]   thick, posterior part of the corpus callosum.

split brain   *See* brain, split.

spongioblast /spun´jĭ-o-blast/ [Gr. *spongia* sponge; *blastos* germ]   primitive cell which is the forerunner of a neuroglial cell.

spot, blind, EYE   area of the optic disk, in the fundus of the eye, where the optic nerve fibers leave the eye and there are no photoreceptors.

spur, scleral, EYE   ridge extending forward from the sclera, at the iridocorneal angle, between the venous sinus of the sclera (canal of Schlemm) and the ciliary body at the origin of the ciliary muscle.

SSA   special somatic afferent.

SSE   special somatic efferent.

Staderini, Rutilio (19th century)   Italian anatomist. The *nucleus of Staderini* is the nucleus intercalatus, one of the parahypoglossal nuclei.

stalk, hypophysial, DIENCEPHALON   slender structure which consists of the infundibular stalk of the neurohypophysis and the pars tuberalis of the adenohypophysis. It connects the median eminence of the tuber cinereum with the infrasellar portion of the pituitary gland.

stalk, infundib´ular, DIENCEPHALON   slender segment of the neurohypophysis, a part of the hypophysial stalk, connecting the median eminence of the tuber cinereum and the pars nervosa of the neurohypophysis.

stalk, olfac´tory, CEREBRUM   slender strand of fibers on the ventral surface of the frontal lobe, extending from the olfactory bulb to its division into medial and lateral olfactory striae, anterior to the olfactory trigone and anterior perforated substance (Fig. C-3C). *See also* tract, olfactory.

stalk, pineal, EPITHALAMUS   short attachment of the pineal body to the posterosuperior corner of the diencephalon. The habenular commissure passes through its cranial leaflet and the posterior commissure through its caudal leaflet (Fig. V-5). Between the two is the pineal recess of the third ventricle.

sta´pes [NA], EAR, [L. stirrup]   one of the three ossicles of the middle ear. The head of the stapes articulates with the incus. Its base, or footplate, fits into and closes the oval window between the middle ear and the internal ear. The stapedius muscle is attached to the posterior surface of the neck of the stapes.

statoco´nia [NA] [*sing.* statoconium], EAR   small calcareous bodies embedded in the gelatinous statoconial membrane overlying the macula utriculi and the macula sacculi in the internal ear. *Syn:* otoconia; ear dust. *See also* otolith.

stat´olith, EAR   *See* otolith.

Steiner, Gabriel (1883-1965)   German neurologist. *Steiner's Wetterwinkel* (or storm center) is the area between the corpus callosum and the caudate nucleus, near the lateral margin of the lateral ventricle. It is a frequent site of demyelination in multiple sclerosis.

stem, brain [truncus encephali, NA]   axial portion of the brain exclusive of the cerebellum and the forebrain, *viz.* the midbrain, pons, and medulla.

stereocilia /ster-e-o-sil´ī-ah/, EAR   stiff, non-motile processes of the hair cells of the maculae utriculi and sacculi and the cristae of the semicircular ducts of the internal ear. These cilia, 60-100 per cell, presumably provide a passive mechanism which restricts bending of the kinocilium in their direction.

Stilling, Benedict (1810-1879)   German anatomist. Before embedding agents were used in the preparation of tissue for histologic study, Stilling prepared and studied serial, frozen sections of the brain and spinal cord and described many features. *Stilling's nucleus* usually refers to a column of nerve cells in the spinal cord, rostral to and continuous with the thoracic nucleus, and sometimes caudal to the nucleus, but the term has also been applied to other cell groups, including the thoracic nucleus itself, the red nucleus, and the hypoglossal nucleus. *Stilling's fibers* are the short association fibers of the cerebellum. The *fleece of Stilling* is the network of fibers that surrounds the dentate nucleus. *Stilling's canal* is the hyaloid canal in the vitreous body of the eye.

stim´ulus, thresh´old   a stimulus strong enough to initiate an action potential.

storm center, CEREBRUM   Steiner's Wetterwinkel. *See* Steiner.

strabismus /strah-biz´mus/   condition resulting from impaired function of an extraocular muscle or the nerve that supplies it, so that one eye deviates laterally (external strabismus) or medially (internal strabismus) and the two eyes do not focus on a single point. *Syn:* squint.

stratum /strat´um, stra´tum/ [*pl.* **strata**] [L. layer or blanket]   *See also* lamina; layer.

stratum al´bum, MIDBRAIN   fiber layer in the superior colliculus.

stratum cinereum /sin-er´e-um/, MIDBRAIN   cellular layer in the superior colliculus.

stratum ependymal´e [NA]   *See* layer, ependymal.

stratum, external sagittal /saj´ī-tal/, CEREBRUM   *See* fasciculus, longitudinal, inferior.

stratum granulo´sum [NA], CEREBELLUM   granular layer of the cerebellar cortex, composed predominantly of small nerve cells.

stratum griseum /gre´ze-um/, MIDBRAIN   cellular layer in the superior colliculus.

stratum lacuno´sum, CEREBRUM   rich plexus of fibers in the cornu ammonis (Fig. C-7).

stratum lemnisci /lem-nī´sī/, MIDBRAIN   layer of nerve cells and fibers in the superior colliculus.

stratum marginal´e [NA]   marginal layer of the neural tube, its outermost layer composed of the processes of the developing nerve cells.

stratum molecular´e, CEREBRUM, CEREBELLUM   superficial layer characteristic of all cortical regions of the brain. It is a synaptic zone composed primarily of nonmyelinated axon terminals and the dendritic terminals with which they synapse. *See also* cortex, cerebral, molecular layer; cornu ammonis (Fig. C-7); gyrus, dentate; cortex, cerebellar (Fig. C-8).

stratum neurono´rum pirifor´mium [NA], CEREBELLUM, [L. *pirum* pear; *forma* form] layer of large (Purkinje) cells in the cerebellar cortex.

stratum op´ticum   **1.** MIDBRAIN   layer of optic nerve fibers in the superior colliculus. **2.** EYE   layer of optic nerve fibers, layer 10, in the retina.

stratum o´riens, CEREBRUM   layer of nerve cells in the cornu ammonis, between the alveus and stratum pyramidalis (Fig. C-7).

stratum pallial´e [NA]   *See* layer, mantle.

stratum plexifor´me [NA], CEREBELLUM   *See* stratum moleculare. *See also* retina, layers 5 and 7.

stratum pyramidal´e, CEREBRUM   most conspicuous layer of nerve cells in the cornu ammonis between the stratum oriens and the stratum radiatum (Fig. C-7).

stratum radiatum /ra-dī-ah´tum/, cerebrum   layer of fine, unmyelinated nerve fibers, in the cornu ammonis between the stratum pyramidale and the stratum lacunosum (Fig. C-7).

stratum zonal´e [NA] [L. *zonale* from Gr. *zone* girdle, one of the zones of a sphere] thin, superficial layer of myelinated fibers **1.** dorsal thalamus   on the dorsal surface of the dorsal thalamus.

2. midbrain   on the surface of the superior colliculus.

stri´a [*pl.* **striae**] [L. furrow]   *See also* stripe; lamina.

striae, cerebel´lar, medulla   *See* striae medullares (of the fourth ventricle).

stria cor´nea, forebrain   *See* stria terminalis.

stria diagonal´is (of Broca) [NA], cerebrum   *See* band, diagonal (of Broca).

stria habenular´is, epithalamus   *See* stria medullaris thalami.

stria, longitudinal, lateral [stria longitudinalis lateralis, NA], cerebrum   strand of nerve fibers which accompanies indusium griseum in the depth of the sulcus of the corpus callosum and is continuous with the fimbria. *Syn:* lateral white stripe of Lancisi; stria tecta.

stria, longitudinal, medial [stria longitudinalis medialis, NA], cerebrum   strand of nerve fibers which accompanies indusium griseum over the corpus callosum close to the median plane and is continuous with the fimbria. *Syn:* medial white stripe of Lancisi.

stria medullar´is acustica /ah-koos´tī-se/, medulla   an early term for the striae medullares (of the fourth ventricle). It is a misnomer. The fibers are not part of the auditory system as originally thought.

striae medullar´es (of the fourth ventricle) [striae medullares (ventriculi quarti), NA], medulla   bands of medullated fibers which cross the floor of the fourth ventricle (Fig. V-4). The fibers arise mainly from cells in the arcuate nuclei adjacent to the pyramids, with some fibers arising from the pontobulbar body; the fibers pass dorsally along the raphe of the medulla to the floor of the fourth ventricle, then crossed and uncrossed fibers pass laterally to enter the cerebellum by way of the inferior cerebellar peduncle. *Syn:* cerebellar stria; fibers of Piccolomini; arcuatocerebellar fasciculus.

stria medullaris thal´ami [NA], epithalamus   bundle of fibers along the dorsal medial border of the dorsal thalamus, from the interventricular foramen to the habenula. It is composed of fibers from the fornix (mostly), stria terminalis, andthe medial forebrain bundle (Figs. H-1, V-5). *Syn:* stria habenularis; stria pinealis.

stria, olfac´tory, intermediate, cerebrum   small, inconstant strand of fibers which sometimes continues from the olfactory tract into the anterior perforated substance.

stria (tract), olfactory, lateral [stria olfactoria lateralis, NA], cerebrum   olfactory tract fibers which arise from mitral cells in the olfactory bulb, course through the olfactory stalk, then turn laterally along the anterolateral margin of the anterior perforated substance to end in the lateral olfactory area (Fig. C-3C).

stria (tract), olfactory, medial [stria olfactoria medialis, NA], cerebrum   olfactory tract fibers which arise from mitral cells in the olfactory bulb, course through the olfactory stalk, then turn medially along the antermedial margin of the anterior perforated substance to end mostly in the medial olfactory area (Fig. C-3C).

stria pineal´is, epithalamus   *See* stria medullaris thalami.

stria semicircularis, forebrain   *See* stria terminalis.

stria tec´ta, CEREBRUM   *See* stria, longitudinal, lateral.

stria terminal´is [NA], FOREBRAIN   nerve fiber bundle which extends along the tail and body of the caudate nucleus, with connections primarily between the two amygdalae and from the amygdala to the diencephalon. *Syn:* stria (tenia) semicircularis; stria cornea.

stria vascular´is [NA], EAR   layer of epithelium on the surface of the spiral ligament, on the side away from the modiolus, which secretes endolymph in the cochlear duct.

stria, vis´ual, CEREBRUM   macroscopic layer of myelinated nerve fibers in layer 4 of the visual cortex (area 17), consisting mainly of terminals of the optic radiation and possibly some association fibers. *Syn:* stripe of Gennari.

stri´ate   marked with striae, e.g., pertaining to the visual cortex of the occipital lobe, which contains the stripe of Gennari.

stria´to- (stri´o-)   combining forms for the efferent connections of the striatum.

stria´tum, CEREBRUM, [L. *striatus* furrowed, striped]   usually the caudate nucleus and putamen, sometimes including the globus pallidus, so named because of the strands of nerve cells interconnecting the caudate nucleus and the putamen across the internal capsule. *See also* corpus striatum; neostriatum; paleostriatum; archistriatum.

striatum, dorsal, CEREBRUM   the caudate nucleus and the putamen. *See* striatum.

striatum olfactor´ium, CEREBRUM   *See* amygdala.

striatum, ventral, CEREBRUM   cellular area ventral to the putamen and extending to the surface of the brain in the anterior perforated substance. It comprises the lateral part of the sublenticular gray, the nucleus accumbens, and the subcommissural part of the substantia innominata.

strings, au´ditory, EAR   component filaments of the basilar membrane which are tightly stretched between the tympanic lip of the osseous spiral lamina on the side of the modiolus and the crest of the spiral ligament of the cochlea. *Syn:* basilar fibers.

strio-   *See* striato-.

striola (striole) /stri-o´lah, stri-ōl´/, EAR   single, curving plane in the macula utriculi, toward which all the hair cells are oriented. When deflected toward the striola, the hair cells are stimulated; when deflected away from the striola, they are inhibited.

striosomes, CEREBRUM   irregularly shaped, ovoid bodies in the striatum, which are shown by histochemical techniques to be cholinesterase-poor.

strip, motor, CEREBRUM   motor area (area 4) in the precentral gyrus of the frontal lobe and in the anterior part of the paracentral lobule.

strip, sensory, CEREBRUM   somesthetic area (areas 3, 1, and 2) in the postcentral gyrus of the parietal lobe and in the posterior part of the paracentral lobule.

stripe   *See* stria.

structure, paranuclear /par-ah-noo´kle-ar/   small, argyrophilic mass, hemispherical or concavoconvex in shape, attached to the nucleolus in the nucleus of nerve cells. Its function is unknown.

subarach´noid   pertaining to the space between the arachnoid and pia mater, which contains cerebrospinal fluid, nerve roots, and blood vessels.

subcommis´sural (subcommissu´ral)   below a commissure, usually the anterior commissure. *See also* organ, subcommissural.

subdu´ral   pertaining to the subdural space between the dura mater and the arachnoid.

subiculum /soo-bik´u-lum/ [*pl.* **subicula**; *adj.* **subicular**], CEREBRUM, [L. dim. of *subex* support]   5-layered cortex of the hippocampal formation, located on the underside of the hippocampal fissure, apposed to the dentate gyrus (Fig. C-7). On one side is the prosubiculum, a transitional area between the subiculum and the cornu ammonis. On the other side the presubiculum lies between it and the entorhinal cortex of the parahippocampal gyrus. The transitional cortex between the subiculum and presubiculum is sometimes designated the parasubiculum.

subnuc´leus caudal´is, MAINLY MEDULLA   caudalmost subdivision of the spinal nucleus of the trigeminal nerve in the closed medulla and upper cervical spinal cord (Fig. T-2). It resembles the dorsal horn in appearance.

subnucleus interpolar´is, MEDULLA   middle subdivision of the spinal nucleus of the trigeminal nerve, located approximately at the level of the middle third of the inferior olive.

subnucleus rostral´is, PONS, MEDULLA   most rostral subdivision of the spinal nucleus of the trigeminal nerve at upper medullar and lower pontine levels.

substance, chromatophil´ic [substantia chromatophilica, NA]   cytoplasmic bodies which contain RNA and iron, and which correspond to the lamellated sacs of rough endoplasmic reticulum (RER) visible at the electron microscopic level. These organelles, of various sizes, are present in the perikaryon of nerve cell bodies, exclusive of the axon hillock, particularly in the large motor neurons of motor nuclei of the brain stem and ventral horn. In unipolar ganglion cells this material is finely granular. *Syn:* Nissl or tigroid bodies, granules or substance. *See also* Nissl; tigroid.

substance, fundamental gray, HYPOTHALAMUS   *See* nucleus, hypothalamic, anterior.

substance P (P for preparation)   a neuropeptide present in small dorsal root ganglion cells and in high concentrations in the superficial layers of the dorsal horn (lamina I and the outer part of lamina II). Presumably it is derived from the axonal terminations of primary afferent nociceptors and is the neurotransmitter for pain. It is also distributed widely in other locations throughout the CNS and PNS, including the substantia nigra and median eminence, and clearly serves multiple physiological functions. *See also* neurotransmitters.

substance, perforated, anterior [substantia perforata anterior (rostralis), NA], CEREBRUM   area between and posterior to the medial and lateral olfactory striae and bounded caudally by the diagonal band of Broca and the optic tract, and includes the ventral pallidum and ventral striatum. The area was so named because of the many small blood vessels that perforate the brain in this region (Fig. C-3C). In animals in which the olfactory system is large this area forms an elevation on the surface and is designated olfactory tubercle. *Syn:* anterior perforated space or area; olfactory area. *See also* trigone, olfactory.

substance, perforated, posterior [substantia perforata posterior (interpeduncularis), NA], MIDBRAIN   floor of the interpeduncular fossa, between the bases of the two cerebral peduncles, through which many small blood vessels, including the posteromedial central arteries, enter the diencephalon (Fig. C-5) and the median arteries of the brain stem enter the rostral midbrain tegmentum.

substance, retic´ular   *See* formation, reticular.

substance, transmit´ter   *See* neurotransmitters.

substance, vis´ceral, sec´ondary [substantia visceralis secundaria, NA], CORD   dorsal horn gray located just dorsal to the lateral horn in cord segments T1-L3 (Fig.

N-6), for relay of impulses from the viscera to nearby visceral motor nuclei and, by way of a bilateral multisynaptic ascending neuron chain (secondary ascending visceral tract), to higher centers.

substan´tia al´ba [NA] [L. *substantia* substance; *alba* white]   white matter of the CNS.

substantia ferrugin´ea, PONS, [L. *ferrugineus* rusty, rust-colored]   *See* locus coeruleus.

substantia gelatino´sa [NA], CORD   nucleus composed of small, closely packed cells in the outer part of the dorsal horn throughout the spinal cord and continuous with the subnucleus caudalis of the medulla, Rexed's lamina II (Fig. N-6). *Syn:* substantia gelatinosa of Rolando.

substantia grisea /gre´zĭ-ah/ [NA] [L. *griseus* gray]   gray matter of the CNS.

substantia innominat´a (of Reichert), CEREBRUM   area in the basal forebrain, adjacent to and including part of the anterior perforated substance. Its caudal part includes the ventral striatum in the sublenticular gray and its rostral part extends forward into the subcommissural region. In its ventral (more superficial) portion is the basal nucleus (of Meynert) consisting of large, deeply staining cells, degeneration of which is thought to underlie the mental deterioration in Alzheimer's disease. *See also* nucleus, basal (of Meynert).

substantia interme´dia central´is [NA], CORD   gray matter surrounding the central canal of the spinal cord; Rexed's lamina 10. *Syn:* dorsal and ventral gray commissures.

substantia intermedia lateral´is [NA], CORD   gray matter of the spinal cord, continuous medially with the substantia intermedia centralis, and extending laterally between the ventral and dorsal horns to include the lateral horn.

substantia ni´gra [NA], MAINLY MIDBRAIN   nucleus of pigmented nerve cells in the dorsal part of the basis pedunculi of the midbrain (Fig. P-1) and in the caudal part of the ventral thalamus (Fig. N-8). It consists of a pars reticulata composed of scattered cells separated by fiber strands, a pars compacta, more dorsally placed, the cells of which are closely packed and are significantly larger than those in other parts, and a small pars lateralis, the oldest part, in the rostral lateral part of the nucleus. In Parkinson's disease insufficient dopamine is released by nigrostriate fibers from cells in the pars compacta. *Syn:* Soemmering's substance.

substantia reticular´is [NA], BRAIN STEM, UPPER CORD   *See* formation, reticular.

subthalamus, DIENCEPHALON   *See* thalamus, ventral.

sulcus /sul´kus/ [NA] [*pl.* **sulci** /sul´sĭ/] [L. groove or furrow]   groove on the surface of the brain or spinal cord. *See also* fissure.

sulcus, anterolateral, MEDULLA, CORD   *See* sulcus, ventrolateral.

sulcus, axial /ak´sĭ-al/, CEREBRUM   any sulcus, such as the calcarine, which develops within the long axis of a developing cortical area and so is located within a functional area.

sulcus, bas´ilar [sulcus basilaris, NA], PONS   median groove on the ventral surface of the pons, for the basilar artery.

sulcus, bulbopon´tine [sulcus bulbopontinus, NA], PONS, MEDULLA   transverse sulcus on the ventral surface of the brain stem under the lowest crossing fibers of the pons, marking the boundary between the medulla oblongata and the pons. *Syn:* inferior pontine sulcus.

sulcus, calcarine /kal´car-in/ [sulcus calcarinus, NA], CEREBRUM   deep groove extending across the medial surface of the occipital lobe and slightly onto the lateral surface (Fig. C-3B). The lips of the calcarine sulcus constitute the visual cortex, Brodmann's area 17. The tissue underlying this sulcus forms a corresponding elevation on the ventricular surface, the calcar avis.

sulcus, callosal /kah-lo ´sal/, CEREBRUM   *See* sulcus (of the) corpus callosum.

sulcus, callosomar ´ginal, CEREBRUM   *See* sulcus, cingulate.

sulcus, central [sulcus centralis, NA], CEREBRUM   sulcus mostly on the lateral surface of the cerebral hemisphere, about midway between the frontal and occipital poles and which separates the frontal and parietal lobes. On the lateral surface it extends anteriorly and inferiorly to a point just above, but not joining, the lateral sulcus (Fig. C-3A,B). Its upper end extends a short distance into the paracentral lobule on the medial surface of the hemisphere. *Syn:* fissure of Rolando.

sulcus, central, of the insula [sulcus centralis insulae, NA], CEREBRUM   sulcus on the surface of the insula which separates the short gyri anterosuperiorly from the long gyri posteroinferiorly.

sulcus, cingulate /sing ´gu-lāt/ [sulcus cinguli (cingulatus), NA], CEREBRUM   sulcus on the medial surface of the cerebrum, separating the cingulate from the medial frontal gyrus and continuous posteriorly with the marginal sulcus (Fig. C-3B). *Syn:* callosomarginal or subfrontal sulcus.

sulcus, circular, of the insula /sir ´ku-lar/ [sulcus circularis insulae, NA], CEREBRUM   sulcus at the margin of the insula, along the line of reflection between the insula and the overlying opercula. *Syn:* sulcus limitans insulae.

sulcus, collat ´eral [sulcus collateralis, NA], CEREBRUM   sulcus on the inferior surface of the cerebrum between the lingual gyrus of the occipital lobe and the parahippocampal gyrus of the temporal lobe medially and the medial occipitotemporal gyrus laterally. Anteriorly it is sometimes continuous with the rhinal sulcus (Fig. C-3B,C). *Syn:* fourth temporal sulcus.

sulcus, complete, CEREBRUM   any cerebral sulcus deep enough that the tissue beneath it forms a corresponding eminence on the ventricular surface, such as the calcarine sulcus and the hippocampal sulcus, or which involves the entire thickness of the cerebral wall, such as the choroid fissure of the cerebrum. *Syn:* total fissure.

sulcus (of the) corpus callosum [sulcus corporis callosi, NA], CEREBRUM   sulcus on the medial surface of the cerebral hemisphere, separating the corpus callosum from the overlying cingulate gyrus (Fig. C-3B). *Syn:* callosal sulcus.

sulcus, dorsolateral (posterolateral) [sulcus dorsolateralis (posterolateralis), NA], MEDULLA, CORD   shallow sulcus on the dorsolateral surface of the spinal cord along the line of attachment of the dorsal roots, and extending rostrally on to the medulla along the lateral margin of the fasciculus cuneatus.

sulcus, fimbrioden ´tate, CEREBRUM   groove on the medial surface of the temporal lobe between the fimbria and the dentate gyrus (Fig. C-7).

sulcus, frontal, inferior [sulcus frontalis inferior, NA], CEREBRUM   sulcus on the lateral surface of the frontal lobe, between the middle frontal gyrus above and the inferior frontal gyrus below (Fig. C-3A).

sulcus, frontal, middle, CEREBRUM   inconstant sulcus on the lateral surface of the frontal lobe, which, in some brains, divides the middle frontal gyrus into superior and inferior parts.

sulcus, frontal, superior [sulcus frontalis superior, NA], CEREBRUM   sulcus on the lateral surface of the frontal lobe, between the superior frontal gyrus above and the middle frontal gyrus below (Fig. C-3A).

sulcus, haben ´ular [sulcus habenulae (habenularis), NA], DIENCEPHALON   short sulcus on the wall of the third ventricle, which separates the habenula of the epithalamus from the dorsal thalamus.

sulcus, hemispher´ic, FOREBRAIN   shallow circular furrow on the surface of the developing brain, which separates the telencephalon from the diencephalon.

sulcus, hippocamp´al [sulcus hippocampi (hippocampalis), NA], CEREBRUM   groove on the medial surface of the temporal lobe, dorsomedial to the parahippocampal gyrus between the dentate gyrus and the subiculum (Fig. C-7).

sulcus, hypothalam´ic [sulcus hypothalamicus, NA], DIENCEPHALON   sulcus on the wall of the third ventricle extending from the interventricular foramen to the cerebral aqueduct and separating the dorsal thalamus dorsally from the hypothalamus ventrally (Fig. V-5).   From its rostral part a branch extends forward into the hypothalamus, toward the optic chiasm. *Syn:* sulcus of Monro.

sulcus, incomplete, CEREBRUM   any shallow sulcus on the surface of the cerebral hemisphere that is not deep enough to form an eminence on the wall of the lateral ventricle.

sulcus, intermediate, dorsal (posterior) [sulcus intermedius dorsalis (posterior), NA], MEDULLA, CORD   sulcus on each side of the dorsal surface of the closed medulla and spinal cord, separating the gracile fasciculus and tubercle from the cuneate fasciculus and tubercle.

sulcus, intrapari´etal [sulcus intraparietalis, NA], CEREBRUM   sulcus on the lateral surface of the parietal lobe, between the superior parietal and inferior parietal lobules (Fig. C-3A).   Because the sulcus is located *within* the parietal lobe, the term *interparietal*, although sometimes used, is a poor choice. *Syn:* Turner's sulcus.

sulcus, lateral [sulcus lateralis, NA], CEREBRUM   horizontally placed groove on the lateral surface of the cerebrum separating the frontal and parietal lobes above from the temporal lobe below.   Two anterior branches extend into the inferior frontal gyrus.   The anterior horizontal ramus separates the orbital and triangular portions of the gyrus and the anterior ascending ramus separates the triangular and opercular portions.   A posterior ramus turns upward for a short distance into the parieto-occipital area (Fig. C-3A). *Syn:* fissure of Sylvius. *See also* Sylvius, Franciscus; triangle, Sylvian; Fig. A-3.

sulcus lim´itans [NA]   shallow groove on the lateral wall on either side of the neural canal, between the alar and basal plates.   This sulcus is retained in the adult brain as a groove on the floor of the fourth ventricle between the medial eminence medially and the vestibular area laterally (Fig. V-4).

sulcus limitans in´sulae, CEREBRUM   *See* sulcus, circular, of the insula.

sulcus, limiting, CEREBRUM   any sulcus which marks the boundary of a functional area.

sulcus, lunate /loo´nāt/ [sulcus lunatus, NA], CEREBRUM   half-moon-shaped sulcus on the lateral surface of the occipital lobe, capping the tip of the calcarine fissure. It is present in some subhuman primate brains and inconstant in man.   When present it marks the limit of the visual cortex. *Syn:* simian fissure; Affenspalte.

sulcus, marginal, CEREBRUM   branch of the cingulate sulcus separating the paracentral lobule from the precuneus on the medial surface of the parietal lobe (Fig. C-3B).

sulcus, median [sulcus medianus, NA], PONS, MEDULLA   sulcus along the median plane, extending the full length of the floor of the fourth ventricle, and which separates the two halves of the rhomboid fossa (Fig. V-4).

sulcus, median, dorsal (posterior) [sulcus medianus dorsalis (posterior), NA], MEDULLA, CORD   shallow sulcus along the mid-dorsal surface of the closed medulla and spinal cord. *Syn:* posteromedian sulcus.

sulcus, median, ventral, MEDULLA, CORD   *See* fissure, median, ventral.

sulcus, mesencephalic, lateral /mez-en-sĕ-fal´ik/, MIDBRAIN   sulcus on the lateral surface of the midbrain, which separates the tegmentum from the base of the cerebral peduncle.

sulcus, occip´ital, lateral, CEREBRUM   inconstant sulcus, horizontally placed on the lateral surface of the occipital lobe. It separates the somewhat variable lateral occipital gyri into superior and inferior groups.

sulcus, occipital, transverse [sulcus occipitalis transversus, NA], CEREBRUM   inconstant sulcus on the superior, lateral surface of the occipital lobe, posterior to the upper end of the parieto-occipital sulcus.

sulcus, occipitopari´etal, CEREBRUM   *See* sulcus, parieto-occipital.

sulcus, occipitotem´poral [sulcus occipitotemporalis, NA], CEREBRUM   sulcus on the inferior surface of the temporal lobe which separates the lateral and medial occipitotemporal gyri (Fig. C-3B,C). *Syn:* formerly inferior temporal sulcus; third temporal sulcus.

sulcus, oculomo´tor, MIDBRAIN   sulcus medial to the base of the cerebral peduncle, near the median plane at the base of the interpeduncular fossa, from which the oculomotor nerve leaves the midbrain.

sulcus, olfac´tory [sulcus olfactorius, NA], CEREBRUM   sulcus on the orbital surface of the frontal lobe between the gyrus rectus medially and the orbital gyri laterally and along which the olfactory bulb and stalk are located (Fig. C-3C).

sulcus, oper´culated, CEREBRUM   any sulcus which separates two structurally different surface areas of cortex but which contains within its depth a third, submerged, intervening type.

sulci, or´bital [sulci orbitales, NA], CEREBRUM   sulci in the form of an H or X on the ventral (orbital) surface of the frontal lobe, which divide the orbital gyri into anterior, medial, posterior, and lateral parts (Fig. C-3C).

sulcus, paracen´tral, CEREBRUM   sulcus on the medial surface of the frontal lobe, separating the paracentral lobule and the medial frontal gyrus (Fig. C-3B).

sulcus, parolfac´tory, anterior, CEREBRUM   small sulcus on the medial surface of the frontal lobe, marking the anterior boundary of the parolfactory area (Fig. C-3B).

sulcus, parolfactory, posterior, CEREBRUM   sulcus on the medial surface of the frontal lobe, between the anterior and the posterior parolfactory gyri (Fig. C-3B).

sulcus, pari´eto-occip´ital [sulcus parieto-occipitalis, NA], CEREBRUM   deep sulcus on the medial surface of the cerebral hemisphere, between the occipital and parietal lobes and extending from the dorsal surface to the calcarine fissure just posterior to the corpus callosum (Fig. C-3A,B). *Syn:* occipitoparietal sulcus.

sulcus, pon´tine, inferior, PONS, MEDULLA   *See* sulcus, bulbopontine.

sulcus, pontine, superior, MIDBRAIN, PONS   transverse sulcus on the ventral surface of the brain stem above the uppermost crossing fibers of the pons, marking the boundary between the pons and midbrain.

sulcus, postcen´tral [sulcus postcentralis, NA], CEREBRUM   sulcus on the lateral surface of the parietal lobe, which roughly parallels the central sulcus and which separates the postcentral gyrus anteriorly from the superior and inferior parietal lobules posteriorly (Fig. C-3A).

sulcus, posterolateral [sulcus posterolateralis (dorsolateralis), NA], MEDULLA, CORD   *See* sulcus, dorsolateral.

sulcus, posteromedian, MEDULLA, CORD   *See* sulcus, median, dorsal.

sulcus, postol´ivary [sulcus retro-olivaris, NA], MEDULLA   sulcus dorsal to the olive on the ventrolateral surface of the medulla.

sulcus, precen´tral [sulcus precentralis, NA], CEREBRUM   sulcus on the lateral surface of the frontal lobe, which roughly parallels the central sulcus and which separates the precentral gyrus posteriorly from the superior, middle, and inferior frontal gyri anteriorly (Fig. C-3A).

sulcus, preol´ivary, MEDULLA   sulcus separating the olive and the pyramid on the ventrolateral surface of the medulla and through which the rootlets of the hypoglossal nerve emerge. It is the rostral continuation of the ventrolateral sulcus of the spinal cord.

sulcus, ret´ro-ol´ivary [sulcus retro-olivaris, NA], MEDULLA   *See* sulcus, postolivary.

sulcus, rhinal /ri´nal/ [sulcus rhinalis, NA], CEREBRUM   sulcus on the ventromedial surface of the temporal lobe, between the uncus and the anterior part of the parahippocampal gyrus medially and the anterior part of the medial occipitotemporal gyrus laterally. Sometimes continuous with the collateral sulcus, it marks the lateral limit of the piriform lobe cortex and the border in this region between the rhinencephalon and neocortex. (Fig. C-3B,C.)

sulcus, scleral /skler´al/ [sulcus sclerae, NA], EYE   slight furrow along the corneoscleral junction of the eye.

sulcus, semicir´cular, FOREBRAIN   sulcus along the lateral margin of the ventricular surface of the dorsal thalamus, separating the thalamus medially from the caudate nucleus laterally. The terminal vein (superior thalamostriate vein) and the stria terminalis (also called stria semicircularis) are located along this sulcus. *Syn:* terminal sulcus.

sulcus, spiral, external [sulcus spiralis externus, NA], EAR   groove in the cochlear duct between the spiral prominence and the spiral organ of the cochlea.

sulcus (tunnel), spiral, internal [sulcus spiralis internus, NA], EAR   groove in the cochlear duct between the vestibular and the tympanic lips of the spiral limbus on one side and the spiral organ on the other.

sulcus, subfron´tal, CEREBRUM   *See* sulcus, cingulate.

sulcus, subpari´etal [sulcus subparietalis, NA], CEREBRUM   posterior continuation of the cingulate sulcus, an inconstant sulcus on the medial surface of the parietal lobe. When present it separates the posterior part of the cingulate gyrus and the precuneus.

sulcus, tem´poral, first, CEREBRUM   old term for the superior temporal sulcus.

sulcus, temporal, fourth, CEREBRUM   old term for the collateral sulcus.

sulcus, temporal, inferior [sulcus temporalis inferior, NA], CEREBRUM   **1.** sulcus on the lateral surface of the temporal lobe between the middle and the inferior temporal gyri (Fig. C-3A). *Syn:* formerly called middle temporal sulcus; second temporal sulcus.

2. old term for the occipitotemporal sulcus on the inferior (ventral) surface of the temporal lobe.

sulcus, temporal, second, CEREBRUM   old term for the inferior temporal sulcus on the lateral surface of the temporal lobe, also formerly called middle temporal sulcus.

sulcus, temporal, superior [sulcus temporalis superior, NA], CEREBRUM   sulcus on the lateral surface of the temporal lobe, between the superior temporal gyrus above and the middle temporal gyrus below (Fig. C-3A). *Syn:* first temporal sulcus.

sulcus, temporal, third, CEREBRUM   old term for the occipitotemporal sulcus, on the ventral (inferior) surface of the temporal lobe, also formerly called inferior temporal sulcus.

sulci, temporal, transverse [sulci temporales transversi, NA], CEREBRUM   sulci on the superior surface of the temporal lobe, within the lateral sulcus. They separate the two transverse temporal gyri from each other and from adjoining cortex.

sulcus, ter´minal, FOREBRAIN   *See* sulcus, semicircular.

sulcus, ventrolateral (anterolateral) [sulcus ventrolateralis (anterolateralis), NA], MEDULLA, CORD   shallow sulcus along the ventrolateral surface of the spinal cord, from which the ventral roots arise, and its rostral continuation on the surface of the medulla, caudal to the olive. It is continuous with the preolivary sulcus, from which the fascicles of the hypoglossal nerve arise.

suprasel´lar   above the sella turcica.

supraspi´nal   above the spinal cord level.

supratentor´ial   above the tentorium cerebelli. The supratentorial part of the brain comprises the cerebral hemispheres and the diencephalon.

surround, EYE   outer, peripheral area around the central zone of the receptive field of a retinal ganglion cell. Stimulation of this part tends to inhibit activity of the central zone which it surrounds. *See also* field, receptive.

SVA   special visceral afferent.

SVE   special visceral efferent.

Sydenham, Thomas (1624-1689)   English physician who first described many diseases. *Sydenham's chorea,* which he called St. Vitus' dance, is an acute chorea of childhood, usually associated with rheumatic fever.

Sylvius, Franciscus (Latin form of François Dubois, de la Bŏe) (1614-1672)   Dutch physician and anatomist. The *fissure of Sylvius* (1641) is the lateral sulcus of the cerebrum. Also named for their association with the Sylvian fissure (lateral sulcus) are the following: The *Sylvian fossa* is a depression on the lateral surface of the developing cerebral hemisphere in the region overlying the area destined to become the insula and, in the adult, the space covered by the opercula. The *Sylvian triangle* (Fig. A-3) is the space in the Sylvian fossa containing the branches of the middle cerebral artery between the insula and the overlying opercula, as revealed by cerebral angiography. The images of the arterial branches as they emerge onto the surface of the hemisphere reveal the position of the lateral sulcus. The upper and lower limits of the triangle are indicated by the sharp turns of the branches along the circular sulcus. The anterior border of the triangle extends from the undivided middle cerebral artery at the limen insulae upward to the first turn of its most anterior opercular branch. Posteriorly the triangle extends to the *Sylvian point,* the posterior limit of the lateral sulcus where the last branches of the middle cerebral artery emerge from the sulcus (Schlesinger, '53). *See also* artery, cerebral, middle.

Sylvius, Jacobus (Latin form of Jacques Dubois) (1478-1555)   French anatomist. The *aqueduct of Sylvius* (1555) is the cerebral aqueduct.

sympathet´ic [Gr. *syn* with; *pathos* suffering]   **1.** pertaining to that division of the ANS whose preganglionic neurons arise in the thoracic and upper lumbar spinal cord segments; the thoracolumbar subdivision of the ANS. *Syn:* orthosympathetic. **2.** old term for autonomic.

sympathetic af´ferent   pertaining to the general visceral afferent fibers which accompany the fibers of the sympathetic division of the ANS.

synapse /sin´aps/ [synapsis, NA] [*v.* **synapse**] [Gr. *syn* together; *haptein* to clasp]   term coined by Sherrington (1897) for the area of close contact between one neuron and another or between a neuron and an effector organ, and specialized for the transmission of an impulse. Endings on neurons are classified according to the parts of the neurons in contact, as: axodendritic (Type I, axon to dendrite); axosomatic (Type II, axon to cell body); axoaxonic (axon to axon, usually ending on an axon hillock, initial axon segment, or close to the axonal termination); and dendrodendritic (dendrite to dendrite). Synapses between adjacent perikarya have also been found. Axodendritic synapses are thought to be excitatory and axosomatic or axoaxonic to be inhibitory. *See also* cleft, synaptic; synaptosome; vesicle, presynaptic.

synaptosome /sin-ap´to-sōm/   pertaining to all the morphologic elements of a synaptic nerve ending: the pre- and postsynaptic components and the intervening cleft material.

syndrome, lateral medullary   disorder resulting from injury in the dorsolateral part of the medulla, usually from infarction of the medullary branches of the posterior inferior cerebellar artery or its parent vessel, the vertebral artery. There is a loss of pain and temperature sense from the contralateral side of the body from injury to the lateral spinothalamic tract. Other signs and symptoms, all on the side of the lesion, include: loss of pain and temperature sense of the face from injury to the spinal tract of V; paralysis of the palate, pharynx, larynx, and upper esophageal muscles, causing dysphagia, dysphonia, and a homolateral loss of the gag reflex from injury to the nucleus ambiguus or its vagus nerve fibers; also a Horner's syndrome, i.e., miosis, ptosis, and anhidrosis from injury to the lateral tecto-tegmentospinal and lateral reticulospinal tracts. There may also be some ataxia if there is injury of the inferior cerebellar peduncle. *Syn:* Wallenberg's syndrome; syndrome of the posterior inferior cerebellar artery.

syndrome, thalamic   disorder consisting of spontaneous paroxysms of intense pain and marked abnormalities in general sensation, involving injury to neurons that transmit pain. Although it may occur following lesions in other parts of the brain, it ordinarily follows thrombosis of a posterolateral central artery, with injury of the ventral posterior nucleus of the dorsal thalamus and its related tracts.

synencephalon, DIENCEPHALON, [Gr. *syn* together; *enkephalos* brain]   caudal part of the diencephalon in which the prerubrum and the pretectum develop.

syringobulbia /sir-ing-go-bul´bī-ah/ [Gr. *syrinx* a tube]   malformation in which there is cavitation (usually slitlike rather than tubular) of the medulla, frequently associated with syringomyelia.

syringocele /sir-ing´go-sēl/, MEDULLA, CORD   *See* canal, central.

syringomye´lia [Gr. *myelos* marrow, hence spinal cord]   malformation in which there is tubular cavitation of the spinal cord extending, sometimes, over many segments. It usually results from such phenomena as trauma, ischemia, tumor, or arachnoiditis. Differentiation from hydromyelia is not always clear.

system, autonomic nervous   *See* system, nervous, autonomic.

system, central nervous   *See* system, nervous, central.

system, centrencephal´ic   central core of brain tissue extending from the spinal cord through the reticular and tegmental portions of the brain stem to the diencephalon, and consisting of multisynaptic ascending and descending neuron chains. It is regarded by some as an integrating system related to arousal, facilitation, and suppression. *See also* formation, reticular.

system, extrapyram´idal   multisynaptic motor system, so named because the pathways do not pass through the pyramids of the medulla. The extrapyramidal system, with connections in the basal ganglia, dorsal thalamus, and ventral thalamus, acts with the pyramidal tract (and cerebellum) in the control of movement and posture. Extrapyramidal disorders include abnormalities of muscle tone and posture, such as dystonia and rigidity, and involuntary movements, such as tremor, chorea, athetosis, and ballism.

system, hypothalamospi´nal   multisynaptic, descending neuron chain from the hypothalamus, mainly its posterior nucleus, with synapses in various tegmental nuclei of the brain stem, for relay to autonomic nuclei of the thoracolumbar spinal cord, by way of the medial, ventral, lateral, and perhaps other reticulospinal tracts. This system is concerned with hypothalamic regulation of the sympathetic division of the ANS. Some fibers from the paraventricular and dorsomedial hypothalamic nuclei are thought to go directly to the spinal cord. *See also* Fig. N-7.

system, lemniscal /lem-nis´kal/   pathways concerned with the transmission of impulses for general somatic sensibility, including: the medial lemniscus, spinal lemniscus (lateral and ventral spinothalamic tracts), and trigeminal lemnisci (dorsal and ventral secondary ascending trigeminal tracts).

system, lim´bic, FOREBRAIN   limbic lobe of the cerebrum and the subcortical nuclei, including parts of the hypothalamus, epithalamus, dorsal thalamus, and possibly the midbrain with which it is related anatomically and functionally. Although the functions of this system are not clearly established, it is generally believed to be related to emotional expression and the control of visceromotor activity. *For a review of this subject, see* Swanson ('87).

system, ner´vous, autonom´ic (ANS) [systema nervosum autonomicum, NA] those neurons which regulate the contraction of smooth and cardiac muscle and the secretion of glands, by way of the general visceral efferent component of cranial and spinal nerves. Its two divisions, parasympathetic and sympathetic, provide double innervation to most organs by way of a two-neuron chain. The first neuron has its cell of origin in the brain or spinal cord and the second in an autonomic ganglion (Fig. S-3, Table S-1). *Syn:* involuntary nervous system.

system, nervous, central (CNS) [systema nervosum centrale, NA]   brain and spinal cord.

system, nervous, peripheral (PNS) [systema nervosum periphericum, NA]   the nerves and ganglia.

system, retic´ular ac´tivating (RAS)   multisynaptic ascending system which, when activated, serves to arouse or to maintain a state of arousal.

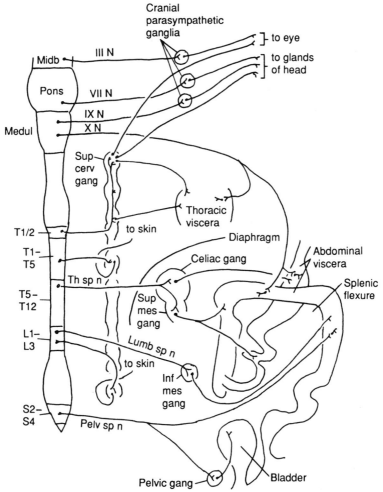

Fig. S-3. Autonomic nervous system, showing the distribution of preganglionic parasympathetic neurons to terminal ganglia, from the brain, for relay to the smooth
muscle and glands of the head, and the thoracic and abdominal viscera including the
colon as far as the splenic flexure and from the sacral spinal cord, for relay to the
descending colon and pelvic organs; and sympathetic neurons from spinal cord
segments T1-L3 to the ganglia of the sympathetic trunk for relay to viscera of the
head, thorax, and skin and, via the splanchnic nerves, to prevertebral ganglia (celiac,
superior and inferior mesenteric ganglia) for relay to the abdominal and pelvic viscera.
Inf mes gang-inferior mesenteric ganglion; Lumb sp n-lumbar splanchnic nerve; Medul-
medulla; Midb-midbrain; Pelv sp n-pelvic splanchnic nerve; Sup cerv gang-superior
cervical ganglion; Sup mes gang-superior mesenteric ganglion; Th sp n-thoracic
splanchnic nerve.

Table S-1
Table of Autonomic Functions

Organ	Sympathetic	Parasympathetic
Skin	Vasoconstriction, secretory to sweat and sebaceous glands, motor to piloerector muscles	Vasodilation (spinal parasympathetic)
Skeletal muscles	Vasodilation?	
Eye	Dilation of pupil, maintenance of open eye	Constriction of pupil, acccommodation of lens
Salivary glands	Vasoconstriction, thick secretion in small amount, low in enzymes	Vasodilation, thin copious secretion, rich in enzymes
Heart	Vasodilation?, increase rate and contractile force of heart	Vasoconstriction?, decrease rate and contractile force of heart
Lungs and bronchi	Vasodilation, dilate bronchioles	Close arterial sphincters, constrict bronchioles
Gastro-intestinal tract	Vasoconstriction?, decrease peristalsis, constrict sphincters	Vasodilation?, increase peristalsis, relax sphincters, increase glandular secretion
Bladder	Vasoconstriction	Relax sphincter, contract detrusor muscle (empty bladder)
Reproduc-tive system	Vasoconstriction in gonads, ejaculation in male	Erection in male

t

T   thoracic.

tac´tile   pertaining to the sense of touch.

taenia /te´nĭ-ah/   *See* tenia.

tanycyte /tan´is-īt/   variety of ependymal cell derived from spongioblasts of the developing nervous system. Such cells retain their embryological characteristics throughout life. They have processes which extend from the ventricular surface to the pial surface, especially in areas where the distance is not great. They may be capable of forming additional ependymal cells and perhaps have other functions. *Syn:* ependymoglial cell; ependymal astrocyte.

tape´tum [NA], CEREBRUM, [L. *tapete* carpet or tapestry]   fibers of the corpus callosum that spread laterally, forming a roof over the inferior horn of the lateral ventricle. *Syn:* Fielding's membrane.

tapetum lucidum /loo´sid-um/ [NA], EYE, [L. *lucidus* clear]   highly reflective iridescent layer located between the vascular layer and the choriocapillary layer in the choroid of the eye of many animals but not of man.

Tapia (Garcia Tapia), Antonio (1875-1950)   Spanish otolaryngologist. *Tapia's syndrome* is a unilateral paralysis of the palate, pharynx, larynx, and tongue and is attributed to a lesion in the medulla involving the hypoglossal nucleus and nucleus ambiguus, or to an extramedullary lesion of the hypoglossal and vagal nerves high in the neck.

Tarin, Pierre (ca. 1725-1761)   French anatomist. *Tarin's fascia* is the dentate gyrus. The *fossa of Tarin* is the interpeduncular fossa.

Tawara, K. Sunao (1873-1938)   Japanese pathologist. The *node of Tawara* or *Aschoff-Tawara* is the atrioventricular node.

Tay, Warren (1843-1927)   English ophthalmologist. In 1881 he described the ocular manifestations in what has become known as *Tay-Sachs disease. See also* Sachs.

tears, crocodile   excessive lacrimation associated with salivation during eating, in patients with faulty recovery from peripheral facial paralysis.

tec´tum [tectum mesencephali, NA], ᴍɪᴅʙʀᴀɪɴ, [L. *tectum* roof]   that part of the midbrain dorsal to a frontal plane through the cerebral aqueduct and comprising the superior and inferior colliculi (Fig. P-1). *Syn:* quadrigeminal plate. *See also* corpora quadrigemina.

tectum, op´tic, ᴍɪᴅʙʀᴀɪɴ   the two superior colliculi.

teeth, au´ditory (of Huschke) [dentes acustici, NA], ᴇᴀʀ   small ridges on the vestibular lip of the spiral limbus of the cochlea.

teg´men tym´pani [NA], ᴇᴀʀ, [L. *tegmen* cover; Gr. *tympanon* drum]   thin layer of bone, part of the petrous part of the temporal bone, forming the roof of the middle ear.

tegmen ventric´uli quar´ti [NA], ᴘᴏɴs, ᴍᴇᴅᴜʟʟᴀ   the anterior and posterior medullary vela, rostral and caudal to the cerebellum, forming a roof over the rostral and caudal parts of the fourth ventricle. *See also* tela choroidea of the fourth ventricle.

tegmen´tum [NA], ᴍɪᴅʙʀᴀɪɴ, ᴘᴏɴs, [L. cover]   dorsal part of the cerebral peduncle of the midbrain between the cerebral aqueduct and tectum dorsally and the basis pedunculi ventrally (Fig. P-1), and the dorsal part of the pons between the fourth ventricle dorsally and the basis pontis ventrally.

te´la choroi´dea [NA] [L. *tela* web; Gr. *chorioeides* like a membrane]   layer of pia mater overlying the ependyma, or both layers which together form a thin membrane separating a part of the ventricular system and the subarachnoid space (Fig. V-5). From it the choroid plexus (capillaries and associated secretory epithelium) projects into the ventricle.

tela choroidea of the fourth ventricle [tela choroidea ventriculi quarti, NA], ᴍᴇᴅᴜʟʟᴀ   pial covering overlying the posterior medullary velum, or both layers, which together constitute a thin membranous roof over the caudal part of the fourth ventricle. On each side vessels of the choroid plexus project into the ventricle.

tela choroidea of the lateral ventricle, ᴄᴇʀᴇʙʀᴜᴍ   pial covering of the ependyma, or both layers, which constitute a thin membrane along the choroid fissure of the cerebrum, separating the inferior horn, collateral trigone, and body of the lateral ventricle from the subarachnoid space, and from which the choroid plexus projects into the ventricle. In the body of the lateral ventricle it is attached medially to the fornix and laterally to the stria terminalis or along the dorsal surface of the dorsal thalamus. In the inferior horn it is attached inferiorly to the fimbria and superiorly along the stria terminalis.

tela choroidea of the third ventricle [tela choroidea ventriculi tertii, NA], ᴅɪᴇɴᴄᴇᴘʜᴀʟᴏɴ   layer of pia mater overlying the ependymal roof of the third ventricle, or both layers. It is attached along the stria medullaris thalami of both sides, and from it a small, double choroid plexus projects into the ventricle (Fig. V-5).

telencephalon /tel-en-sef´al-on/, ғᴏʀᴇʙʀᴀɪɴ, [Gr. *telos* end; *enkephalos* brain]   most rostral subdivision of the embryonic brain, derived from the prosencephalon from which the cerebral hemispheres develop. *See also* cerebrum.

telencephalon im´par, ғᴏʀᴇʙʀᴀɪɴ, [L. *impar* unequal]   *See* telencephalon medium.

telencephalon medium, ғᴏʀᴇʙʀᴀɪɴ, [L. *medius* middle]   that area anterior to a plane from the base of the interventricular foramen to the upper border of the optic chiasm and adjacent to the anterior part of the third ventricle. It includes the area preoptica (now thought likely to be a diencephalic rather than a telencephalic derivative), the lamina terminalis, and, where present, the paraphysis. *Syn:*

telencephalon impar.

teloden´dron [NA] [Gr. *dendron* tree]   terminal branching of an axon. *Syn:* terminal arborization.

temp´oral   pertaining to the temporal bone or to the temporal lobe, its cortex or related structures.

te´nia (taenia) [Gr. *tainia* band or tape]   **1.** [NA], FOREBRAIN, MEDULLA   slight thickening along the line of attachment of the choroid plexus where a thin membrane merges with the substance of the brain.
2. band of nerve fibers.

tenia (taenia) acus´tica, MEDULLA   old term for the stria medullaris of the fourth ventricle; a misnomer, as it is not a part of the auditory system.

tenia (taenia) choroi´dea [NA], CEREBRUM   slight thickening of the tissue along the line of attachment of the choroid plexus to the stria terminalis in the body and inferior horn of the lateral ventricle. *See also* tenia (of the) fourth ventricle and tenia thalami.

tenia (taenia) diagonal´is, CEREBRUM   *See* band, diagonal (of Broca).

tenia (taenia) fim´briae, CEREBRUM   that part of the tenia fornicis along the line of attachment of the choroid plexus to the fimbria, in the inferior horn of the lateral ventricle.

tenia (taenia) for´nicis [NA], CEREBRUM   slight thickening of the tissue along the line of attachment of the choroid plexus to the fimbria-fornix in the inferior horn, collateral trigone, and body of the lateral ventricle.

tenia (taenia) (of the) fourth ventricle [tenia (taenia) ventriculi quarti, NA], MEDULLA   slight thickening of the tissue of the roof of the fourth ventricle, along the line of attachment of the choroid plexus of the fourth ventricle at the edge of the medulla. *Syn:* ligula. *See also* tenia choroidea.

tenia (taenia) semicircular´is, FOREBRAIN   *See* stria terminalis.

tenia (taenia) tec´ta, CEREBRUM   *See* stria, longitudinal, lateral.

tenia (taenia) thal´ami [NA], DIENCEPHALON   slight thickening of the tissue along the line of attachment of the choroid plexus of the third ventricle to the stria medullaris of the dorsal thalamus. *See also* tenia choroidea.

Tenon, Jacques René (1724-1816)   French ophthalmologist. *Tenon's capsule* is the fascia bulbi of the eye.

Tensilon   trademark for a solution of edrophonium chloride, a short-acting, anticholinesterase drug used in testing for myasthenia gravis.

tentor´ium cerebel´li [NA] [L. *tentorium* tent]   dural fold interposed between the cerebrum and the cerebellum and forming a roof over the posterior cranial fossa (Fig. F-1).

tetraple´gia   paralysis of all four limbs. *Syn:* quadriplegia.

thalamec´tomy   operation in which a part of the dorsal thalamus is excised.

thalamenceph´alon   that part of the diencephalon consisting particularly of the dorsal thalamus.

thal´amocele (thalamocoele)   *See* ventricle, third.

thal´amus, DIENCEPHALON [Gr. *thalamos* inner chamber, bedroom]   term used as a synonym for dorsal thalamus. *See also* thalamus, ventral.

thalamus, dorsal [thalamus dorsalis, NA], DIENCEPHALON   that part of the diencephalon located on either side of the third ventricle just above the hypothalamic sulcus and bounded laterally by the posterior limb of the internal capsule (Fig. C-1). It consists of a series of nuclear groups, separated from one another by thin layers of myelinated nerve fibers, the internal and external medullary laminae (Fig. N-8). *See also* nuclei, thalamic; metathalamus.

thalamus, op´tic, DIENCEPHALON   old term for dorsal thalamus.

thalamus, ventral [thalamus ventralis, NA], DIENCEPHALON   that part of the diencephalon located ventral to the dorsal thalamus and caudolateral to the hypothalamus, and consisting of the subthalamic nucleus, the zona incerta and nucleus of the field of Forel, the entopeduncular nucleus, and the rostral extensions of the red nucleus and substantia nigra (Fig. N-8). *Syn:* subthalamus. The ventral thalamus is not to be confused with the ventral nuclei of the dorsal thalamus.

theca /the´kah/ [L. case or sheath]   the meningeal sac of the spinal cord.

theca lenticular´is, CEREBRUM   innermost layer of fine fibers of the external capsule, on the outer surface of the putamen.

theory, neuron   *See* doctrine, neuron.

thermorecep´tor   receptor sensitive to warming of the skin which stops responding when the skin is cooled, or a receptor which does the opposite, firing when the skin is cooled and ceasing to fire when the skin is warmed.

thoracic (T)   pertaining to one or more of the 12 thoracic spinal cord segments, nerves, or vertebrae. *Syn:* dorsal.

thorns, dendrit´ic   *See* spines, dendritic.

TIA   transient ischemic attack.

ti´groid   pertaining to the granules in the cytoplasm of nerve cell bodies, chromatophilic substance, misnamed as tigers have stripes and not spots.

Tinel, Jules (1879-1952)   French neurologist who treated French casualties during World War I. He reported that when patients with peripheral nerve injuries noted a tingling sensation in the distribution of an injured peripheral nerve, it was indicative of regeneration of the injured fibers, *Tinel's sign* (1915). The same finding was also reported by Hoffmann for German soldiers in the same year.

tinni´tus   ringing in the ears; head noises; the perception of sound in the absence of an acoustic stimulus. It may be a ringing, whistling, buzzing, or roaring sound or may be more complex sounds and vary over time.

tomog´raphy [Gr. *tome* a cutting; *graphein* to write]   procedure whereby images of selected planes of the CNS or other internal organs are recorded.

    computerized axial tomography (CAT) or **computed tomography (CT)**   utilizes X-ray transmission data.

    single photon emission computerized tomography (SPECT) uses radioactive tracers, glucose or oxygen, tagged with a radioactive molecule, to measure the brain's metabolic function as it processes information and so reveals the location of metabolically active brain areas.

    positron emission tomography (PET), which detects positrons, is a similar but more powerful procedure. It also reveals the location of metabolically active brain areas, including those involved in thinking.

    magnetic resonance imaging (MRI)   procedure that uses strong magnets to detect minute radio signals given off by brain molecules, thus determining their location and providing precise images of the internal structure of the brain. Also known as nuclear magnetic resonance (NMR).

    magnetoencephalog´raphy (MEG)   procedure that measures the infinitesimal magnetic fields that accompany the electrical activity generated by neuronal firing. It provides precise images of the internal structure of the brain, and can even detect thoughts as they occur. MEG is faster and potentially more accurate than either PET or SPECT.

tone, muscle the constant, slight tension of muscle, normally evident as slight resistance when a limb is moved passively, dependent in part on stretch reflexes. *See also* loop, gamma (Fig. L-1) *and* reflex, stretch (Fig. R-5).

tonotop´ic pertaining to the frequency (pitch) pattern demonstrated in various parts of the auditory pathway.

ton´sil [tonsilla cerebelli, NA], CEREBELLUM segment on the inferior surface of the cerebellar hemisphere (Figs. C-2, N-2). Because of its location, on each side of the median plane dorsal to the medulla, sudden herniation of this mass into the foramen magnum may compress the adjacent medulla during and cause sudden death. *Syn:* ventral paraflocculus of comparative neuroanatomy.

Tooth, Howard Henry (1856-1925) English physician. He described peroneal muscular atrophy in his doctoral thesis in 1886, the same year as a paper on this subject by Charcot and Marie. The disorder is now known as *Charcot-Marie-Tooth* disease.

tor´cular heroph´ili [L. wine-press of Herophilus] old term for the confluence of the sinuses.

torsion (of the eyeball) /tor´shun/ rotation of the eyeball on its anatomical axis.

torticol´lis [L. *tortus* twisted; *collum* neck] wry neck, with contraction of the neck muscles, so that the head is held in an unnatural position.

trabecula, arach´noid /trah-bek´u-lī/ [trabecula arachnoidea, NA] [*pl.* **trabeculae**] [L. dim. of *trabs* a beam] one of the thin, filamentous strands interconnecting the arachnoid and the pia mater across the subarachnoid space.

tra´cer, fluores´cent protein used to mark the cell bodies of neurons. When injected into the terminal site of nerve processes, it is carried by retrograde transport to the cell body where it can be visualized by fluorescent microscopy. Some tracers, such as Nuclear Yellow and Diamidino Yellow, mark the cytoplasm of the perikarya, and some, such as True Blue and Fast Blue, mark the nucleus of the cells. *For more information, including the use of such tracers, see* Heimer and Záborszky ('89). *See also* neurotransmitters.

tract [tractus, NA] [L. a drawing out] bundle of nerve fibers within the CNS, usually having a common origin and a common termination. *See also* bundle; column; fasciculus; fibers.

tract, aber´rant pyram´idal *See* fibers, pyramidal, aberrant.

tract, acoustico-optic /ah-koos´tī-ko-op´tik/ tract arising from cells in the nucleus of the inferior colliculus and terminating in the superior colliculus. These fibers ascend through the periaqueductal gray of the midbrain.

tract, amygdalohypothalam´ic, ventral, FOREBRAIN *See* bundle, longitudinal association, of the amygdala.

tract, anulo-ol´ivary *See* tract, tegmental, central.

tract, ar´cuate, dorsal external (superficial) *See* fibers, arcuate, dorsal external.

tract, arcuate, ventral external (superficial) *See* fibers, arcuate, ventral external.

tract, arcuatocerebel´lar fibers arising from cells in the arcuate nucleus of the medulla which pass by way of ventral external arcuate fibers or the striae medullares of the fourth ventricle through the inferior cerebellar peduncle to the cerebellum.

tract, bulbospi´nal any tract arising in the brain stem and terminating in the spinal cord.

tract, central tegmen´tal [tractus tegmentalis centralis, NA] fiber bundle located in the tegmentum of the brain stem. It contains fibers which are part of a descending chain of neurons from the basal ganglia (pallido-incerto-tegmento-rubro-olivary fibers) and, in its caudal portion, fibers from the cerebellum (dento-olivary fibers), which end mainly in the inferior olivary nucleus (Fig. O-1). It also includes fibers that end in the reticular gray, nucleus ambiguus, and, to some extent, the spinal cord (Bebin, '56). *See also* Nathan and Smith ('82). *Syn:* anulo-olivary tract; thalamo-olivary tract (a misnomer); medial tract of the tegmentum.

tract, cerebel´lar, direct   old term for the dorsal spinocerebellar tract.

tract, cerebellomotor´ius   *See* fibers, cerebellomotorius.

tract, cerebellospi´nal   fibers originally considered a spinal portion of the uncinate fasciculus. Although most cerebellospinal connections synapse in the vestibular nuclei and those entering the spinal cord arise from vestibular nuclei and descend in the medial vestibulospinal tract (medial longitudinal fasciculus, Fig. F-2), some fibers from the fastigial nuclei have been shown to go directly to the spinal cord and terminate in cord segments C2-C3.

tract, cerebrospi´nal   *See* tract, corticospinal.

tract, cerebrospinal, direct   *See* tract, corticospinal, ventral.

tract, colliculospi´nal   old term for the (medial) tectospinal tract.

tract, com´ma, CORD   *See* fasciculus interfascicularis.

tract, corticobul´bar [tractus corticonuclearis, NA]   *See* tract, corticonuclear.

tract, corticomesencephal´ic   *See* tract, corticotectal.

tract, corticonuc´lear (corticobul´bar) [tractus corticonuclearis, NA]   that part of the pyramidal tract which descends through the genu of the internal capsule (Fig. C-1) and terminates in motor nuclei of the brain stem. Some fibers leave the main bundle in the brain stem to descend through the medial lemniscus (*see* fibers, pyramidal, aberrant). A variable number of fibers are also said to reach the pyramidal decussation, cross the median plane, and ascend to end in the nucleus ambiguus (Pick's bundle).

tract, corticopon´tine   either of two tracts arising from cells in the cerebral cortex and terminating on cells of the pontine gray in the basis pontis, for relay to the cerebellum. Some fibers arise from the frontal lobe; others arise from more posterior regions, particularly, in man, the temporal lobe. In man probably few, if any, corticopontine fibers arise from the occipital lobe. *See also* tract, corticopontine, frontal *and* temporal.

tract, corticopontine, fron´tal (frontopon´tine) [tractus frontopontinus, NA]   tract arising from cells in the association cortex of the frontal lobe and terminating in the rostral and medial portions of the pontine gray. In its course this tract passes through the anterior limb of the internal capsule (Fig. C-1) and the medial one-fifth of the pes pedunculi before entering the basis pontis. *Syn:* Arnold's tract.

tract, corticopontine, occip´ital (occcipitopon´tine)   tract said to arise from cells in the cortex of the occipital lobe and terminating in the pontine gray, although its presence in man has been questioned. *See also* tract, corticopontine.

tract, corticopontine, pari´etal (parietopon´tine)   tract arising from cells in the parietal cortex and terminating in the pontine gray. In the monkey it is a large tract but in man its presence has been questioned. *See also* tract, corticopontine.

tract, corticopontine, temporal (temporopon´tine) [fibrae temporopontinae, NA]   tract composed of fibers which arise from posterior portions of the cerebral cortex, mainly the superior, middle, and inferior temporal gyri. This tract passes through the sublenticular (Fig. C-1) and, to some extent, the postlenticular part of the posterior limb of the internal capsule, then the lateral one-fifth of the pes pedunculi of the midbrain, to enter the basis pontis and terminate on cells of the lateral pontine gray for relay to the cerebellum. *Syn:* tract of Türck. *See also* tract, corticopontine.

tract, corticoru´bral [fibrae corticorubrales, NA]   tract arising from cells mostly in the frontal cortex (premotor area, area 6). The fibers descend through the anterior part of the posterior limb of the internal capsule (Fig. C-1) and end, without crossing the median plane, in the red nucleus of the midbrain.

tract, corticospi´nal [tractus corticospinalis, NA]   that part of the pyramidal tract which descends into and terminates in the spinal cord. It passes through the thalamolenticular part of the posterior limb of the internal capsule (Fig. C-1), and the bases of the midbrain and pons. At the junction of the medulla oblongata and spinal cord 70% to 90% of the fibers cross the median plane in the pyramidal decussation to enter the spinal cord as the lateral corticospinal tract. Most of the remaining fibers continue into the spinal cord as the ventral corticospinal tract. Some uncrossed fibers descend with the lateral corticospinal tract and some (the anterolateral corticospinal, or Barnes', tract) descend on the ventrolateral surface of the spinal cord. *Syn:* cerebrospinal tract. *See also* tract, pyramidal. *For the variations in position and relations of the lateral and ventral corticospinal tracts, see* Nathan *et al.* ('90).

tract, corticospinal, anterior [tractus corticospinalis anterior, NA]   *See* tract, corticospinal, ventral.

tract, corticospinal, anterolateral   corticospinal tract fibers which do not cross the median plane in the pyramidal decussation but descend directly into the superficial, ventrolateral part of the spinal cord, near the fibers of the olivospinal tract. *Syn:* Barnes' tract.

tract, corticospinal, lateral [tractus corticospinalis (pyramidalis) lateralis, NA]   those corticospinal tract fibers which cross the median plane in the pyramidal decussation (and some uncrossed fibers) and descend in the dorsal part of the lateral funiculus of the spinal cord (Figs. B-2, T-3). About 55% of the fibers, located in the medial part of the tract, end in the cervical enlargement for relay to the upper extremity. Most of the remaining fibers continue caudally to synapse in the lumbosacral enlargement for relay to the lower extremity. *Syn:* crossed pyramidal tract.

tract, corticospinal, ventral [tractus corticospinalis (pyramidalis) ventralis (anterior), NA]   those corticospinal tract fibers which do not cross in the pyramidal decussation but descend into the ventral funiculus of the spinal cord and terminate in the ventral horn at cervical and thoracic cord levels. Most, but not all, fibers cross in the ventral white commissure at their level of termination and end in the medial cell groups of the ventral horn for relay to the axial muscles of the body. *Syn:* anterior or direct corticospinal or cerebrospinal tract; anterior tract of Türck; uncrossed pyramidal tract.

tract, corticotec´tal   either of two tracts, the internal and external corticotectal tracts, which arise from cells in the cerebral cortex and terminate in the superior colliculus.

tract, corticotectal, external   fibers which arise from cells in the auditory-visual association cortex in the temporo-occipital transition area, and terminate in the superior colliculus via its stratum zonale (Fig. R-3).

tract, corticotectal, internal   fibers which arise from cells in area 18 of the occipital cortex and area 19 of the preoccipital cortex, and terminate in the contralateral superior colliculus via its stratum album intermediale. These fibers are concerned with following (optokinetic) eye movements in the vertical plane. Those which arise from the lower part of area 18 and the upper part of area 19 terminate in the rostral part of the superior colliculus for upward eye movements. Those which arise from the upper part of area 18 and the lower part of area 19 terminate in the caudal part of the superior colliculus for downward eye movements (Crosby *et al.*, '62; Crosby and Schneider, '82). Some corticotectal fibers presumably function in accommodation (Fig. R-2). *See also* Parinaud for the Parinaud syndrome.

tract, cuneatocerebel´lar   fibers which arise from cells in the accessory cuneate nucleus and pass, as dorsal external arcuate fibers, through the inferior cerebellar peduncle to terminate in the cerebellar vermis. They carry proprioceptive and tactile impulses from the homolateral upper extremity and neck.

tract, cuneocerebellar   *See* tract, cuneatocerebellar.

tract, Deiterospinal /di-ter-o-spi´nal/   *See* tract, vestibulospinal.

tract, dentato-ol´ivary (dento-ol´ivary)   *See* fibers, dentato-olivary.

tract, dentatoru´bral (dentoru´bral) [fibrae dentatorubrales, NA]   fibers which arise from cells in the dentate nucleus of the cerebellum, ascend through the superior cerebellar peduncle, cross the median plane in the caudal part of the midbrain tegmentum, and end in the red nucleus, for relay caudally to motor nuclei of the brain stem and spinal cord or rostrally, with the dentatothalamic tract, to the dorsal thalamus.

tract, dentatothalam´ic (dentothalam´ic) [tractus dentatothalamicus, NA]   fibers which arise from cells in the dentate nucleus of the cerebellum, ascend through the superior cerebellar peduncle, cross the median plane in the caudal part of the midbrain tegmentum, and end mostly in the ventrolateral nucleus and partly in the ventral anterior nucleus of the dorsal thalamus.

tract, descending, of V   *See* tract, spinal, of the trigeminal nerve (of V).

tract, dorsal secondary ascending, of V   *See* tract, trigeminal, dorsal secondary ascending (of V).

tract (fascic´ulus), dorsolateral (of Lissauer) [tractus dorsolateralis, NA], CORD   tract located superficial to the tip of the dorsal horn. Its fibers terminate in the substantia gelatinosa. Most fibers (75%) are propriospinal, arising from the substantia gelatinosa. The medial part of the tract also contains the short ascending and descending (one or two segments) processes of dorsal root fibers for pain and temperature from the dermatomes of the related spinal nerves. Other fibers descending in the lateral part of the tract carry impulses for pain inhibition. *See also* Fig. T-2. *Syn:* zona terminalis. *For a review of this topic, see* Kerr ('75).

tract, floc´culo-oculomo´tor   tract arising from Purkinje cells in the flocculus of the cerebellum and terminating, with or without synapse in the dentate nucleus, in the oculomotor nucleus of the midbrain. In the rostral part of its course it is contained in the medial longitudinal fasciculus (Fig. F-2). It is concerned with the maintenance of tone in the ocular and levator palpebrae muscles. *Syn:* fibers of Wallenberg-Klimoff.

tract, frontopon´tine   *See* tract, corticopontine, frontal.

tract, geniculocal´carine, FOREBRAIN   *See* radiation, optic.

tract, geniculotem´poral, FOREBRAIN   *See* radiation, acoustic.

tract, habenulodiencephal´ic, DIENCEPHALON   tract arising from cells in the habenula and terminating in the dorsomedial nucleus of the dorsal thalamus (Fig. H-1).

tract, habenulo-interpedun´cular [tractus habenulo-interpeduncularis, NA], DIENCEPHALON, MIDBRAIN   major discharge bundle from the habenula of the epithalamus. It arches forward and down, passes through the edge of the red nucleus and terminates in the interpeduncular nucleus of the midbrain (Fig. H-1). *Syn:* fasciculus retroflexus; habenulopeduncular tract; fasciculus or tract of Meynert.

tract, habenulotegmen´tal   tract which arises from the habenula and descends to end in the dorsal tegmental nucleus of the midbrain and upper pons (Fig. H-1).

tract, hypothalamohypophysi´al (hypothalamohypophys´ial) [tractus hypothalamo-hypophysalis, NA], DIENCEPHALON   supraopticohypophysial and paraventriculo-hypophysial fibers, which carry certain neurosecretory hormones from cell bodies in the hypothalamic nuclei into the neurohypophysis where they are released. *See also* factors, releasing.

tract, hypothalamopedun´cular   small tract which arises from the medial mamillary nucleus and ends in the interpeduncular nucleus (Fig. H-1). *Syn:* mamillopeduncular or mamillo-interpeduncular tract.

tract, hypothalamospi´nal   fibers from the paraventricular and the dorsomedial hypothalamic nuclei which are said to descend directly to end in the spinal cord. Some end in laminae I and II of the dorsal horn; some end in the intermediolateral nucleus of the lateral horn. *See also* system, hypothalamospinal. *For additional information, see* Carpenter and Sutin ('83, p. 565).

tract, interstitiospinal /in-ter-stĭ-she-o-spi´nal/   fibers which arise from the interstitial nucleus of the medial longitudinal fasciculus and descend in the medial longitudinal fasciculus to terminate in the ventral horn of the cervical spinal cord.

tract, mamillopedun´cular (mamillo-interpeduncular)   *See* tract, hypothalamopeduncular.

tract, mamillotegmen´tal [fasciculus mamillotegmentalis, NA], DIENCEPHALON   tract which arises from cells in the medial mamillary nucleus, with the mamillothalamic tract, as part of a common bundle, fasciculus mamillaris princeps. It arches dorsally in the hypothalamus and then caudally to end in the dorsal and ventral tegmental nuclei of the midbrain. It also contains some ascending fibers interconnecting these nuclei. *Syn:* Gudden's tract.

tract, mamillothalam´ic [fasciculus mamillothalamicus, NA], DIENCEPHALON   tract which arises with the mamillotegmental tract from cells in the medial mamillary nucleus. Most fibers, from the medial mamillary nucleus, ascend through the internal medullary lamina of the dorsal thalamus and end in the anterior nuclear group of the dorsal thalamus, mainly the anteroventral nucleus. Some fibers, from the lateral mamillary nucleus, cross the median plane and end in the small, contralateral anterodorsal nucleus. A few descending fibers from the anterior nuclei to the mamillary body have also been described. *Syn:* bundle of Vicq d'Azyr.

tract, medial, of the tegmentum   *See* tract, central tegmental.

tract (root), mesencephal´ic, of the trigeminal nerve (of V) [tractus mesencephalicus trigeminalis, NA]   bundle of nerve fibers located primarily in the pontine isthmus ventrolateral to the fourth ventricle and in the midbrain lateral to the periaqueductal gray. It consists of the single processes of unipolar cells in the mesencephalic nucleus of V. These fibers bifurcate as they leave the root, one branch extending peripherally as a dendrite and the other, an axon, terminating in the related motor nucleus. Most fibers enter the trigeminal nerve to supply proprioceptive nerve endings in the chewing muscles, the temporomandibular joint, and the periodontal membrane, and function in jaw reflexes. Some fibers (Probst's tract) are thought to descend caudally into the upper cervical spinal cord and to inhibit the action of muscles that lower the mandible. Other fibers supply proprioceptive endings in the extraocular muscles.

tract, neospinothalam´ic   subdivision of the lateral spinothalamic tract, particularly those fibers concerned with the transmission of sharp pain from the body. *For a discussion of this subject, see* Taren *et al.* ('82, pp. 1499-1505). *See also* Fig. T-3.

tract, nigrostri´ate   fibers which arise from cells in the substantia nigra, pars compacta. Supplemented by fibers from the ventral tegmental area, they pass, in fascicles, rostrally and laterally through the internal capsule to end in the caudate nucleus and putamen where they release dopamine and are inhibitory. *Syn:* comb bundle.

tract, occipitopon´tine   *See* tract, corticopontine, occipital.

tract, olfac´tory [tractus olfactorius, NA], CEREBRUM   bundle of nerve fibers arising from the olfactory bulb and extending posteriorly in the olfactory stalk on the ventral surface of the frontal lobe. It divides into medial and lateral olfactory striae as it joins the overlying hemisphere.

tract, olivocerebel´lar [tractus olivocerebellaris, NA]   main efferent bundle from the inferior olivary complex. Its fibers, predominantly crossed, enter the cerebellum by way of the inferior cerebellar peduncle and terminate as climbing fibers on Purkinje cells (piriform cells) in the cerebellar cortex (Fig. O-1). Those from the lateral part of the inferior olivary nucleus end in the lateral part of the posterior lobe of the cerebellar hemisphere; those from the medial part end in the medial part of the hemisphere. From the dorsal lamella of the nucleus, fibers go to the rostral part of the cerebellar hemisphere; those from the ventral lamella go to the caudal part of the hemisphere. The dorsal accessory olivary nucleus projects to the rostral part of the vermis; the medial accessory nucleus projects to the vermis and to the flocculus. Some fibers from the accessory olivary nuclei also end directly in the fastigial nucleus.

tract, olivococh´lear [tractus olivocochlearis, NA]   *See* bundle, olivocochlear.

tract, olivospi´nal [tractus olivospinalis, NA]   tract said to be composed of fibers which arise in the inferior olivary nucleus, mostly crossing the median plane at the level of their origin and descending along the ventrolateral border of the spinal cord to end on motor cells of the cervical spinal cord. The reality of this tract has been questioned. *Syn:* Helweg's tract.

tract, op´tic [tractus opticus, NA], DIENCEPHALON   bundle of nerve fibers of the visual system from the optic chiasm to the lateral geniculate nucleus, with some fibers synapsing in the midbrain for reflex connections (Figs. R-2, R-7).

tract, paleospinothalam´ic   multisynaptic ascending neuron chain located in the lateral funiculus of the spinal cord just lateral to the ventral horn, sometimes considered the deepest portion of the lateral spinothalamic tract. Its fibers arise from cells in the secondary visceral substance (gray) of both sides and carry visceral impulses including visceral pain and dull somatic pain. It ascends with multiple connections at various spinal cord and brain stem levels and terminates in the dorsal thalamus in the intralaminar nuclei, particularly the centromedian nucleus, and in the dorsomedial nucleus. *Syn:* secondary ascending visceral tract. *For a discussion of this subject, see* Taren *et al.* ('82, pp. 1499-1505). *See also* Fig.

T-3.

tract, pallidohypothalam´ic, FOREBRAIN   tract said to arise from cells of the globus pallidus, mainly the medial segment, and end chiefly in the ventromedial nucleus of the hypothalamus, and to be a part of the discharge path for emotional expression.

tract, paraventriculohypophysi´al [tractus paraventriculohypophysialis, NA], DIENCEPHALON   tract composed of fibers arising from neurosecretory cells in the paraventricular nucleus of the hypothalamus. Most fibers carry oxytocin, others carry antidiuretic hormone, for release in the neurohypophysis. *See also* oxytocin.

tract, parietopon´tine   *See* tract, corticopontine, parietal.

tract, pedunculotegmen´tal   tract which arises from cells in the interpeduncular nucleus and ends in the dorsal tegmental nucleus. It is one link in the discharge system of the habenula (Fig. H-1).

tract, pontocerebel´lar   tract arising from cells in the pontine gray in the base of the pons. The fibers, which constitute the second link in a 2-neuron chain from the cerebral cortex to the cerebellum, are mostly crossed but a few are uncrossed. They enter the cerebellum via the middle cerebellar peduncle and end as mossy fibers in the granular layer of the cerebellar cortex mainly in the hemisphere of the posterior lobe.

tract, posterior spinocerebel´lar   *See* tract, spinocerebellar, dorsal.

tract, propriospi´nal, CORD   *See* fasciculus proprius.

tract, pyram´idal [fasciculus pyramidalis, NA]   tract whose cell bodies are located in the cerebral cortex and whose axons terminate directly or indirectly in motor nuclei of the brain stem and spinal cord, by way of corticonuclear and corticospinal tract fibers respectively. These fibers arise partly from the giant pyramidal (Betz) cells of area 4, and partly from other cells in the frontal lobe. Other fibers, from sensory cortex in the pyramidal lobe, end in sensory nuclei of the brain stem and spinal cord, particularly the spinal nucleus of V and the nucleus proprius. The pyramidal tract was so named because its fibers compose the pyramids of the medulla and not because they arise from pyramidal cells in the cerebral cortex. *See also* tract, corticospinal *and* corticobulbar.

tract, pyramidal, crossed   *See* tract, corticospinal, lateral.

tract, pyramidal, lateral   *See* tract, corticospinal, lateral.

tract, pyramidal, uncrossed   *See* tract, corticospinal, ventral.

tract, quintothalam´ic   either of two tracts, the ventral or the dorsal secondary ascending trigeminal tract. *Syn:* trigeminal lemniscus.

tract, reticulospi´nal [tractus reticulospinalis, NA] [L. *reticulum* small net, dim. of *rete*]   any of several tracts whose fibers arise from cells in tegmental or reticular nuclei (reticular formation) of the brain stem and which descend into the spinal cord. These tracts, in other species and presumably in man, have multiple functions, including motor coordination and the regulation of muscle tone. They also serve to regulate autonomic functions mediated through the spinal cord (Fig. T-1). *For additional information, see* Crosby *et al.* ('62, pp. 104-105, 184-186). *See also* tract, reticulospinal, lateral, medial, ventral, *and* ventrolateral; *and* tract, vesicopressor.

tract, reticulospinal, lateral   tract arising from cells in the lateral and medial reticular gray of the medulla and perhaps other brain stem levels. It descends into the spinal cord in the lateral funiculus next to the gray matter between the dorsal and ventral horns. Some fibers end in the lateral horn at spinal cord levels T1 and T2, and carry impulses for sweating of the homolateral side of the face, neck, and upper shoulder (Figs. B-2, T-1).

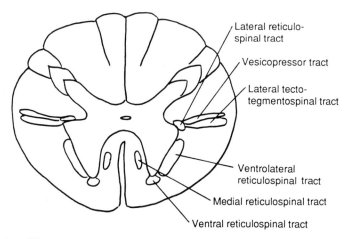

Fig. T-1.   Diagram to show the position in the cervical spinal cord of tracts for autonomic and respiratory control: vesicopressor tract for micturition; lateral tectotegmentospinal tract for maintenance of an open eye and dilation of the pupil; lateral reticulospinal tract for sweating of the face, neck, and shoulder; ventrolateral reticulospinal tract for automatic breathing; medial reticulospinal tract for correlation of parasympathetic and sympathetic control, and the maintenance of heart rate and blood pressure; and ventral reticulospinal tract for sweating of the body.

tract, reticulospinal, medial   tract arising from cells of the reticular gray of the midbrain, pons, and medulla. It descends in the ventral funiculus of the spinal cord with the medial vestibulospinal and the medial tectospinal tracts to end in the lateral and, presumably, ventral horns of the spinal cord. Its autonomic function consists of coordinating the sympathetic activities of the spinal cord with the parasympathetic functions of the brain stem. A lesion in the cervical spinal cord, presumably involving section of this tract bilaterally, results in a decrease in heart rate and a lowering of blood pressure (Fig. T-1). *See also* reflex, carotid sinus.

tract, reticulospinal, ventral   tract which arises from cells in the ventrolateral tegmental nucleus at rostral pontine and caudal midbrain levels, with some fibers crossing at the level of their origin. It descends in the ventral funiculus of the spinal cord and, with some fibers crossing at spinal levels, ends in the lateral horn for sweating of the body. A unilateral lesion does not usually produce a complete loss of sweating on either side of the body but may produce a diminution of sweating on both sides. Other fibers, inhibitory in nature, are also thought to be included in this tract, fibers which cause the detrusor muscle of the bladder to relax and inhibit micturition (Kuru, '65) (Fig. T-1).

tract, reticulospinal, ventrolateral   tract which arises from respiratory centers in the brain stem, in particular the medial reticular gray of the medulla. The fibers descend in a position ventrolateral to the ventral horn of the spinal cord. They end bilaterally on ventral horn cells which supply respiratory muscles and probably to some extent in preganglionic nuclei for relay to the bronchial muscles. Bilateral lesions of this tract in the spinal cord above the origin of the phrenic nucleus result in a loss of automatic breathing, especially important during sleep (Taren *et al.* ('82, p. 1507) (Fig. T-1).

tract, retinohypothalam´ic, DIENCEPHALON   optic tract fibers that terminate in the suprachiasmatic nucleus of the hypothalamus, a connection present in the rat and probably in mammals in general. It is thought to function in relation to certain neuroendocrine activities, particularly those that are light-dependent, including the control of circadian rhythms (Fig. N-7).

tract, rubrospi´nal [tractus rubrospinalis, NA]   tract beginning in the red nucleus of the midbrain and terminating in the spinal cord, at cervical levels in man (Nathan and Smith, '82). Fibers of this tract facilitate the contraction of flexor muscles, in man particularly of the upper extremity. Activation of these fibers may account for the flexion of the upper extremity in decorticate rigidity in man. *Syn:* Monakow's tract.

tract, secondary ascending vis´ceral   *See* tract, paleospinothalamic.

tract, solitary [tractus solitarius, NA]   *See* fasciculus solitarius.

tract, solitariospi´nal (of Cajal)   descending fibers in the medial reticulospinal tract which carry impulses from the nucleus parasolitarius directly or after synapse in the reticular gray.

tract, spinal, of the trigeminal nerve (of V) [tractus spinalis nervi trigemini, NA]   tract composed mainly of descending tactile, pain, and temperature fibers from the face and oral cavity by way of the trigeminal nerve, supplemented by fibers from the soft palate, posterior third of the tongue, and adjoining pharynx via nerve IX, perhaps from the larynx via nerve X, and from the external ear via nerves V, VII, IX, and X (Figs. O-2, R-3, R-4, R-6). Some tactile fibers, from levels below the entering fibers of nerve V, ascend in the spinal tract. The tract is located in the dorsolateral part of the caudal pons and the medulla, and overlaps the dorsolateral fasciculus of the spinal cord (Fig. T-2). Its fibers terminate in the spinal nucleus of the trigeminal nerve in the pons, medulla, and upper three or four cervical spinal cord segments. *See also* onion-skin pattern; reflexes, vagal *and* Fig. R-9.

tract, spinocerebel´lar, direct   old term for the dorsal spinocerebellar tract.

tract, spinocerebellar, dorsal (posterior) [tractus spinocerebellaris dorsalis (posterior), NA]   uncrossed tract arising from cells in the thoracic nucleus and carrying proprioceptive and tactile impulses primarily from the lower extremities to the cerebellar vermis, ending mainly in the central lobule, culmen, declive, pyramis, and uvula. In the spinal cord it is located on the surface in the dorsal part of the lateral funiculus, then shifts dorsally to overly the spinal tract of V in the medulla before entering the inferior cerebellar peduncle (Fig. T-2). *Syn:* direct spinocerebellar tract; tract of Flechsig.

tract, spinocerebellar, indirect   any of several connections from the spinal cord to the cerebellum with a synapse in the brain stem, such as the spino-olivary and olivocerebellar relay and the spinoreticular and reticulocerebellar relay. At times the term has also been used to mean the ventral spinocerebellar tract.

tract, spinocerebellar, ventral (anterior) [tractus spinocerebellaris ventralis (anterior), NA]   tract which arises bilaterally from cells in the nucleus proprius and ascends on the ventrolateral surface of the spinal cord. It loops over the superior cerebellar peduncle and ends bilaterally in the cerebellum. Presumably the fibers which cross in the cord cross again in the cerebellum. The tract carries impulses from neurotendinous and tactile endings of the body and terminates as mossy fibers in the vermis (central lobule and culmen) and adjoining part of the hemisphere of the anterior lobe, also in the posterior lobe vermis (pyramis and uvula) and in the fastigial nucleus. *Syn:* indirect spinocerebellar tract; fasciculus or tract of Gowers; superficial anterolateral fasciculus.

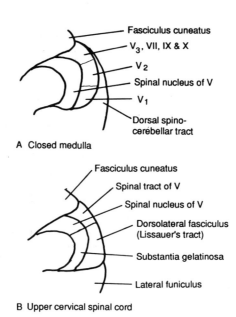

A Closed medulla

B Upper cervical spinal cord

Fig. T-2. Diagram to show the position and relations of the spinal tract and nucleus of V (subnucleus caudalis) in the closed medulla (A) and upper cervical spinal cord (B), and the position of fibers of the facial (VII), glossopharyngeal (IX), and vagus (X) nerves and the ophthalmic (V_1), maxillary (V_2), and mandibular (V_3) branches of the trigeminal nerve in the spinal tract of V. As the dorsal spinocerebellar tract ascends, it shifts dorsally from the lateral funiculus of the spinal cord to a position external to the spinal tract of V. *See also* Fig. N-1.

tract, spinocer´vical, CORD   uncrossed spinal cord tract described for cat the and certain other mammalian species. It is said to arise mainly from Rexed lamina IV and ascend in the dorsolateral part of the lateral funiculus to terminate in the lateral cervical nucleus. Although it appears to mediate impulses of cutaneous origin, its role in the transmission of sensory information is unclear.

tract, spino-ol´ivary [tractus spino-olivaris, NA]   tract composed of fibers arising apparently from cells in the nucleus proprius at cervical spinal cord levels. The fibers cross the median plane through the ventral white commissure and ascend to the inferior olive along the ventrolateral border of the spinal cord. They are thought to carry proprioceptive and tactile impulses. *Syn:* Bechterew's bundle.

tract, spinoretic´ular [tractus spinoreticularis, NA]   tract composed of fibers from all spinal cord levels, which ascend in the ventral part of the lateral funiculus. Those ending in the reticular formation of the medulla are mostly uncrossed. Some of these end in the lateral reticular nucleus for relay to the cerebellum. Some fibers distribute bilaterally to the reticular formation of the pons and a few to the pons-midbrain transition area. These fibers are part of the multisynaptic ascending reticular system.

tract, spinospi´nal, CORD   *See* fasciculus proprius.

tract, spinotec´tal [tractus spinotectalis, NA]   tract carrying impulses, set off by various kinds of stimuli, from the spinal cord to the superior colliculus.

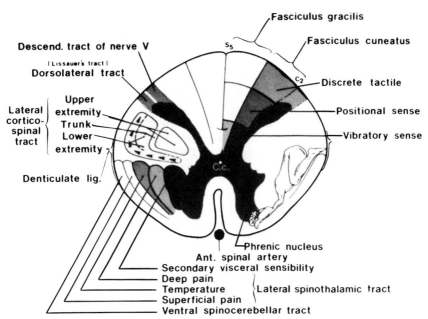

Fig. T-3.   Diagram of a cross section through the C2 level of the spinal cord to illustrate on one side the relative positions of the fibers carrying visceral and somatic pain and temperature in the ventral part of the lateral funiculus. The inverted homunculus on the other side suggests the general anatomical relationships within the lateral spinothalamic tract. The modality pattern in the dorsal funiculus is also shown. From R.C. Schneider, E.A. Kahn, E.C. Crosby, and J.A. Taren, eds. *Correlative Neurosurgery,* 3rd ed., 1982. Courtesy of Charles C. Thomas, Publisher, Springfield, Illinois.

tract, spinothalam´ic, lateral [tractus spinothalamicus lateralis, NA]   tract which arises from cells in the dorsal horn of the spinal cord. It consists of secondary neurons carrying pain and temperature impulses from the body to the ventral posterolateral nucleus of the dorsal thalamus. In the spinal cord it is located in the ventral half of the lateral funiculus and at cervical levels extends into the ventral funiculus (Fig. B-2). Fibers from more caudal regions are in the dorsolateral part of the tract; those from more rostral regions are in the ventromedial part. Fibers for sharp, cutaneous pain (the neospinothalamic tract) are most superficial. Those for temperature sensibility ascend deep to those for sharp pain. Those for dull pain and visceral pain (the paleospinothalamic tract), which arise bilaterally and ascend most deeply, synapse in course and end in the dorsomedial and the intralaminar nuclei of the dorsal thalamus. (Fig. T-3.) *See also* tract, secondary ascending visceral.

tract, spinothalamic, ventral (anterior) [tractus spinothalamicus ventralis (anterior), NA]   tract composed of secondary neurons for general (light) tactile sensibility, its fibers arising primarily from dorsal horn cells of the spinal cord and to some extent from cells in the ventral horn. They cross the median plane in the ventral white commissure (as many as six to eight segments above the level of origin of their primary neurons), and ascend near the ventral and ventrolateral surface of the spinal cord. Although some fibers synapse in the brain stem, most fibers end in the posterolateral ventral nucleus of the contralateral dorsal thalamus. *Syn:* tract of Dejerine.

tract, spinovestib´ular   tract composed of fibers which arise from cells of the nucleus proprius in the dorsal horn of the upper cervical and perhaps other spinal cord segments, cross the median plane in the ventral white commissure, ascend in the ventral funiculus of the spinal cord, and end in the inferior vestibular nucleus. It carries proprioceptive impulses from nerve endings in the neck and is a link for certain neck reflexes and eye movements.

tract, supraopticohypophysi´al (supraopticohypophys´ial) [tractus supraoptico-hypophysialis, NA], DIENCEPHALON   tract composed of fibers arising from neurosecretory cells in the supraoptic nucleus of the hypothalamus. Most fibers carry antidiuretic hormone (ADH), others carry oxytocin, for release in the neurohypophysis. *See also* antidiuretic hormone.

tract, tectobul´bar [tractus tectobulbaris, NA]   tract which arises with and accompanies the fibers of the (medial) tectospinal tract but which ends in motor nuclei of the brain stem.

tract, tectocerebel´lar   tract arising largely from the nucleus of the inferior colliculus, which descends through the anterior medullary velum and ends in the vermis. It probably carries auditory impulses to the cerebellum.

tract, tectohaben´ular   tract which arises in the superior colliculus and ends in the habenula (Fig. H-1). Other fibers arise in the habenula and end in the superior colliculus.

tract, tectopon´tine   tract from the superior colliculus to the base of the pons, probably carrying visual impulses for relay to the cerebellum.

tract, tectospi´nal (medial) [tractus tectospinalis, NA]   tract which, in other species and presumably in man, is composed of fibers which arise in the superior colliculus, enter the stratum album profundum, and curve around the periaque-ductal gray. It crosses the median plane in the dorsal tegmental decussation of the midbrain and turns caudally in a position just ventrolateral to the medial longitudinal fasciculus to reach the cervical spinal cord. Its fibers end by way of intercalated neurons mainly on ventral horn cells which supply neck muscles and, to some extent, on cells which supply upper extremity muscles. *Syn:* predorsal bundle of Edinger. *See also* tract, tectotegmentospinal, lateral.

tract, tectotegmentospi´nal, lateral   fibers arising from cells in the superior colliculus which, after a partial decussation in the commissure of the superior colliculus, synapse in the nearby dorsolateral tegmentum. From there fibers descend into the lateral funiculus of the spinal cord and terminate in the lateral horn mainly at the T1 segment, for relay to the homolateral superior cervical ganglion and distribution to the dilator muscle fibers of the iris and to the sweat glands of the face, neck, and shoulder (Figs. B-2, R-3, T-1).

tract, tegmen´tal, central [tractus tegmentalis centralis, NA]   *See* tract, central tegmental.

tract, tegmental, dorsal   *See* fasciculus, longitudinal, dorsal.

tract, tem´poral corticopon´tine (temporopon´tine)   *See* tract, corticopontine, temporal.

tract, temporoparietopon´tine   *See* tract, corticopontine, temporal.

tract, temporopon´tine   *See* tract, corticopontine, temporal.

tract, thalamobul´bar (thalamo-ol´ivary)   old term, a misnomer, for the central tegmental tract, which does not arise from the thalamus.

tract, thalamostri´ate, FOREBRAIN   fibers which arise from cells in the intralaminar nuclei of the dorsal thalamus, mainly the centromedian nucleus, and which terminate in the caudate nucleus and the putamen of the basal ganglia.

tract, trigeminal, central /tri-jem´in-al/   *See* tract, trigeminal, dorsal *and* ventral secondary ascending (of V).

tract, trigeminal, dorsal central   *See* tract, trigeminal, dorsal secondary ascending (of V).

tract, trigeminal, dorsal secondary ascending (of V)   tract arising from cells in the pontine trigeminal nucleus. Its fibers, some of which cross the median plane in the pons, end bilaterally in the ventral posteromedial nucleus of the dorsal thalamus. The tract carries tactile impulses, including fine tactile discrimination, from the face. *Syn:* dorsal trigeminal lemniscus; dorsal central trigeminal tract.

tract, trigeminal, mesencephalic /mez-en-sĕ-fal´ik/   *See* tract, mesencephalic, of the trigeminal nerve (of V).

tract, trigeminal, spinal   *See* tract, spinal, of the trigeminal nerve (of V).

tract, trigeminal, ventral central   *See* tract, trigeminal, ventral secondary ascending (of V).

tract, trigeminal, ventral secondary ascending (of V)   fibers which carry impulses for pain and temperature from the face and oral cavity from the spinal nucleus of V in the closed medulla and from the dorsal horn in cervical spinal cord segments C1-C4 (Figs. O-2, R-3) and nondiscriminatory (general) tactile sensibility from the pontine and spinal nuclei of V. After crossing the median plane, the fibers ascend obliquely to end in the ventral posteromedial nucleus of the dorsal thalamus. *Syn:* ventral central trigeminal or quintothalamic tract; ventral trigeminal lemniscus.

tract, trigeminospi´nal   *See* tract, spinal, of the trigeminal nerve (of V).

tract, trigeminothalam´ic   *See* tracts, trigeminal, dorsal *and* ventral secondary ascending (of V). *Syn:* trigeminal lemniscus.

tract, u´veal, EYE   *See* uvea.

tract, ventral secondary ascending, of V   *See* tract, trigeminal, ventral secondary ascending (of V).

tract, vesicopres´sor   fibers which arise from cells in the midbrain, pons, and medulla, and descend in the lateral funiculus of the spinal cord in a position just ventral to the lateral corticospinal tract, to end in the sacral spinal cord (Kuru, '65;

Foley, '70). These fibers, sometimes regarded as part of the lateral reticulospinal tract, end bilaterally and presumably underlie automatic emptying of the bladder (Fig. T-1). Other fibers, which descend within the lateral corticospinal tract, end bilaterally for voluntary control of the bladder and to initiate micturition (Crosby et al., '62).

tract, vestibulospi´nal [tractus vestibulospinalis, NA]   tract whose fibers arise from large cells in the lateral vestibular nucleus, descend without decussation into the spinal cord in a position ventral to the ventral horn, and end on ventral horn cells throughout the cord, especially on cells that supply the lower extremity. The tract facilitates contraction of extensor muscles and is concerned mainly with postural adjustments. *Syn:* lateral or ventrolateral vestibulospinal tract; Deiterospinal tract.

tract, vestibulospinal, lateral   *See* tract, vestibulospinal.

tract, vestibulospinal, medial   fibers which arise from cells in the homolateral and contralateral inferior, medial, and lateral vestibular nuclei and descend in the medial longitudinal fasciculus (Fig. F-2) to end mainly on cells in the accessory nuclei of the cervical spinal cord, for positioning of the head.

tract, vestibulospinal, ventrolateral   *See* tract, vestibulospinal.

tractot´omy   cutting of a CNS tract, especially for the relief of pain.

transmit´ter, neurohu´moral   *See* neurotransmitters.

transmitter substance   *See* neurotransmitters.

trap´ezoid [Gr. *trapeza* table; *eidos* shape]   a 4-sided figure with two parallel sides. *For* trapezoid body *and* fibers, *see the nouns.*

trem´or [L. from *tremere* to shake]   involuntary oscillating movements which may occur when the limbs are at rest (Parkinson tremor, also called "static," "resting," "pill-rolling," or sometimes "non-intention" tremor), or during voluntary movement (cerebellar tremor, also called "ataxic," "intention," or sometimes "action" tremor) or when the limbs are held in an outstretched position (postural or action tremor). *For additional information on this and related disorders, see* Adams and Victor ('89, pp. 78-92). *See also* cerebellum; Parkinson.

triangle   *See also* trigone.

triangle (trigone) (of the) lateral ventricle, CEREBRUM   *See* trigone, collateral.

triangle, mesencephal´ic, MIDBRAIN   *See* trigone, lemniscal.

triangle, Syl´vian, CEREBRUM   *See* Sylvius, Franciscus for terms related to the lateral sulcus (Sylvian fissure) *and* Fig. A-3.

tri´gone   *See also* triangle.

trigone, collat´eral [trigonum collaterale, NA], CEREBRUM   part of the lateral ventricle which connects the posterior part of the body of the ventricle with the inferior horn and with the posterior horn, and which contains the glomus choroideum of the choroid plexus (Fig. V-3). *Syn:* atrium, triangle, or vestibule of the lateral ventricle.

trigone, haben´ular [trigonum habenulae (habenularis), NA], EPITHALAMUS   small, triangular area on the superior, posterior part of the wall of the third ventricle, overlying the habenula.

trigone, hypoglos´sal [trigonum hypoglossale (nervi hypoglossi), NA], MEDULLA   elevation on the floor of the fourth ventricle, medial to the vagal trigone, in the caudal part of the medial eminence, and overlying the nucleus of the hypoglossal nerve (Fig. V-4).

trigone, lemniscal /lem-nis´kal/ [trigonum lemnisci, NA], MIDBRAIN   area on the lateral surface of the midbrain, bounded anteriorly by the fibers of the pes pedunculi, posteroinferiorly by the lateral lemniscus, and posterosuperiorly by the brachium of the inferior colliculus. The lateral spinothalamic tract passes rostrally just under the surface in this region, and at this location can be interrupted by mesencephalic tractotomy for the relief of pain (Walker, '42). *Syn:* (lateral) mesencephalic triangle; triangle of Reil.

trigone, olfac´tory [trigonum olfactorium, NA], CEREBRUM   triangular area between the diverging medial and lateral olfactory striae, anterior to the anterior perforated substance.

trigone, pontocerebel´lar [trigonum pontocerebellare, NA]   area in the region of the cerebellopontine angle, bounded by the base of the pons, the inferior cerebellar peduncle, and the flocculus of the cerebellum.

trigone, va´gal [trigonum vagale (nervi vagi), NA], MEDULLA   elevation on the floor of the fourth ventricle, lateral to the hypoglossal trigone in the caudal part of the medial eminence, and overlying the dorsal efferent nucleus of the vagus nerve (Fig. V-4). *Syn:* ala cinerea; Arnold's area.

trigonum   *See* triangle; trigone.

trochlear /trok´le-ar/ [L. *trochlea* pulley]   *For* trochlear nerve *and* nucleus, *see the nouns.*

Trolard, Paulin (1842-1910)   French anatomist. The *lateral lakes of Trolard* are lacunae extending outward from the superior sagittal sinus. The *vein of Trolard* is the superior anastomotic vein on the lateral surface of the cerebral hemisphere.

True Blue   trademark for a fluorescent tracer used to mark the cytoplasm of nerve cell bodies. *See also* tracer, fluorescent.

trunc´us enceph´ali [NA]   *See* stem, brain.

trunk, sympathet´ic   ganglionated nerve cord, one on each side of the vertebral column from the base of the skull into the pelvis. The ganglia of the sympathetic trunk receive preganglionic sympathetic fibers from the spinal cord, by way of the white rami of the thoracic and upper lumbar spinal nerves, for relay to the skin, head, and thoracic viscera. Some preganglionic fibers pass through the thoracic and lumbar sympathetic ganglia without synapse and continue as splanchnic nerves to end in prevertebral ganglia for relay to abdominal and pelvic viscera. Afferent fibers from the organs innervated accompany the sympathetic fibers. *See also* ramus, gray *and* white; ganglia (of the) sympathetic trunk, *and* prevertebral; *and* system, nervous, autonomic; Fig. S-3; Table S-1. *Syn:* sympathetic chain.

Tsai, Chiao (b. 1898)   neuroanatomist at the University of Chicago. The *ventral tegmental area of Tsai* is that portion of the tegmental gray in the rostral part of the midbrain, ventral to the red nucleus. It is traversed by descending fibers from the hypothalamus and by fibers of the oculomotor nerve.

tube, au´ditory [tuba auditiva (auditoria), NA], EAR, [L. *tuba* a straight trumpet]   channel which connects the middle ear with the nasopharynx and which functions in the equalization of air pressure in the middle ear and outside the tympanic membrane. *Syn:* Eustachian tube.

tube, neural /nu´ral/ [tubus neuralis, NA] [L. *tubus* tube or canal]   embryonic tube derived from the neural plate, from which the CNS develops. It is formed at the end of the third week of gestation. From its lumen, the neural canal, outward, it consists of four zones: the ventricular and subventricular zones (ependymal layer), the intermediate zone (mantle layer), and the marginal zone or layer (Angevine *et al.*, '70).

tu´ber cinereum /sin-er´e-um/ [NA], HYPOTHALAMUS   slight elevation on the ventral surface of the diencephalon, between the mamillary bodies posteriorly and the optic chiasm anteriorly (Figs. C-3C, V-5).

tuber ver´mis [NA], cerebellum, [L. knot or swelling] subdivision of the cerebellar vermis between the folium vermis and the pyramis (Figs. C-2, V-6). *See also* vermis cerebelli.

tu´bercle, acoustic /ah-koo´stik/, medulla small swelling containing the dorsal cochlear nucleus, on the dorsolateral surface of the medulla, at the attachment of the cochlear nerve.

tubercle, anterior, of the thalamus [tuberculum anterius thalami, NA], dorsal thalamus elevation on the dorsal, anterior part of the wall of the third ventricle, overlying the anterior nuclei of the dorsal thalamus (Fig. V-5).

tubercle, cuneate /ku´ne-ăt/ [tuberculum cuneatum, NA], medulla elevation on the dorsolateral surface of the medulla overlying the nucleus cuneatus (Fig. V-4).

tubercle, gracile /gras´ĕl/ [tuberculum gracile, NA], medulla protuberance on the dorsal surface of the medulla, overlying the nucleus gracilis (Fig. V-4). *Syn:* clava.

tubercle, intercolum´nar, cerebrum *See* organ, subfornical.

tubercle, olfac´tory [tuberculum olfactorium], cerebrum eminence in animals which have a large olfactory system, in the region designated anterior perforated substance in man.

tubercles, quadrigem´inal, midbrain corpora quadrigemina, *viz.* the superior and inferior colliculi.

tubercle, trigem´inal [tuberculum trigeminale, NA], medulla elevation on the lateral surface of the medulla overlying the spinal nucleus and tract of V. *Syn:* tuberculum cinereum; eminentia trigemini.

tuberculum cinereum /sin-er´e-um/, medulla *See* tubercle, trigeminal.

tunnel, inner, ear spiral canal which extends the full length of the cochlear duct between the inner and outer pillars of the spiral organ. *Syn:* tunnel of Corti.

tunnel, spiral, internal, ear *See* sulcus, spiral, internal.

Türck, Ludwig (1810-1868) Austrian neurologist who made many fundamental neurologic discoveries. From his study of secondary degeneration he determined the direction of conduction of a number of tracts. The *anterior tract* or *column of Türck* is the ventral corticospinal tract and the *tract of Türck* is the temporal corticopontine tract.

Turner, Sir William Aldren (1832-1916) British neurologist, Professor of Anatomy at the University of Edinburgh, noted for his studies of cerebral morphology. *Turner's sulcus* is the intraparietal sulcus.

'tweenbrain *See* diencephalon.

tympan´um, ear, [L. from Gr. *tympanon* drum] the tympanic cavity of the middle ear.

ty´rosine neuropeptide which is the precursor of the thyroid hormones, the catecholamines (dopamine, norepinephrine, and epinephrine), and melanin. *Syn:* oxyphenylaminopropionic acid. *See also* neurotransmitters.

u

U-fibers, CEREBRUM *See* fibers, arcuate, *def.* 2.

um´bo [umbo membranae tympani, NA], EAR, [L. knob] projection at the center of the inner surface of the tympanic membrane where the tip of the manubrium of the malleus is attached.

uncinate /un´sin-āt/ hook-like. *See* uncus; fasciculus, uncinate.

uncus /ung´kus/ [NA], CEREBRUM, [L. hook] segment of the parahippocampal gyrus turned back at its anterior end, forming a protuberance on the medial side of the temporal lobe over the amygdala (Fig. C-3B,C). An irritative lesion in this area causes olfactory hallucinations (uncinate fits). *Syn:* uncinate gyrus.

unit, motor lower motor neuron and all the muscle fibers which it supplies.

u´tricle [utriculus, NA], EAR, [L. little uterus] subdivision of the membranous labyrinth, an ovoid, slightly flattened sac in the superoposterior region of the vestibule of the bony labyrinth. It is connected with the semicircular ducts and, by the utriculosaccular duct, with the endolymphatic duct and the saccule. The macula utriculi, its sensory portion, is in an approximately horizontal position and is stimulated by changes in head position, such as tilting or nodding the head, or by linear acceleration.

u´vea, EYE, [L. *uva* grape] vascular tunic of the eye, consisting of the choroid and the ciliary body (but not including their epithelium) and the iris. *Syn:* uveal tract.

uvula ver´mis /u´vu-lah/ [NA], CEREBELLUM, [L. *uvula* little grape] segment of the cerebellar vermis, so named because of its resemblance to the uvula of the soft palate. It is separated from the nodule by the postnodular fissure and from the pyramis by the prepyramidal fissure (Figs. C-2, V-6). *See also* vermis cerebelli.

V

VA   ventral anterior nucleus of the dorsal thalamus.

va´gus [L. wandering]   *See* nerve, vagus.

Valentin, Gabriel Gustav (1810-1883)   German-Swiss physiologist. The *ganglion of Valentin* is a thickening in the superior dental plexus, above the root of the second premolar tooth at the junction of the middle and posterior superior alveolar nerves. It is not a true ganglion but consists of interlacing bundles of nerve fibers and contains no nerve cells. The *nerve of Valentin* is a strand of nerve fibers that interconnects the pterygopalatine ganglion and the abducens nerve.

vallecula cerebelli /val-ek´u-lah/ [NA], CEREBELLUM, [L. *vallecula* little valley]   deep median fossa between the two cerebellar hemispheres on the inferior surface of the cerebellum (Fig. C-2).

Varolio, Constanzo (1543-1575)   Italian anatomist known mainly for his studies of the brain. In 1573 he described the pons, and it was named *pons Varolii* for him. He gave the hippocampus its name.

vas prom´inens [NA], EAR   large capillary loops within the spiral prominence in the outer wall of the cochlear duct.

vas spira´le [NA], EAR   small artery which runs the length of the cochlea in the basilar membrane beneath the inner tunnel of the spiral organ.

vasa corona /kor-o´nah/, CORD   plexus of small arterial vessels on the lateral and ventral surfaces of the spinal cord whose penetrating branches supply a narrow zone of the underlying white matter.

vasa nervor´um   small blood vessels within peripheral nerve trunks.

vasopres´sin   antidiuretic hormone (ADH). This neurohormone, administered in amounts larger than necessary for antidiuretic activity, will increase vasoconstriction and raise blood pressure, hence its name. *For a review of the recent advances in this field, see* Gash and Boer ('87).

Vater, Abraham (1684-1751)   German anatomist who first noted the large encapsulated nerve endings, the *corpuscles of Vater-Pacini,* later rediscovered and described by Pacini. *See also* Pacini.

vegetative nervous system   *See* system, nervous, autonomic.

veins   *For additional information on the veins of the human brain and spinal cord, see* Stephens and Stillwell ('69), and Salamon and Huang ('76).

vein, anastomot′ic, greater, CEREBRUM   *See* vein, anastomotic, superior.

vein, anastomotic, inferior [vena anastomotica inferior, NA], CEREBRUM   anastomotic vein on the lateral surface of the cerebral hemisphere, connecting the superficial middle cerebral vein and the transverse sinus. *Syn:* posterior or lesser anastomotic vein; vein of Labbé.

vein, anastomotic, lesser, CEREBRUM   *See* vein, anastomotic, inferior.

vein, anastomotic, posterior, CEREBRUM   *See* vein, anastomotic, inferior.

vein, anastomotic, superior [vena anastomotica superior, NA], CEREBRUM   anastomotic vein on the lateral surface of the cerebral hemisphere, connecting the superficial middle cerebral vein and the superior sagittal sinus. *Syn:* greater anastomotic vein; vein of Trolard.

vein, ba′sal (of Rosenthal) [vena basalis, NA], CEREBRUM   vein formed by the union of the anterior vein of the corpus callosum, the deep middle cerebral vein, and the anterior cerebral vein. It courses posteriorly around the brain stem, and empties into the great cerebral vein. It and its tributaries drain the cortex of the insula

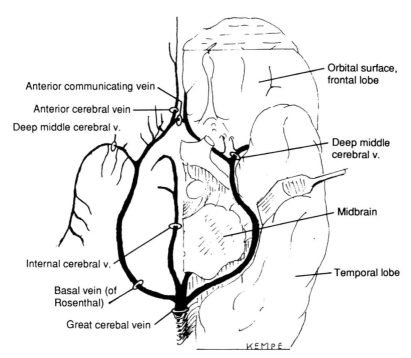

Fig. V-1.   Basal veins and their tributaries, as seen from below. The basal veins and the internal cerebral veins join the great cerebral vein at the entrance to the straight sinus. Drawing courtesy of Dr. L.G. Kempe.

and medial surface of the anterior and parietal lobes, as well as certain internal structures of the forebrain and to some extent the midbrain and cerebellum (Figs. V-1, V-2). *Syn:* basal cerebral vein.

vein, cer´ebral, anterior, CEREBRUM   small vein which accompanies the anterior cerebral artery. It drains the orbital surface of the frontal lobe and the anterior portions of the corpus callosum and cingulate gyrus then, with the deep middle cerebral vein, joins the basal vein (Fig. V-1).

vein, cerebral, ba´sal, CEREBRUM   *See* vein, basal.

veins, cerebral, deep [venae profundae cerebri, NA], FOREBRAIN   system of veins which drain the internal structures of the forebrain, and which empty into the internal cerebral veins and, in part, the basal veins.

vein, cerebral, deep middle [vena media profunda cerebri, NA], CEREBRUM   vein deep within the lateral sulcus. It receives blood from the insular and the inferior thalamostriate veins, then joins the anterior cerebral vein to form the basal vein (Fig. V-1). *See also* veins, cerebral, middle.

vein, cerebral, great (of Galen) [vena magna cerebri, NA], FOREBRAIN   short, median vein formed by the fusion of the two internal cerebral veins, just above the pineal body. It empties into the straight sinus. Its main tributaries are the internal cerebral and basal veins, but it also receives branches from the occipital and cerebellar surfaces, above and below the tentorium cerebelli (Figs. V-1, V-2).

veins, cerebral, inferior [venae inferiores cerebri, NA], CEREBRUM   superficial veins which drain the lower part of the lateral surface of the occipital and temporal lobes and which empty into the transverse sinus.

vein, cerebral, internal [vena interna cerebri, NA], FOREBRAIN   vein formed at the venous angle by the juncture of the superior thalamostriate (terminal) vein and the septal vein, joined by several small veins including some from the lentiform and caudate nuclei and the choroid plexus of the lateral ventricle. It passes posteriorly in the velum interpositum along the roof of the third ventricle and joins its counterpart of the other side to enter the great cerebral vein (Figs. V-1, V-2). *Syn:* lesser or small vein of Galen.

veins, cerebral, middle, CEREBRUM   two veins, the superficial and deep middle cerebral veins, located along the surface or deep within the lateral sulcus of the cerebrum. Anterior to the lateral sulcus, the superficial vein continues anteriorly into the cavernous or sphenoparietal sinus; the deep vein turns posteriorly and empties into the basal vein, which joins the great cerebral vein (Fig. V-1). *Syn:* Sylvian vein.

veins, cerebral, superior [venae superiores cerebri, NA], CEREBRUM   superficial veins which run upward on the surface of the cerebral hemispheres to empty into the superior sagittal sinus.

vein, cerebral, superficial middle [vena media superficialis cerebri, NA], CEREBRUM   vein which runs anteriorly along the surface of the lateral sulcus. Its tributaries drain the inner and superficial surfaces of the opercula and have anastomotic connections with the superior and transverse dural sinuses. It turns medially along the sphenoid ridge and empties into the cavernous or the sphenoparietal sinus. *See also* veins, cerebral, middle.

vein, chor´oid, superior, CEREBRUM   main vein of the choroid plexus of the lateral ventricle which, with the superior thalamostriate vein, joins the internal cerebral vein at the venous angle (Fig. V-2).

vein, choroid, inferior, CEREBRUM   small vein that drains part of the choroid plexus of

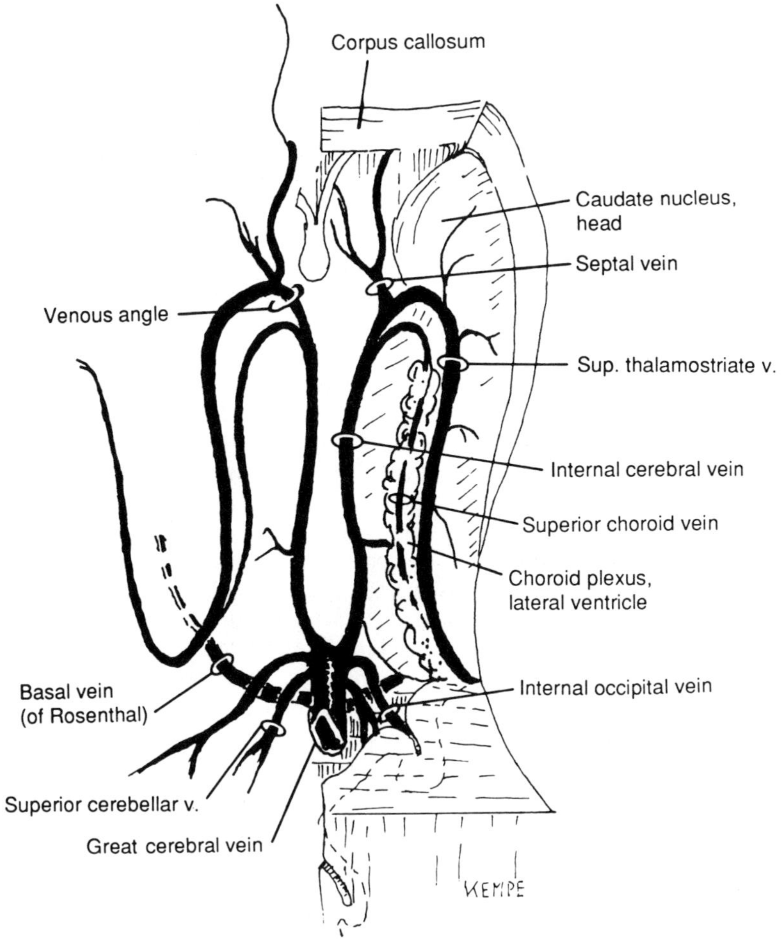

Fig. V-2. Great cerebral vein and its tributaries, as seen from above. Drawing courtesy of Dr. L.G. Kempe.

the lateral ventricle and empties into the basal vein.

vein, communicating, anterior, CEREBRUM anastomotic vein between the two anterior cerebral veins on the base of the cerebrum (Fig. V-1).

vein, communicating, posterior anastomotic vein in the interpeduncular fossa, which interconnects tributaries of the two basal veins across the median plane. It varies in size from fairly large to indistinguishable. *Syn:* Charpy's anastomotic vein.

veins, diplo ´ic [venae diploicae, NA] plexus of veins between the inner and outer tables of the calvaria, and which communicates with the intracranial and extracranial venous systems. *Syn:* veins of Breschet.

veins, em ´issary [venae emissariae, NA] any veins which by connections through the skull connect a dural sinus and the extracranial venous system. The largest of these is the superior ophthalmic vein which interconnects the angular vein of the face and the cavernous sinus.

veins, in´sular [venae insulares, NA], CEREBRUM   veins which drain the insula and empty into the deep middle cerebral vein.

vein, jug´ular, internal [vena jugularis interna, NA]   large vein which begins at the posterior compartment of the jugular foramen in the base of the skull. It drains blood from the brain, mainly from the sigmoid sinus, with contributions from the inferior petrosal and occipital sinuses. In the neck it receives branches from the face and neck and descends in the carotid sheath to empty into the brachycephalic vein.

veins, lenticulostri´ate, CEREBRUM   superior and inferior thalamostriate veins.

vein, occip´ital, internal, CEREBRUM   tributary of the basal or the great cerebral vein, it drains the medial and inferior surfaces of the occipital lobe (Fig. V-2).

veins, ophthal´mic   two valveless veins, superior and inferior, which pass through the superior orbital fissure and join the cavernous sinus. Because they (especially the superior) also join the veins of the face, these veins may transmit infectious agents from the face into the cavernous sinus and thence to the brain.

vein, sep´tal, CEREBRUM   subependymal vein in the septum pellucidum in the medial wall of the anterior horn of the lateral ventricle. It empties into the internal cerebral vein at the venous angle (Fig. V-2).

veins, spi´nal, anterior/posterior [venae spinales anteriores/posteriores, NA], CORD   longitudinally arranged, valveless veins, usually six in number, on the surface of the spinal cord. Three anterior spinal veins lie along the anterior median fissure and next to the emerging ventral roots on either side. Three posterior spinal veins lie along the mid-dorsal plane, and next to the attaching dorsal roots on either side. They empty into the internal vertebral venous plexus.

veins, stri´ate, FOREBRAIN   *See* veins, thalamostriate, inferior *and* superior.

vein, striothalam´ic, FOREBRAIN   *See* vein, thalamostriate, superior.

vein, ter´minal [vena terminalis, NA], FOREBRAIN   *See* vein, thalamostriate, superior.

veins, thalam´ic, DORSAL THALAMUS   veins which drain the dorsal thalamus and are tributaries of the internal cerebral vein.

veins, thalamostri´ate, inferior [venae thalamostriatae inferiores, NA], FOREBRAIN   veins which drain the inferior part of the corpus striatum then join the deep middle cerebral vein, a tributary of the basal vein. *Syn:* inferior striate or lenticulostriate veins.

vein, thalamostriate, superior [vena thalamostriata superior (vena terminalis), NA], FOREBRAIN   vein which accompanies the tail of the caudate nucleus and the stria terminalis along the roof of the inferior horn of the lateral ventricle, then turns forward and continues along the junction of the body of the caudate nucleus and the dorsal thalamus on the floor of the body of the lateral ventricle to the interventricular foramen, where it joins the internal cerebral vein at the venous angle (Fig. V-2). *Syn:* striothalamic vein; terminal vein.

veins, transcer´ebral, CEREBRUM   connecting vessels between the cortical veins on the surface of the cerebral hemispheres and the internal cerebral system of veins.

veins, ver´tebral   system of valveless epidural and perivertebral veins associated with the vertebral column. They have many connections with other valveless veins including those of the brain and spinal cord on the one hand and those of the thorax, abdomen, and pelvis on the other. Among other things this plexus plays an important role in metastasis from the body to the brain (Batson, '57).

veins, vorticose /vor´tĭ-kōs/, EYE   large veins of the uveal tract. The veins of the vascular layer of the choroid of the eye converge and empty into these vessels which, in turn, pass through the sclera and drain into the ophthalmic veins of the orbit.

ve´lum interpos´itum [NA], FOREBRAIN   pia mater and connective tissue occupying the space between the corpus callosum dorsally and the dorsal thalamus, roof of the third ventricle, and pineal body ventrally, and through which the internal cerebral veins pass.

velum, med´ullary, anterior (rostral or **superior)** [velum medullare anterius (rostralis, superius), NA], PONS, CEREBELLUM, [L. *velum* veil or covering]   thin layer of tissue between the two superior cerebellar peduncles, forming a roof over the rostral part of the fourth ventricle (Fig. V-4). The caudal part of this structure contains the lingula of the cerebellar vermis. *Syn:* valve of Vieussens.

velum, medullary, posterior (caudal or **inferior)** [velum medullare posterius (caudalis, inferius), NA], MEDULLA   membranous roof over the caudal part of the fourth ventricle. *Syn:* tela choroidea of the fourth ventricle.

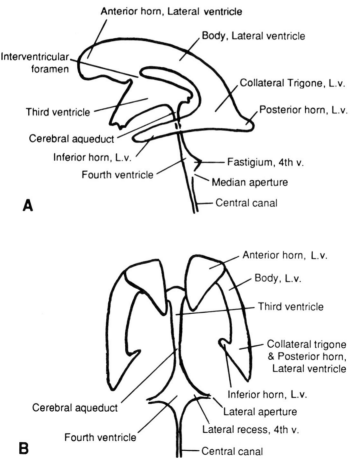

Fig. V-3.   Ventricular system, showing the parts of the lateral (L.v.), third, and fourth (4th v.) ventricles, and their connections. A. lateral view. B. anteroposterior view.

velum, medullary, rostral, PONS, CEREBELLUM   *See* velum, medullary, anterior.

velum, medullary, superior, PONS, CEREBELLUM   *See* velum, medullary, anterior.

velum terminal´e, CEREBRUM   **1.** *See* lamina terminalis.

   2. membrane which, with the choroid plexus in the inferior horn of the lateral ventricle, closes the choroid fissure of the cerebral hemisphere. On one side it attaches to the fimbria and on the other to the stria terminalis.

ven´tricle [ventriculus, NA] [L. *ventriculus,* dim. of *venter* belly]   one of the irregularly shaped cavities within the CNS, which contain cerebrospinal fluid.

ventricle, fifth, CEREBRUM   *See* cavum septi pellucidi.

ventricle, first, CEREBRUM   either of the two lateral ventricles.

ventricle (of the) for´nix, CEREBRUM   horizontal cleft which sometimes occurs between the corpus callosum and the underlying hippocampal commissure.

ventricle, fourth [ventriculus quartus, NA], HINDBRAIN   cavity bounded ventrally by the pons and open medulla and dorsally by the anterior medullary velum, cerebellum, and posterior medullary velum. Its floor is the rhomboid fossa. The dorsal apical portion is called the fastigium. Rostrally the ventricle communicates with the cerebral aqueduct of the midbrain and caudally with the central canal of the closed medulla. It also communicates with the subarachnoid space by way of the two lateral apertures and one median aperture through which cerebrospinal fluid leaves the ventricular system (Figs. C-6, V-3, V-4, V-6).

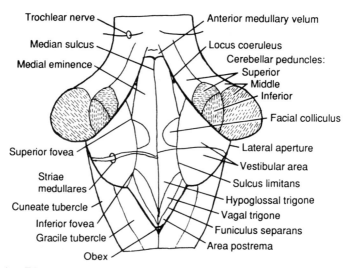

Fig. V-4.   Diagram to show the features of the rhomboid fossa and the structures neighboring the fourth ventricle. Rostral to a plane through the lateral apertures the pons is the floor of the fourth ventricle. Caudal to that level it is the open medulla.

ventricle, lateral [ventriculus lateralis, NA], CEREBRUM   irregularly shaped cavity within each cerebral hemisphere. It consists of an anterior horn in the frontal lobe, a body mostly in the parietal lobe, a posterior horn in the occipital lobe, an inferior horn in the temporal lobe, and a collateral trigone at the junction of the body and the posterior and inferior horns. It communicates with the third ventricle through the interventricular foramen (Fig. V-3).

ventricle, olfac´tory, cerebrum   cavity within the olfactory bulb, present in man during fetal life, and in certain subhuman species throughout life. When present it communicates with the anterior horn of the lateral ventricle.

ventricle, second, cerebrum   either of the two lateral ventricles.

ventricle, sixth, cerebrum   posterior extension of the cavum septi pellucidi. *Syn:* ventricle of Verga; cavum Vergae.

ventricle, ter´minal [ventriculus terminalis, NA], cord   moderately dilated part of the central canal in the caudal segments of the spinal cord. *Syn:* ventricle of Krause.

ventricle, third [ventriculus tertius, NA], diencephalon   median cavity between the two halves of the diencephalon and extending rostrally to the lamina terminalis. It communicates with each lateral ventricle through an interventricular foramen and caudally is continuous with the cerebral aqueduct of the midbrain (Figs. C-6, N-8, V-3, V-5). *Syn:* thalamocele.

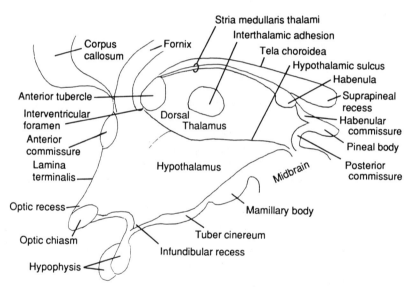

Fig. V-5.   Third ventricle, showing its parts and the structures which bound it. The fornix and the anterior part of the dorsal thalamus have been separated to show the anterior tubercle. The suprapineal recess of the third ventricle is a pocket of the tela choroidea which extends posteriorly over the pineal body.

ventric´ulus im´par telencephal´icus, cerebrum   part of the third ventricle, anterior to a plane extending from the interventricular foramen to the preoptic recess and the anterior margin of the optic chiasm. *Syn:* cavum Monroi.

Verga, Andrea (1811-1895)   Italian anatomist and psychiatrist. The *ventricle of Verga* or *cavum Vergae* is the posterior extension of the cavity of the septum pellucidum, sometimes also called the sixth ventricle.

ver´mis cerebel´li [NA], CEREBELLUM, [L. *vermis* worm]   median portion of the cerebellum between the two cerebellar hemispheres (Figs. C-2, N-2, V-6). *See also* cerebellum, lobes. *For additional information on this subject, see* Crosby *et al.* ('62, pp. 188-192). The subdivisions of the vermis, in rostral to caudal order, are as follows:

anterior lobe:

lingula /ling´gu-lah/ [NA] [L. dim. of *lingua* tongue]   most rostral segment of the vermis located in the anterior medullary velum and sometimes also including the adjacent segment of the vermis. It is not continuous with the cerebellar hemispheres. *Syn:* lobule I.

central lobule [lobulus centralis, NA]   segment consisting of one or two parts on the anterior, superior surface of the vermis. It is separated from the lingula anteriorly by the precentral fissure and from the culmen posteriorly by the postcentral fissure. It is continuous laterally with the ala centralis of the cerebellar hemisphere. *Syn:* lobules II, III.

culmen /kul´men/ [L. hill]   segment on the superior surface of the vermis, separated from the central lobule anteriorly by the postcentral fissure and from the declive posteriorly by the primary fissure. It is continuous laterally with the anterior quadrangular lobule of the cerebellar hemisphere. *Syn:* culmen monticuli; lobules IV, V.

posterior lobe:

declive /de-klīv´/ [NA] [L. *declivis* sloping downward]   segment on the superior surface of the vermis, separated from the culmen anteriorly by the primary fissure and from folium vermis posteriorly by the postclival fissure. It is continuous laterally with the posterior quadrantic lobule of the hemisphere. *Syn:* declivus; clivus; lobule VI.

fo´lium ver´mis [NA] [L. *folium* leaf]   single folium that lies between the declive above and anteriorly and the tuber vermis inferiorly, and marks the posterior limit of the arbor vitae. It is continuous laterally with the much expanded superior semilunar lobule of the cerebellar hemisphere. *Syn:* lobule VII in part.

tu´ber vermis [NA]   segment on the posterior inferior surface of the vermis, between the folium vermis and horizontal fissure above and the pyramis and postpyramidal fissure anterior and inferior to it. It is continuous laterally with the inferior semilunar and gracile lobules of the hemisphere. With the folium vermis and pyramis it lies at the base of the vallecula cerebelli. *Syn:* lobule VII in part.

pyr´amis vermis [NA]   segment on the inferior surface of the vermis, separated from the uvula anteriorly by the prepyramidal fissure and from the tuber posterior and superior to it by the postpyramidal fissure. It is continuous laterally with the biventer of the hemisphere. *Syn:* lobule VIII.

u´vula vermis [NA]   segment on the inferior surface of the vermis, separated from the nodule anterior and superior to it by the postnodular fissure, and from the pyramis posterior to it by the prepyramidal fissure. It is continuous laterally with the tonsil of the hemisphere. *Syn:* lobule IX.

flocculonod´ular lobe:

nod´ule [nodulus, NA]   most caudal segment of the vermis, overlying the posterior medullary velum and separated from the uvula posterior and inferior to it by the postnodular fissure. It is connected to the flocculus of the hemisphere by the peduncle of the flocculus. *Syn:* lobule X.

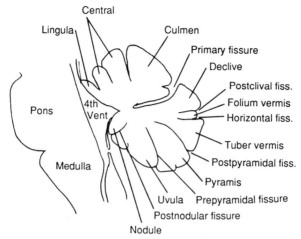

Fig. V-6. Vermis cerebelli. Diagram to show the parts of the vermis and the fissures which separate them. The primary fissure separates the anterior and posterior lobes of the cerebellum and the postnodular fissure separates the posterior and flocculonodular lobes.

ver´tigo [L. *vertere* to turn]   sensation of turning, as if the external world were moving or revolving around the patient, or as if he himself were moving or revolving in space.

Vesalius, Andreas (1514-1564)   great Flemish anatomist, born in Brussels, at one time army surgeon for Charles V, later professor of surgery and anatomy at Padua. His monumental work, *De humani corporis fabrica,* containing descriptions and illustrations based on his dissections of the human brain, provided a turning point in the knowledge of the nervous system.

ves´icle, auditory   *See* vesicle, otic.

vesicle, brain, primary   traditional term, now discredited for the mammalian brain, for the three early subdivisions of the developing brain, from rostral to caudal: the prosencephalon or forebrain, the mesencephalon or midbrain, and the rhombencephalon or hindbrain. *For a discussion of this subject, see* O'Rahilly and Gardner ('79).

vesicle, brain, secondary   traditional term, now discredited for the mammalian brain, for the five subdivisions derived from the so-called primary brain vesicles (q.v.): telencephalon and diencephalon, from the prosencephalon; the undivided mesencephalon; and the metencephalon and myelencephalon, from the rhombencephalon.

vesicle, op´tic [vesicula optica, NA], EYE   evagination of the wall on each side of the embryonic forebrain. They first appear as depressions, optic sulci, about the middle of the third prenatal week and give rise to the optic cup and then the retina and the epithelial layers of the choroid and iris.

vesicle, o´tic [vesicula otica, NA], EAR   closed sac derived from the superficial ectoderm, from which the membranous labyrinth develops. *Syn:* otocyst; auditory vesicle.

vesicle, presynap´tic [vesicula presynaptica, NA]   one of the small membranous structures within the presynaptic terminal of an axon. They store neurotransmitter substance until it is released during synaptic transmission to act upon the postsynaptic cell. Spherical vesicles with clear centers are thought to be excitatory and flattened vesicles to be inhibitory. Those with dense centers appear to be adrenergic. *See also* plate, motor end. *For a review of this topic, see* Peters *et al.* ('76, pp. 145-153).

ves´tibule   1. [vestibulum, NA], ᴇᴀʀ   central cavity of the bony (perilymphatic) labyrinth, which contains the utricle and saccule. It is continuous with the scala vestibuli and the scala tympani of the cochlea anteriorly, and with the semicircular canals which lie above and lateral to it.

2. ᴄᴇʀᴇʙʀᴜᴍ   *See* trigone, collateral.

vestibulocerebel´lum   portion of the cerebellum, particularly the flocculonodular lobe, dominated by impulses relayed from the vestibular apparatus. *Syn:* archi-cerebellum.

Vialet, N. (late 19th century)   the *fasciculus of Vialet* consists of association fibers which connect the inferior lip of the calcarine fissure with the inferolateral occipital cortex. It is one of the transverse occipital fasciculi.

Vicq d'Azyr, Félix (1748-1794)   French neuroanatomist of Paris. The *bundle of Vicq d'Azyr* (1781) is the mamillothalamic tract. The *stripe of Vicq d'Azyr* is a layer of nerve fibers in layer II of the cerebral cortex. The *body of Vicq d'Azyr* is the substantia nigra.

Vidius, Vidus (Latin form of **Guido Guidi**) (1500-1569)   Italian physician of Pisa, for some years physician to Francis I of France, later Professor of Medicine at Pisa, Italy. The *Vidian nerve* is the nerve of the pterygoid canal, and the canal is called the *Vidian canal.*

Vieussens, Raymond de (1641-1716)   French physician and anatomist of Montpellier. He described many structures of the CNS and PNS, including the ansa hypoglossi (1685), celiac plexus, pyramids, olives, and centrum ovale. The *valve of Vieussens* is the anterior medullary velum; *the anulus* or *ansa of Vieussens* (1706) is the ansa subclavia; and *Vieussens' ventricle* is the cavum septi pellucidi. The celiac ganglion is also sometimes called *Vieussens' ganglion.*

vil´li, arach´noid   small projections which invaginate the dura mater and project into the dural venous sinuses, usually along the superior sagittal sinus, and through which cerebrospinal fluid enters the venous system. Clusters of these villi constitute the arachnoid granulations.

vinculum /ving´ku-lum/, ᴍᴇᴅᴜʟʟᴀ, [L. band or ligament]   bridge of gray matter connecting the spinal nucleus of V and the central gray of the medulla.

Virchow, Rudolf Ludwig Carl (1821-1902)   German pathologist, a pupil of Johannes Müller's. He is known as the founder of cellular pathology. In 1851 he noted the perivascular spaces around blood vessels entering the CNS in sections of fixed tissue. These spaces were later described in greater detail by Robin and known as the *spaces of Virchow-Robin.*

visual purple, ᴇʏᴇ   *See* rhodopsin.

VL   ventral lateral nucleus of the dorsal thalamus.

Vogt, Cécile Mugnier (1875-1962)   distinguished French neurologist and neuro-pathologist, later of Germany. She and her husband, Oskar Vogt, were noted for their work on the architectonics of the cerebral cortex and for their studies of neuroanatomy as a substratum for neurologic disorders.

Vogt, Oskar (1870-1959)   eminent German neurologist and psychiatrist, for years

Director of the Kaiser Wilhelm Institute for Brain Research. Later he and his wife, Cécile, established their own brain research institute in southern Germany. In addition to other contributions the Vogts together laid the foundation for the study of cerebral cortex architecture.

vomerona´sal [L. *vomer* ploughshare]   The vomer is a trapezoid-shaped bone of the nasal septum. *For* vomeronasal nerve *and* organ, *see the nouns.*

VP   ventral posterior nucleus of the dorsal thalamus.

VPL   ventral posterolateral nucleus of the dorsal thalamus.

VPM   ventral posteromedial nucleus of the dorsal thalamus.

W

Wald, George (b. 1906)   American neurophysiologist, noted for his research on the photochemistry and biochemistry of visual pigments. In 1967 he, R. Granit, and H.K. Hartline shared the Nobel Prize in physiology and medicine for their discoveries concerning physiological and chemical processes in the retina.

Waldeyer, Heinrich Wilhelm Gottfried von (1836-1921)   German anatomist and pathologist. *Waldeyer's nucleus* is the nucleus proprius (Rexed laminae III & IV) of the spinal cord. *Waldeyer's cell layer* is the layer of marginal cells (Rexed lamina I) on the surface of the dorsal horn of the spinal cord.

Wallenberg, Adolf (1862-1949)   German physician and neuroanatomist of Danzig, later a resident of the United States. *Wallenberg's syndrome* (1895) is the lateral medullary syndrome. The *fibers of Wallenberg-Klimoff* constitute the flocculo-oculomotor tract.

Waller, Augustus Volney (1816-1870)   English physiologist who demonstrated that the nerve fiber depends on its cell body for its nutrition and functional integrity; he showed that nerve fibers separated from their cell bodies undergo complete degeneration, called secondary degeneration, or *Wallerian degeneration.*

Weber, Sir Hermann David (1823-1918)   English physician. *Weber's syndrome* consists of a dilated pupil and paralysis of the muscles supplied by the oculomotor nerve on the side of the lesion and a contralateral hemiplegia, resulting from a lesion of the oculomotor nerve and the pyramidal tract in the base of the midbrain. According to the *Weber-Fechner law,* the intensity of a sensation increases proportionately with the logarithm of stimulus intensity.

Weigert, Carl (1845-1904)   German pathologist who introduced a number of staining procedures, particularly one for myelin sheaths (1882).

Wenzel, Joseph W. (1768-1808)   German anatomist. *Wenzel's ventricle* is the cavity of the septum pellucidum, cavum septi pellucidi.

Werdnig, Guido (1844-1919)   Austrian neurologist of Graz. In 1891 he described infantile spinal muscular atrophy, a familial degenerative disease of muscle in children, usually fatal by four years of age. J. Hoffmann also described this disorder (1893), now commonly called *Werdnig-Hoffmann disease*. *See also* dystrophy, muscular.

Wernekinck, Friedrich Christian Gregor (1798-1835)   German anatomist. The *decussation* or *commissure of Wernekinck* is the decussation of the superior cerebellar peduncles in the caudal part of the midbrain tegmentum.

Wernicke, Karl (1848-1904)   German psychiatrist of Berlin, who described several neurologic disorders. *Wernicke's aphasia* is sensory aphasia with impaired understanding of spoken and written words. Although patients with this disorder tend to be "fluent" and use many words, they speak and write incorrectly, and their ideas are not effectively conveyed. The underlying lesion is in the posterior part of the left superior temporal gyrus and the angular gyrus of the parietal lobe in the dominant hemisphere, *Wernicke's area*. *Wernicke's disease* is characterized by ophthalmoplegia and nystagmus, ataxia, and mental confusion in patients with nutritional deficiencies, particularly of thiamine, and with lesions in the hypothalamus and midbrain, near the third ventricle and cerebral aqueduct. *Wernicke's field* or *zone* is the area triangularis just lateral to the lateral geniculate nucleus and pulvinar. The planum temporale was also called the *field of Wernicke*. *Wernicke's fasciculus* is the lateral occipital fasciculus.

Westphal, Carl Friedrich Otto (1833-1890)   German neurologist and psychiatrist of Berlin. The *Edinger-Westphal nucleus* is the parasympathetic nucleus of the oculomotor nerve.

Whytt, Robert (1714-1766)   Scottish physician noted for his studies of reflexes. *Whytt's reflex* (1751) is the light reflex.

Wiesel, Torsten Nils (b. 1924)   Swedish neurophysiologist, active in the United States. He and D. Hubel are noted for their studies of the visual system, its synaptic organization and ocular dominance columns. In 1981 they shared the Nobel Prize in physiology and medicine for their discovery that vision in later life is dependent on adequate sight stimulation in infancy.

Wilder, Burt Green (1841-1925)   American anatomist. The *interventricular antrum of Wilder* is the anterior part of the third ventricle with which the interventricular foramina communicate.

Willis, Thomas (1621-1675)   English physician of London, noted for his contributions to the anatomy of the brain. In 1664 he reclassified the cranial nerves and described the cerebral arterial circle *(circle of Willis)* on the base of the brain and the spinal accessory nerve *(accessory nerve of Willis)*. At one time the ophthalmic branch of the trigeminal nerve was called the *nerve of Willis*. *Willis paracusis*, or false paracusis, is characterized by the ability to hear better in a noisy environment than in quiet surroundings.

Wilson, Samuel Alexander Kinnier (1878-1937)   eminent British neurologist, born in the United States. He practiced at the National Hospital for Nervous Diseases in London for most of his professional life. *Wilson's disease* (1912) is hepaticolenticular degeneration, a disorder of copper metabolism, inherited as an autosomal recessive. The *pencils of Wilson* are small fascicles of nerve fibers which arise from cells in the caudate nucleus and putamen and pass into, through, or along the globus pallidus.

window, cochlear, ᴇᴀʀ   *See* window, round.

window, oval [fenestra ovalis (vestibuli), NA], ᴇᴀʀ   opening between the scala vestibuli of the cochlea and the tympanic cavity of the middle ear, closed by the footplate of the stapes.

window, round [fenestra rotunda (cochleae), NA], ᴇᴀʀ   opening between the scala tympani of the cochlea and the tympanic cavity of the middle ear, closed by the secondary tympanic membrane.

window, vestibular, ᴇᴀʀ   *See* window, oval.

Wrisberg, Heinrich August (1739-1808)   German anatomist of Göttingen. Both the medial cutaneous nerve of the arm and the nervus intermedius have been called the *nerve of Wrisberg.* The *ganglion of Wrisberg* is the cardiac ganglion.

Z

Zinn, Johann Gottfried (1727-1759)   German anatomist and physician of Göttingen who published a classical treatise on the eye in 1755. The *anulus of Zinn* is the fibrous ring from which the four rectus muscles of the eye arise. The *zonule of Zinn* is the ciliary zonule.

zo´na arcua´ta [NA], EAR   inner part of the basilar membrane under the inner tunnel of the cochlea, between the tympanic lip of the spiral limbus and the outer pillars of the spiral organ. *Syn:* zona perforata.

zona incer´ta [NA], VENTRAL THALAMUS   nucleus located between the dorsal thalamus and thalamic fasciculus dorsally and the lenticular fasciculus and subthalamic nucleus ventrally (Fig. N-8). It is a way station for fibers from the striatum in the extrapyramidal system.

zona pectina´ta [NA], EAR   outer part of the basilar membrane of the cochlea, between the outer pillars of the spiral organ and the crest of the spiral ligament.

zona perfora´ta, EAR   zona arcuata of the basilar membrane of the cochlea.

zona terminal´is [NA], CORD   *See* tract, dorsolateral.

zone, intermediate   layer which forms between the ventricular and the marginal zones of the neural tube. It is composed at first of immature neurons which do not divide. As they develop, cell arrangements in this zone may remain relatively simple or become exceedingly complex and take on the variation characteristic of the adult gray matter. This zone corresponds to the mantle layer of the classic terminology (Angevine *et al.*, '70).

zone, marginal   outer cell-sparse layer of the neural tube, first recognizable shortly after the formation of the ventricular zone. In the early stages of development it is composed of the outermost cytoplasmic parts of the ventricular cells. Later it contains the processes of the developing nerve cells and corresponds to the marginal layer of the classic terminology (Angevine *et al.*, '70).

zone, subventric´ular   layer of the neural tube consisting of small, round-to-oval cells at the junction of the ventricular and intermediate zones of the neural tube (Angevine *et al.*, '70).

zone, ventric´ular   layer of the neural tube adjacent to the neural canal or, in the early stages of development, occupying the entire thickness of the tube. It contains the mitotic and intermitotic forms of pseudostratified columnar cells. These cells are the forerunners of neurons and macroglia. The ventricular and subventricular zones correspond to the ependymal layer of the neural tube of the classical terminology (Angevine *et al.*, '70).

zon´ule, cil´iary [zonula ciliaris, NA], EYE   the suspensory ligament of the lens. It consists of a system of fibers which holds the lens in place. The fibers, which arise from the epithelium of the ciliary body, attach to the capsule of the lens. *Syn:* zonule of Zinn.

Zuckerkandl, Emil (1849-1910)   Austrian anatomist of Graz and Vienna. *Zuckerkandl's bodies* are the chromaffin paraganglia along the abdominal aorta. *Zuckerkandl's convolution* is the subcallosal gyrus. *Zuckerkandl's olfactory radiation* is the diagonal band (of Broca).

References

Adams, R.D. and M. Victor 1989 *Principles of Neurology*, 4th ed. McGraw-Hill, New York, 1286 pp.

Adelman, G., ed. 1987 *Encyclopedia of Neuroscience*, 2 Vols. Birkhäuser, Boston. Contains concise accounts on a wide range of topics, summarizing the historical and current knowledge of each subject.

Altner, H. and H. Zimmermann 1972 The saccus vasculosus in *The Structure and Function of Nervous Tissue, 5:* 293-328, G.H. Bourne, ed. Academic Press, New York.

Alves, A.M. and R. Ceballos 1971 The syndrome(s) of akinetic mutism. *Int. Surg., 56:* 392-401.

Amaral, D.G. and H.M. Sinnamon 1977 The locus ceruleus: neurobiology of a central noradrenergic nucleus. *Prog. Neurobiol., 9:* 147-196.

Andy, O.J. and H. Stephan 1968 The septum in the human brain. *J. Comp. Neur., 133:* 383-409.

Angevine, J.B. Jr., D. Bodian, A.J. Coulombre, *et al.* 1970 Embryonic vertebrate central nervous system: Revised terminology. *Anat. Rec., 166:* 257-262.

Area postrema 1984 A composite of two symposiums presented by The American Physiological Society in 1983. *Fed. Proc., 43:* 2937-2971.

Ariëns Kappers, C.U. 1914 Phenomena of neurobiotaxis in the central nervous system. *Trans. XVII Int. Congr. Med. London,* 1913, Section 1, Part II: 109-122.

Ariëns Kappers, C.U., G.C. Huber, and E.C. Crosby 1936 *The Comparative Anatomy of the Nervous System of Vertebrates, Including Man,* 2 Vols. The Macmillan Publishing Co., New York.

Ariëns Kappers, J. 1955 The development of the paraphysis cerebri in man with comments on its relationship to the intercolumnar tubercle and its significance for the origin of cystic tumors in the third ventricle. *J. Comp. Neur., 102:* 425-509.

Barr, M.L. and E.G. Bertram 1949 A morphological distinction between neurones of the male and female, and the behaviour of the nucleolar satellite during accelerated nucleoprotein synthesis. *Nature, 163:* 676-677.

Batson, O.V. 1944 Anatomical principles concerned in the study of cerebral blood flow. *Fed. Proc., 3:* 139-144.

Batson, O.V. 1957 The vertebral vein system. Caldwell lecture, 1956. *Amer. J. Roentgenol. Radium Therapy Nucl. Med., 78:* 195-212.

Beattie, J.M., W.E.C. Dickson, and A.M. Drennan 1948 *A Textbook of Pathology, General and Special,* vol. 2, 5th ed. William Heinemann, London.

Bebin, J. 1956 The central tegmental bundle. An anatomical and experimental study in the monkey. *J. Comp. Neur., 105:* 287-332.

Benson, D. F. 1979 *Aphasia, Alexia, and Agraphia.* Churchill Livingstone, New York, 213 pp. A concisely and clearly written text with an extensive bibliography.

Brown, J.R. 1967 Examination for ataxia in children. *Proc. Mayo Clinic, 34:* 570-573.

Bueker, E.D. 1948 Implantation of tumors in the hind limb field of the embryonic chick and the developmental response of the lumbosacral nervous system. *Anat. Rec., 102:* 369-389.

Cajal, S. Ramón y 1909, 1911 *Histologie du Système Nerveux de l'Homme et des Vertébrés,* 2 Vols. Maloine. Reprinted 1952, 1955 by Instituto Ramón y Cajal, Madrid.

Carpenter, M.B. and J. Sutin 1983 *Human Neuroanatomy,* 8th ed. The Williams and Wilkins Co., Baltimore, 872 pp.

Corner, G.W. 1943 Spelling of the adjective "hypophyseal." *Science, 97:* 67-68.

Critchley, M. 1966 The enigma of Gerstmann's syndrome. *Brain, 89:* 183-198.

Crosby, E.C., T. Humphrey, and E.W. Lauer 1962 *Correlative Anatomy of the Nervous System.* The Macmillan Publishing Co., New York, 731 pp. Comprehensive text of human neuroanatomy, including extensive documentation.

Crosby, E.C. and R.C. Schneider 1982 Cortical areas related to voluntary and following eye movements. Chapt. 15, Sect. G, pp. 736-790 in *Comparative Correlative Neuroanatomy of the Vertebrate Telencephalon,* E.C. Crosby and H.N. Schnitzlein, eds. (next reference).

Crosby, E.C. and H.N. Schnitzlein, eds. 1982 *Comparative Correlative Neuroanatomy of the Vertebrate Telencephalon.* The Macmillan Publishing Co., New York, 830 pp. Includes human as well as subhuman forms.

Erlich, S.S. and M.L.J. Apuzzo 1985 The pineal gland: anatomy, physiology, and clinical significance. *J. Neurosurg., 63:* 321-341.

Emson, P.C., ed. 1983 *Chemical Neuroanatomy.* Raven Press, New York, 560 pp.

Fawcett, D.W. 1986 *Bloom and Fawcett, A Textbook of Histology,* 11th ed. W.B. Saunders Co., Philadelphia, 1017 pp.

Foley, A.L. 1970 A descending vesicopressor pathway in the monkey. *Proc. Soc. Exptl. Biol. Med., 133:* 25-29.

Forel, A.H. 1877 Untersuchungen über die Haubenregion und ihre oberen Verknüpfungen im Gehirne des Menschen und einiger Säugetiere. *Arch. Psychiat. Nervenkr., 7:* 393-495.

Fulton, J. 1946 *Harvey Cushing, a Biography.* Charles C. Thomas, Springfield, 754 pp.

Gash, D.M. and G.J. Boer 1987 *Vasopressin, Principles and Properties.* Plenum Press, New York, 635 pp.

Ghanbari, H.A., B.E. Miller, H.J. Haigler, *et al.* 1990 Biochemical assay of

Alzheimer's disease--associated protein(s) in human brain tissue. *J.A.M.A., 263:* 2907-2910.

Goldstein, A. 1987 Dynorphin (dynorphin peptides), pp. 346-347, in *Encyclopedia of Neuroscience,* G. Adelman, ed., *op. cit.*

Gorski, R.A., R.E. Harlan, C.D. Jacobson, *et al.* 1980 Evidence for the existence of a sexually dimorphic nucleus in the preoptic area of the rat. *J. Comp. Neur., 193:* 529-539.

Greenfield, J.G., W. Blackwood, W.H. McMenemy, *et al.* 1958 *Neuropathology,* Edward Arnold, London, 640 pp.

Harris, G.W. and B.T. Donovan 1966 *The Pituitary Gland,* 3 Vols. Butterworths, London.

Hayashi, M. 1924 Einige wichtige Tatsachen aus der ontogenetischen Entwicklung des menschlichen Kleinhirn. *Dt. Z. Nervenheilk., 81:* 74-82.

Haymaker, W. 1969 *Bing's Local Diagnosis in Neurological Diseases,* 15th ed. The C.V. Mosby Co., St. Louis, 599 pp.

Haymaker, W., E. Anderson and W.J.H. Nauta, eds. 1969 *The Hypothalamus.* Charles C. Thomas, Springfield, 805 pp.

Heimer, L. and M.J. Robards 1981 *Neuroanatomical Tract-Tracing Methods.* Plenum Press, New York, 567 pp. This book and the 1989 edition (next reference) contain descriptions for many procedures of value to the neuroscience investigator, in addition to those which have been specifically cited in the text.

Heimer, L. and L. Záborsky 1989 *Neuroanatomical Tract-Tracing Methods 2, Recent Progress.* Plenum Press, New York, 408 pp.

Herrick, C.J. 1915 *An Introduction to Neurology.* W.B. Saunders Co., Philadelphia, 355 pp.

Infantile Autism 1987 No. 299.0 in *American Psychiatric Association Diagnostic and Statistical Manual of Mental Disorders,* 3rd ed., revised, p. 456. Washington, D.C. American Psychiatric Association.

Johnston, M.C., A. Bhakdinaronk, and Y.C. Reid 1973 An expanded role of the neural crest in oral and pharyngeal development. Chapt. 3, pp. 37-52 in *Oral Sensation and Perception--Development in the Fetus and Infant,* J.F. Bosma, ed. DHEW Pub. No. (NIH) 73-546.

Kerr, F.W. 1975 Neuroanatomical substrates of nociception in the spinal cord. *Pain, 1:* 325-356.

Kristensson, K. and Y. Olsson 1971 Retrograde axonal transport of protein. *Brain Research, 29:* 363-365.

Kuhlenbeck, H. 1969 Boundaries of the hypothalamus. Chapt. 2, Sect. III, pp. 21-28, in *The Hypothalamus,* W. Haymaker, *et al.,* eds., *op. cit.*

Kuré, K.G. Saégusa, K. Kawaguchi, and K. Shiraishi 1930 On the parasympathetic (spinal parasympathetic) fibres in the dorsal roots and their cells of origin in the spinal cord. *Quart. J. Exp. Physiol., 20:* 51-66.

Kuru, M. 1965 Nervous control of micturition. *Phys. Rev., 45:* 425-494.

Lattes, R. 1950 Nonchromaffin paraganglioma of ganglion nodosum, carotid body, and aortic-arch bodies. *Cancer, 3:* 667-694.

Levi-Montalcini, R. and V. Hamburger 1951 Selective growth-stimulating effects of mouse sarcoma on the sensory and sympathetic system of the chick embryo. *J. Exptl. Zool., 116:* 321-362.

List, C.F. and R.C. Schneider 1982 Developmental anomalies of the craniovertebral border. Chapt. 28, pp. 882-908, in *Correlative Neurosurgery,* R.C. Schneider, E.A.

Kahn, *et al.*, eds. (see below).

Lockard, I. 1982 The blood-brain barrier: an alternative hypothesis. *J. Theor. Biol., 97:* 167-176.

Lorente de Nó, R. 1934 Studies on the structure of the cerebral cortex II. Continuation of the study of the ammonic system. *J. Psych. Neurol., 46:* 113-177.

Lowenstein, O. and J. Wersäll 1959 A functional interpretation of the electron microscopic structure of the sensory hairs in the cristae of the elasmobranch *Raja clavata* in terms of directional sensitivity. *Nature, 184:* 1807-1808.

Melzack, R. and P.D. Wall 1965 Pain mechanisms: a new theory. *Science, 150:* 971-979.

Mettler, F.A. 1948 *Neuroanatomy.* The C.V. Mosby Co., St. Louis. See especially for the correlation of older and newer terminology.

Mobley, W.C., A.C. Server, D.N. Ishii, *et al.* 1977 Nerve growth factor. *N. Eng. J. Med., 297:* 1096-1104, 1149-1158, 1211-1218.

Müller, F. and R. O'Rahilly 1989 Mediobasal prosencephalic defects, including holoprosencephaly and cyclopia, in relation to the development of the human forebrain. *Am. J. Anat., 185:* 391-414.

Nathan, P.W. 1976 The gate-control theory of pain. A critical review. *Brain, 99:* 123-158.

Nathan, P.W. and M.C. Smith 1982 The rubrospinal and central tegmental tracts in man. *Brain, 105:* 223-269.

Nathan, P.W., M.C. Smith, and P. Deacon 1990 The corticospinal tracts in man, course and location of fibres at different segmental levels. *Brain, 113:* 303-324.

Nomina Anatomica 1983 5th ed., revised by the International Anatomical Nomenclature Committee and approved by the Eleventh International Congress of Anatomists at Mexico City, 1980. *Nomina Histologica,* 2nd ed., and *Nomina Embryologica,* 2nd ed., prepared by subcommittees of the International Anatomical Nomenclature Committee. The Williams & Wilkins Co., Baltimore.

O'Rahilly, R. 1989 Anatomical terminology, then and now. *Acta Anat., 134:* 291-300.

O'Rahilly, R. and E. Gardner 1979 The initial development of the human brain. *Acta Anat., 104:* 123-133.

Papez, J.W. 1937 A proposed mechanism of emotion. *Arch. Neurol. Psychiatr., 38:* 725-734.

Paxinos, G., ed. 1990 *The Human Nervous System.* Academic Press, San Diego, 1195 pp. This volume contains a wealth of anatomical information derived from studies of the nervous system, using histochemical procedures.

Pearse, A.G.E. 1977 The diffuse neuroendocrine system and the APUD concept: related "endocrine" peptides in brain, intestine, pituitary, placenta, and anuran cutaneous glands. *Med. Biol., 55:* 115-125.

Penfield, W. and H. Jasper 1954 *Epilepsy and the Functional Anatomy of the Human Brain.* Little, Brown and Co., Boston, 896 pp.

Peters, A., S.L. Palay, and H. deF. Webster 1976 *The Fine Structure of the Nervous System: The Neurons and Supporting Cells.* W.B. Saunders Co., Philadelphia, 406 pp.

Rakic, P. 1972 Mode of cell migration to the superficial layers of monkey neocortex. *J. Comp. Neur., 145:* 61-84.

Rakic, P. and R.L. Sidman 1970 Histogenesis of cortical layers in human cerebellum, particularly the lamina dissecans. *J. Comp. Neur., 139:* 473-500.

Rexed, B. 1964 Some aspects of the cytoarchitectonics and synaptology of the spinal cord, in *Prog. Brain Res.* Vol. II, pp. 58-92. *Organization of the Spinal Cord,* J. C. Eccles and J. P. Schadé, eds., Elsevier Publishing Co., Amsterdam,

Richter, E. 1965 *Die Entwicklung des Globus Pallidus und des Corpus Subthalamicum.* Springer-Verlag, Berlin.

Rioch, D. McK., G.B. Wislocki, J.L. O'Leary, *et al.* 1940 A précis of preoptic, hypothalamic and hypophysial terminology. Chapt. 1 in *The Hypothalamus and Central Levels of Autonomic Function, Res. Publ. Ass. Nerv. Ment. Dis., 20:* 3-30.

Rose, M. 1927 Die sog. Riechrinde beim Menschen und beim Affen. II. Teil und Mensch. *J. Pschol. Neur. (Lpz.), 34:* 261-401.

Salamon, G. and Y.P. Huang 1976 *Radiologic Anatomy of the Brain.* Springer-Verlag, Berlin, 404 pp. The blood vessels of the brain and many other anatomical features are described and beautifully illustrated.

Schlesinger, B. 1953 The insulo-opercular arteries of the brain, with special reference to angiography of striothalamic tumors. *Am. J. Roentgenol., 70:* 555-563.

Schneider, R.C. and E.C. Crosby 1982 Surgery of cerebral hemispheres and cerebellum in the balancing of abnormal tonus and movement. Chapt. 24, pp. 702-765 in *Correlative Neurosurgery,* R.C. Schneider, E.A. Kahn, *et al.*, eds., (next reference).

Schneider, R.C., E.A. Kahn, E.C. Crosby, and J.A. Taren, eds. 1982 *Correlative Neurosurgery,* 3rd ed., 2 Vols. Charles C. Thomas, Springfield. These volumes contain considerable neuroanatomical information correlated with neurosurgical topics.

Schwartz, J.C. and H. Pollard 1987 Histamine, in *Encyclopedia of Neuroscience,* G. Adelman, ed., pp. 495-497, *op. cit.*

Shantha, T.R. and G.H. Bourne 1968 The perineural epithelium--a new concept. Chapt. 10, pp. 379-459 in *The Structure and Function of Nervous Tissue,* Vol. 1, G.H. Bourne, ed., Academic Press, New York.

Steinbusch H.W.M. and R. Nieuwenhuys 1983 The raphe nuclei of the rat brainstem: a cytoarchitectonic and immunohistochemical study, pp. 131-207, in *Chemical Neuroanatomy,* P.C. Emson, ed., *op. cit.*

Stephens, R.B. and D.L. Stillwell 1969 *Arteries and Veins of the Human Brain.* Charles C. Thomas, Springfield. Invaluable book with text, many illustrations, and extensive documentation.

Steward, O. 1981 Horseradish peroxidase and fluorescent substances and their combination with other techniques. Chapt. 8, pp. 279-310 in *Neuroanatomical Tract-Tracing Methods,* L. Heimer and M.J. Robards, eds., *op. cit.*

Swanson, L.W. 1987 Limbic system, pp. 589-591, in *Encyclopedia of Neuroscience,* G. Adelman, ed., *op.cit.*

Tagliavini, F. 1987 The basal nucleus of Meynert, pp. 115-116, in *Encyclopedia of Neuroscience,* G. Adelman, ed., *op.cit.*

Taren, J.A., E.A. Kahn, and T. Humphrey 1982 Mechanisms and surgical control of chronic pain. Chapt. 39, pp. 1499-1560, in *Correlative Neurosurgery,* R.C. Schneider, E.A. Kahn, *et al.*, eds., *op. cit.*

Terzian, H. and G. D. Ore 1955 Syndrome of Klüver and Bucy, reproduced in man by bilateral removal of the temporal lobes. *Neurology, 5:* 373-380.

Walker, A.E. 1942 Relief of pain by mesencephalic tractotomy. *Arch. Neur. Psych., 48:* 865-883.

Worthington, W.C. Jr. and R.C. Cathcart 1963 Ependymal cilia: distribution and activity in the adult human brain. *Science, 139:* 221-222.

Záborszky, L. and L. Heimer 1989 Combinations of tracer techniques, especially HRP and PHA-L, with transmitter identification for correlated light and electron microscopic studies. Chapt. 4, pp. 49-96 in *Neuroanatomical Tract-Tracing Methods 2, Recent Progress,* L. Heimer and L. Záborsky, eds., *op. cit.*

Additional references for biographical and historical information, and other valuable sources of information:

Appenzeller, O. 1990 *The Autonomic Nervous System: An Introduction to Basic and Clinical Concepts,* 4th ed. Elsevier Biomedical Press, Amsterdam, 722 pp.

Beighton, P. and G. Beighton 1986 *The Man Behind the Syndrome.* Springer-Verlag, Berlin, 240 pp.

Dobson, J. 1962 *Anatomical Eponyms,* 2nd ed. E. & S. Livingstone Ltd., Edinburgh, 235 pp.

Haymaker, W. and F. Schiller 1970 *The Founders of Neurology,* 2nd ed. Charles C. Thomas, Springfield, 616 pp.

Hoppenfeld, S. 1976 *Physical Examination of the Spine and Extremities.* Appleton-Century-Crofts, New York, 276 pp. Valuable for its clear presentation of the descriptions and illustrations of the deep reflexes.

McHenry, L.C. 1969 *Garrison's History of Medicine.* Charles C. Thomas, Springfield, 552 pp.

Pepper, O.H.P. 1949 *Medical Etymology.* W.B. Saunders Co., Philadelphia, 263 pp.

Skinner, H.A. 1961 *The Origin of Medical Terms,* 2nd ed. The Williams & Wilkins Co., Baltimore, 438 pp.

Taveras, J.M. and E.H. Wood 1964 *Diagnostic Neuroradiology.* The Williams and Wilkins Co., Baltimore, 960 pp.